D0161524

THE ENCYCLOPEDIA OF

DIABETES

THE ENCYCLOPEDIA OF

DIABETES

William A. Petit, Jr., M.D., F.A.C.P., F.A.C.E.
and
Christine Adamec

Facts On File, Inc.

The Encyclopedia of Diabetes

Copyright © 2002 by William A. Petit, Jr., and Christine Adamec

Facts On File, Inc.
132 West 31st Street
New York NY 10001

Library of Congress Cataloging-in-Publication Data
Petit, William A.
The encyclopedia of diabetes / by William A. Petit, Jr., and Christine Adamec.
p. cm.—(The Facts on File library of health and living)
Includes bibliographical references and index.
ISBN 0-8160-4498-8 (hardcover : alk. paper)
1. Diabetes—Encyclopedias. I. Adamec, Christine A., 1949– II. Title. III. Series.
RC660.P424 2002
616.4′62.003—dc21   2001051257

Facts On File books are available at special discounts when purchased in bulk quantities for businesses, associations, institutions, or sales promotions. Please call our Special Sales Department in New York at (212) 967-8800 or (800) 322-8755.

You can find Facts On File on the World Wide Web at http://www.factsonfile.com

Text and cover design by Cathy Rincon

Printed in the United States of America

VB FOF 10 9 8 7 6 5 4 3 2 1

This book is printed on acid-free paper.

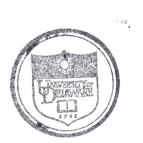

CONTENTS

FOREWORD

If people with diabetes will make important lifestyle changes and adhere to treatment recommended by their physicians and discussed in this book, they *will* live longer, happier, and healthier lives. This has been clearly proven by studies such as the Diabetes Control and Complications Trial (DCCT) and the United Kingdom Prospective Diabetes Study (UKPDS), and it is my mission to convey this information to as many people as possible.

Diabetes may well be the Black Plague of the 21st century, in terms of both pervasiveness and pain. This plague upon us involves insulin resistance and Type 2 diabetes mellitus and is a growing threat to people all over the globe. Although diabetes can be treated very effectively today and many complications can be prevented, slowed down, or treated, it is also a very insidious disease that people suffer from for a long, long time. While they struggle with their diabetes, the disease costs them time, money, pain, aggravation and, sometimes, major sorrow and death.

Ignorance of the disease and how to manage it has cost thousands of people their limbs as well as their eyesight. Yet, in most cases, this loss of sight and these amputations, as well as the other complications of diabetes, can be avoided by regular self-care and medical management.

Experts predict that there may be 30 million new cases in China alone by 2025. All of these patients worldwide will require therapy in the form of billions of dollars of medications, testing, and office/clinic visits. As of 2000, it was estimated that diabetes costs the United States alone $130 billion in direct and indirect costs.

Diabetes may well be the paradigm for all chronic diseases. It is a metabolic syndrome that affects every organ system in the body. Diabetes is also innately involved with the blood vessels and the heart. In fact, heart and blood vessel disease causes 80 percent of the deaths among patients with diabetes.

Fortunately, the past 10 years have seen a renaissance of the treatment of diabetes, ranging from home blood glucose monitors, to human insulin, disposable syringes, new medications, and the insulin pump. Startling genetic breakthroughs and astonishing pancreas and islet cell transplants have clearly shown that the tide is finally turning, even as the disease claims more and more people.

My goal as a clinician is to educate people about diabetes. For those who do not have diabetes, I want to educate them so that they can do everything in their power to try to prevent the development of the disease and to help others who are living with diabetes. The education for those who *do* have diabetes consists of teaching them that they need to keep their blood glucose levels as close to normal as is safely possible. I urge those of you with diabetes to not smoke, encourage you to exercise regularly and keep your cholesterol and blood pressure levels as low as possible to avoid developing diabetic complications. If people with diabetes follow this plan and avoid the irreversible complications, then when we finally do have a cure, these patients can partake of this cure and enjoy *wellness!*

Diabetes requires a lot of education. This cannot be done by one person and necessarily involves a team centered around patients and their families, a team that includes physicians, nurses, dietitians, and many other folks. The education is also ongoing. You cannot learn it "all" and then "graduate." As physicians learn more, the treatment paradigms and therapeutic focus changes and evolves, and we share this knowledge with our patients.

Diabetes requires advocacy. People with diabetes are too quiet and diabetes does not obtain nearly the level of federal funding that it deserves based on the destructive toll it takes upon our society.

The Encyclopedia of Diabetes is a beginning and a means to educate readers. It is not meant to be read cover to cover, although, as I recall from medical school, there are some readers who are wired in a compulsive manner and will read through it, from A to Z.

Maybe you have had diabetes for 20 years or perhaps you were diagnosed today. You may have a family member or friend with diabetes, and you are trying to educate yourself. We hope that this book will give you a good place to start in your quest for information about diabetes. We have tried to cover enough information to be useful as a first source and reference and a good overview of diabetes. In some areas, we cover a lot of what you need to know. In other areas, we can only scratch the surface and give you leads to other written and computer based resources. Please provide us feedback. We hope to update and improve this *Encyclopedia of Diabetes* as research and knowledge progresses.

Keep learning and keep asking questions. Go back and take a class again, and call your local educators for a review. Call, fax, and e-mail your Congressman whenever the issue of diabetes funding is in front of them—as well as when other issues affecting diabetes come up, such as drug laws, Medicare, insurance regulations, disability laws, and stem cell research. Join your local American Diabetes Association and help us move forward to improve your life and the lives of all those affected by diabetes!

—William A. Petit, Jr., M.D.
Fellow of the American College of Physicians,
Fellow of the American College of
Endocrinology

ACKNOWLEDGMENTS

Many people have assisted us with their advice, recommending research or even readings and additions to entries.

Special thanks to Marie Mercer, reference librarian, at the DeGroodt Public Library in Palm Bay, Florida, for her assistance in locating difficult-to-find material and her advice on seeking references. Grateful thanks also to Mary Jordan, Interlibrary Loan Librarian at the Central Library Facility in Cocoa, Florida.

Thanks also to Michael Bliss, professor at the University of Toronto, Richard Landon, director of the Thomas Fisher Rare Book Library at the University of Toronto, and Jennifer Toews, also of the Thomas Fisher Rare Book Library, for their assistance in identifying the rare photographs of children with diabetes.

Special and grateful thanks to our editor, James Chambers, for his excellent editing of our manuscript.

William Petit, Jr., would like to thank the entire staff at the Joslin Diabetes Center affiliate at New Britain General Hospital in New Britain, Connecticut, especially the following individuals: Mary Armetta; James Bernene, M.D.; Latha Dulipsingh, M.D.; Youseff Khawaja, M.D.; Jean Kostak; Karen McAvoy; Lee Metchick, M.D.; Patricia O'Connell; and Joseph Rosenblatt, M.D. Also, extra thanks to his wife Jennifer Hawke-Petit, and to daughters Hayley and Michaela.

Thanks also to his staff in Plainville and New Britain, Connecticut, including Robin Romero, Barbara Bartolucci, Milly Cruz, Aracelis Munoz, Mona Huggard, LPN, and Doreen Rackliffe, PA-C.

Christine Adamec would especially like to thank her husband, John Adamec and her children, Jane and Stephen, for their patience and support during this project.

A HISTORY OF DIABETES:
FROM ANCIENT TIMES TO THE TWENTY-FIRST CENTURY

Most decidedly *not* just a modern problem, diabetes was known and feared as a killing disease and an illness without hope for thousands of years. Nothing that physicians tried, no medications, concoctions, treatments, or diets, could prevent an early and inevitable death. It was not until the 20th century that medical researchers developed miraculous lifesaving and life-prolonging treatments. The discovery of insulin in 1921 was the key to diabetes salvation for millions of patients worldwide, then and now.

As a result of further medical research performed in the early part of the 21st century, and that continues on even as we write, researchers are making astonishing medical breakthroughs that will eventually lead to cures for many people with diabetes. For example, in 2000, the successful transplantation of islets of Langerhans cells from the pancreases of recently deceased people by physician A. M. James Shapiro in Canada has presented, for the first time, the possibility of a cure for diabetes. Thus far, this treatment has led to an apparent complete remission of the disease in a handful of patients. The National Institutes of Health has planned a worldwide test of the "Edmonton Protocol" used by Dr. Shapiro.

Other breakthroughs, such as complete pancreas transplants or joint pancreas-kidney transplants, although still rare, also offer hope for a cure. Genetic manipulation may bring new hope for future sufferers of diabetes.

Today, many people with diabetes and their families envision a bright future. They would probably feel even more optimistic and appreciative if they learned about how people with diabetes fared with the disease and were treated for it by physicians in the past.

Diabetes in Ancient Times

The first recorded mention of a medical condition that was distinguishable as diabetes was found in an ancient papyrus, discovered in 1862 by German Egyptologist George Ebers. The Ebers papyrus, which dates back to about 1500 B.C.E., revealed translations of several different prescriptive directions for concoctions that purportedly could "remove the urine, which runs too often."

In the early part of the first millennium, Celsus, a Roman writer who lived during the times of Hippocrates, translated Greek writings on medicine. He also wrote a summary of medicine and surgery. Wrote Celsus, for physicians whose patients apparently had diabetes, "The food should be astringent, the wine dry and undiluted . . . and in quantity the minimum required to allay thirst." Celsus also recommended exercise for these patients, advice still offered today for people with diabetes.

Although his contributions to the written medical knowledge of the time were major, Celsus made one serious mistake about diabetes. He claimed that people with diabetes urinated more than they drank. Strangely, this view was accepted for hundreds of years, until finally, in the 16th century, Girolamo Cardano measured the amount of fluid consumed by a diabetic patient and then compared it to the amount of urine produced. They were roughly equivalent; thus, Cardano refuted the long-accepted medical error.

In about the second century C.E., the ancient Ionian Greeks gave the illness its name of "diabetes," which translated to "pass through" or "siphon." They had observed that individuals afflicted with the disease drank copious quantities of fluid and that they also urinated a great deal. Generally, the name "diabetes" is specifically attributed to the Greek physician, Aretaeus of Cappadocia, who described the illness in this way in a translation of his medical treatise, "Of the Causes and Signs of Acute and Chronic Diseases,"

> Diabetes is a wasting of the flesh and limbs into urine from a cause similar to dropsy. The patient never ceasing to make water and the discharge is as incessant as a sluice let off. The patient does not survive long for the marasmus is rapid and death speedy. The thirst is ungovernable, the copious potations are more than equalled by the profuse urinary discharge, for more urine flows away . . . The epithet diabetes has been assigned from the disorder being something like passing of water by a syphon . . .

Aretaeus made one major mistake, however. He believed that diabetes was caused by a snakebite.

The great Greek physician Galen was also familiar with diabetes. Galen said diabetes was "a weakness of the kidneys which cannot hold back water." Some Greek physicians urged exercise as a therapy for diabetes, especially horseback riding, which was regarded as an especially good way to rid the body of excessive urination.

Japanese and Chinese physicians were also aware of the disease. Ghang-ke wrote about diabetes around 229 C.E., stating that diabetic urine was copious and sweet, and that it attracted dogs.

In the fifth and sixth century C.E., Susruta, a prestigious physician from India, wrote about his observations on diabetes. He noted that the urine of a person with diabetes had a honey-like taste, one that attracted ants and other insects. Dr. Susruta was also one of the first known physicians to recognize that there were actually two primary types of diabetes, including one that afflicted very thin people and another form that was more commonly seen among obese and more sedentary individuals.

Today we call one form of diabetes "Type 1" (generally seen in thin or average-sized children and adults) and we call the other form "Type 2" diabetes (the more commonly diagnosed form of diabetes in the West today among obese and sedentary middle-aged and older individuals.)

During this period, Dr. Susruta advised moderation in diet and recommended exercise for his overweight patients with diabetes, recommendations that are still offered today for people with Type 2 diabetes—albeit that they are also supplemented with oral medications.

Avicenna (980–1027 C.E.), an Arabian physician, attempted to codify all known medical knowledge. He was deemed a great medical writer of his time. Avicenna wrote of his knowledge of diabetes, "The kidneys attract humors from the liver in greater quantities than they are able to retain. The urine leaves a residue like honey." Avicenna also noted that his patients with diabetes had extreme thirst, were nervous and unable to work, and experienced sexual dysfunction.

Avicenna was also aware of diabetic gangrene, although he knew that it could not be treated at that time, and thus, the affected patients invariably worsened and died.

Diabetes from the Seventeenth through the Nineteenth Centuries

Thomas Willis, a 17th-century Oxford University physician, believed that diabetes was a disease of the blood. He said that the sugar found in the blood was later apparent in the urine of the person with diabetes. Willis also noted that the illness had been rare in ancient times but that diabetes was on the rise because of "good fellowship and gustling down chiefly of unallayed wine." Clearly, Willis was referring to what we now call Type 2 diabetes.

About 100 years later, Matthew Dobson first demonstrated the presence of "saccharine matter" in both the urine and the blood in experiments performed in 1772. Dobson let urine stand until it dried, after which he observed a substance that closely resembled brown sugar. Dobson also left blood standing and found that the remaining serum was sweet. He concluded that "the saccharine matter was not formed in the secretory organ (the kidneys), but previously existed in the serum of the blood." It was not until 1815, however, that French chemist M. E. Chevreul definitively identified the substance found in the urine of people with diabetes as glucose.

William Cullen, a professor of chemistry and medicine in Glasgow and Edinburgh, Scotland, in the late 18th century, stated his thesis that diabetes was essentially a disease of the nervous system. We now know that diabetes is actually an endocrine disorder, although it can also have profound effects on the nervous system as well, particularly after many years. However, Dr. Cullen is credited for adding the term "mellitus" to the word diabetes.

In 1853, Ernst Stadelmann discovered that the diabetic coma was a consequence of a greatly increased accumulation of acids, and was what we now call "diabetic ketoacidosis" or DKA.

However, it was Bernhard Naunyn, Stadelmann's teacher, who was the first to employ the term "acidosis." Naunyn was a very strong proponent of diet as a means to control diabetes. He wrote 10 principles of treatment, some of which are still applicable today. Here are his first seven principles:

1. The Alpha and Omega in the area of diabetes is dietetic treatment, and not drugs.

2. It must be known that diabetic glycosuria increases with time while the tolerance of the patient decreases.

3. When the diabetic is free from sugar, his tolerance usually increases. Therefore, aim to render the patient sugar free and keep him aglycosuric.

4. Limitation of the total diet with resulting disencumbrance of the entire metabolism brings about a favorable result.

5. Reduction of carbohydrates or proteins for the removal of glycosuria.

6. Sugar producing foods are the carbohydrates and proteins.

7. We should determine the exact qualitative and quantitative diet for every diabetic who comes under treatment.

In 1857, Claude Bernard isolated a substance he then called "glycogen" and illustrated the role that the liver played in the metabolism of glucose. He demonstrated through his experiments what some physicians had previously believed: that individuals with diabetes had excessive sugar in the blood, followed by excessive sugar in the urine. At this time, however, it was still unknown that the pancreas was the key organ involved in diabetes.

Then in 1869, German researcher Paul Langerhans wrote a dissertation about special clusters of cells that he identified within the pancreas. He was particularly intrigued by one type of cell in the pancreas. Wrote Langerhans: "This cell is a small irregularly polygonal structure with brilliant cytoplasm; free of any granule with distinct round nuclei of moderate size. The cells lie together in considerable numbers diffusely scattered in the parenchyma of the gland." Although the cells had been identified, the importance of the pancreas to the development of diabetes remained a mystery to researchers and physicians.

In 1889, Oskar Minkowski performed experiments on removing the pancreases of dogs, thus inducing diabetes in the animals and definitively proving the significance of the pancreas. As with many great discoveries, Minkowski did not start out to study diabetes, nor did he suspect that the pancreas was the key. Instead, his colleague, Joseph von Mering, wanted to know if and how the pancreas affected the digestion of fat, and what would happen if the pancreas was removed.

Minkowski removed the pancreas from a dog and the next day a laboratory technician complained that the dog, which had been completely house-trained, was now constantly urinating everywhere. Minkowski, who had been trained by Dr. Carl H. von Noorden to test for diabetes whenever he identified polyuria, found that the dog's urine was laden with glucose. Minkowski realized the significance of this study—that the pancreas was the primary organ involved in diabetes. However, he did not discover the secret of how to resolve diabetes.

Minkowski and many others sought to find what substance it was that made the difference between diabetes and no diabetes, but none of them succeeded. Years later, when another colleague complained to him that it was really *he* who first discovered insulin, not Doctors Frederick G. Banting and Charles H. Best, Minkowski said, "I, too, wish I had discovered insulin." Minkowski received one of the early batches of insulin from Banting and Best, and he told his students that if he could not be the father of insulin, he was happy to be the grandfather.

Author J. O. Liebowitz, in his article on the historical perspective of diabetes, wrote that the finding from Minkowski's experiment was the "greatest single contribution to experimental research on diabetes" and further, "From here on a straight line can be drawn to the epoch-making work of Banting and Best."

In 1893, Edouard Laguesse noted the importance of the cells that had been identified by Langerhans, and, in honor of Langerhans, he dubbed them the "islands of Langerhans." (These cells are now called "islets of Langerhans.")

Medical Treatments for Diabetes before the Discovery of Insulin

There was little relief for people with diabetes before the 20th century, but there were plenty of ideas on how to treat it. Opium was a drug of treatment for people with diabetes from the 17th-century recommendation of Thomas Willis to use a "syrup of poppies" and onward through the late 19th century. Most doctors didn't believe that opium cured or even much helped the person with diabetes; however, they did believe that it made this distressing disease more tolerable. Doctors also relied on bloodlettings in the 19th century, believing that they would be of some medical value. (Getting rid of the "bad blood" was the plan.) As we now know, they were mistaken in this belief.

During this period, surgeons rarely performed amputations on patients diagnosed with gangrene, which was considered an inevitable death sentence. Many patients did develop ulcerations and infections that led to gangrene and thus, many died. In his article for a 1972 issue of *Medical History*, Frank Allan described his own childhood memories of people he knew who had diabetes prior to the discovery of insulin. He described a man in his fifties who began to have pain in his toe that was severe and constant and that prevented him from sleeping. Allan said,

> Then to his horror it began to turn black. His family doctor called it gangrene and confirmed the diagnosis of diabetes which he himself had feared, since a brother and several members of his family had been diabetic. A surgeon, consulted in the hope that the gangrenous toe could be amputated, was unwilling to operate. He stated that, with diabetes, healing would fail to occur. The man was bedridden for months as the gangrene extended into his foot. Finally death came to end his suffering.

Dr. Banting, the discoverer of insulin, commented on the nontreatment of gangrene prior to the discovery of insulin, in a paper published in 1937 in *Science*. Banting said, "Another complication of diabetes that was met with in the older patients was gangrene. In the pre-insulin days operation was dangerous and the patients usually died following the operation. Now diabetics can be safely operated upon because insulin controls the blood sugar and acetone production."

Before Banting and Best's discovery of insulin, some unusual pancreatic experimentation occurred by doctors attempting to help their patients with diabetes. For example, in 1906, following on the work of Minkowski, Scottish scientists Rennie and Fraser reported on their experiments with extracts from the islets of fish they had purchased at the Aberdeen Fish Market. They selected a daily supply of fish for their experiments, seeking out species known to have unusually large islets. Their results were reported in *The Biochemical Journal.*

The doctors boiled part of the pancreas, specifically the islets of Langerhans from the fish, and subsequently administered this compound to patients who were very ill with diabetes; for example, one patient who was given the fish extract was nearly blind and he was also very weak.

According to the doctor's notes, this patient showed improvement after receiving the compound, producing much less urine and reporting to them that he felt better. Their own tests revealed that his urinary glucose levels were considerably decreased. When the substance was withheld, however, the patient's urine volume increased and he felt much worse.

Unfortunately, the doctors rapidly ran out of fish and they were unable to procure any more in the fish market. As a result, they could no longer provide the compounded substance that they had created to their patient, who rapidly deteriorated. Other patients had also received the extract and had shown improvement, but a prolonged trial was not possible at that time. Several patients died or became very sick and the doctors lost track of one patient who refused to participate in their study any longer. The doctors did not continue their research.

Most Cases of Diabetes Prior to the 1930s Were Type 1 Diabetes: Today Most Cases Are Type 2 Diabetes

Although physicians have been able to identify diabetes for thousands of years, their treatments were largely ineffectual and most individuals with diabetes sickened and died. It is safe to assume that most of these patients had Type 1 diabetes.

There are two key reasons for this assumption. First, most people prior to the mid-20th century were not obese nor were they sedentary. Hence, they were less likely to develop Type 2 diabetes. Secondly, several generations ago, the life span of most people was far shorter and few lived to be elderly or even middle-aged, when the onset of Type 2 diabetes is most commonly observed.

As a result, frustrated physicians concentrated on striving to help their very ill patients with Type 1 diabetes, despite the fact that few treatments were effective until the discovery of insulin.

Pre-Insulin Era Attempts to Treat Diabetes with Diet

Some well-intentioned physicians put their patients on starvation or semi-starvation diets, ordering them to subsist for days on foods such as oatmeal alone, or to follow a broad array of other rigorous and difficult dietetic recommendations.

Some recommendations were actually harmful; some physicians mistakenly assumed that the body needed much *more* sugar and they mistakenly urged their already hyperglycemic patients to eat large quantities of heavily sweet foods. One account was reported of a physician who had diabetes himself and who decided to follow the regimen of the heavy consumption of sweets. He quickly died.

Other physicians urged the consumption of alcohol to their patients as a means to stave off acidosis and to theoretically help with digestion. (In sharp contrast to today's medical recommendations, which are to avoid alcohol altogether or to drink very moderately.) Lacking the arsenal of medications available today, doctors had to rely on whatever methods they found that seemed to work, if only for a while.

In the latter part of the 18th century, British physician John Rollo was firm in his belief that diabetes should be treated by dietary changes and restrictions, and he was credited as one of the pioneers of this idea. Rollo recommended a diet that was high on protein and fat, with entrees such as blood pudding, and lime water with milk to wash it down. On this diet, vegetables were eliminated. Rollo, as with many other physicians of the time, also favored the use of opium with diabetic patients.

Another 18th-century physician, Apollinaire Bourchardat, took the idea of using diet to control diabetes even further. In addition to inventing diagnostic tests for diabetes, Bouchardat also came up with the recipe for gluten bread. Unlike Rollo, he encouraged his patients to eat green vegetables. Bourchardat also recommended days of fasting and undereating for his patients. He had noted that in times of severe scarcity of food, sugar in the urine of those afflicted with diabetes had virtually vanished and their conditions had improved. Bourchardat was also a strong proponent of exercise.

In the 19th century, Italian physician Arnaldo Cantani was noted for his dietary regimen, which was composed of days of fasting, followed by meat consumption. According to some experts, if Dr. Cantani didn't believe his patients were adhering to his regimen, he locked them up in his clinic and forced them to comply.

Dr. Frederick Allen was famous for writing about and recommending the "Allen Starvation Diet," which he began propounding in 1912, based on his research. He believed that the islets of Langerhans deteriorated because they were overworked and thus, he concluded that less food would not strain them so much and they would have the opportunity to rest. The diet was comprised of several days of fasting followed by a semistarvation diet.

Introduced in 1895 and alluded to earlier, another popular diet was the oatmeal diet, the brainchild of Dr. Carl H. von Noorden in Frankfort, Germany. Dr. von Noorden believed that oatmeal had special qualities that somehow alleviated the symptoms of diabetes.

In another diet that was popular during the early 20th century, Dr. Karl Petren, a Swedish physician, recommended very high fat diets for his patients who had diabetes.

Guelpa of Paris made regular fasting popular in Europe in 1896. He used periodic fasting to "disintoxicate" the patient with diabetes, along with saline laxatives. Other physicians, however, questioned this advice and stated their belief that fasting could lead to diabetic coma.

Although such diets may sound strange or wrongheaded to modern readers, it is important to keep in mind that prior to the discovery of insulin, physicians' attempts to control the diet of the person with diabetes were really the *only* treatment (other than the administration of opium) found to give any temporary relief to the majority of their patients with Type 1 diabetes.

The Discovery of Insulin

Everything changed with the discovery of insulin in 1921. It was a medical paradigm shift and ultimately a lifesaver for millions of people. For people interested in diabetes, it was the equivalent of the discovery of fire or the wheel.

It all began with Dr. Frederick Banting, who built on the knowledge of others but who also made a grand leap forward, and the one that made all the difference. Banting, a co-discoverer with Dr. Best of insulin therapy, was a Canadian physician who was fascinated by research on diabetes. Dr. Banting also had a more personal interest in finding a way to prolong life for people afflicted with diabetes. A little girl from his childhood in Alliston, Ontario, had died of diabetes many years ago, and this had continued to affect him deeply, as he sought to find a treatment or cure.

Dr. Best also had a personal drive to resolve the problem of diabetes. Best wrote in an article published in 1956 in *Diabetes*,

My own interest in diabetes began when my father's sister, who had gone from Nova Scotia to train as a nurse at the Massachusetts General Hospital, came to help my father in his small hospital on the Maine-New Brunswick border. She had developed diabetes some years previously and although her life was prolonged by the treatment administered by Dr. Joslin [a noted figure in the early 20th century], she died a few years before insulin became available.

In 1921, Dr. Banting, a recently returned wounded and decorated war veteran of the "Great War" (World War I), was planning to practice orthopedic surgery. He had received an appointment to the faculty of the University of Western Ontario in London, Canada. While preparing a lecture on physiology, Banting happened to read an article by Moses Barron in the November 1920 issue of *Surgery, Gynecology and Obstetrics*. The article discussed the physiology of the pancreas and also commented on the deterioration that occurred when the pancreatic ducts of an animal were cut. Banting read and reread the article, transfixed.

Inspired, Banting then and there developed the idea of using a hormone extracted from the pancreas of an animal to treat diabetes in humans. Consumed by his idea, Banting traveled to the University of Toronto to ask Dr. J. J. R. MacLeod, a prominent diabetes researcher, for permission to use his laboratory so that he could do pancreatic experiments on dogs. Dr. Banting was not a medical researcher nor had he ever performed any research on diabetes. To his credit, MacLeod agreed to the request and asked Charles Best, a medical student at the time, to assist Dr. Banting in the laboratory. MacLeod went home for the summer to his native Scotland, with no idea of the drama that would follow the experiments of Banting and Best.

During an unseasonably sweltering summer and spending most of their time in the small laboratory, Banting and Best performed their experiments and successfully treated a diabetic dog with their insulin extract.

Best later wrote, "Every time one of our diabetic dogs responded to insulin we hoped that the effect on patients would be just as dramatic.

When, in the autumn of 1921, we had demonstrated on 75 successive occasions in 10 completely depancreatized dogs, the invariably definitely and frequently very impressive lowering of blood sugar after the administration of our pancreatic extracts, we considered that the phase of the discovering was complete."

The first human trial on 14-year-old Leonard Thompson, who weighed 64 pounds at the time, was disappointing. Thompson developed abscesses at the sites of the injections and he became very sick, although his glucose levels dropped. Then biochemist James Collip, who had assisted Banting and Best, developed a refined extract, which he tested on Thompson. It worked amazingly well and Thompson's glucose levels plunged from 520 to 120 mg/dL within a day. Thompson lived another 15 years, dying of an unrelated ailment.

At first, however, Collip was unwilling to share the information about his refining process with Banting or Best. Through the course of the very stressful process of the experiments, relations between Collip with Banting and Best had become extremely strained. According to a later account by Best, when Collip announced that he was leaving to go patent the process himself, Best told him he was *not* leaving until Banting heard the news. Best then put a chair in front of the door, sat in it, and physically blocked Collip from leaving. When Banting came back and heard of Collip's plan, he was very upset. There are differing accounts of what happened next and whether or not a scuffle ensued between Banting and Collip. The men somehow resolved their differences and they subsequently worked together.

Banting and Best made their first report of their exciting discovery at a meeting of the American Physiological Society in December 1921 in New Haven, Connecticut. At first they met with considerable skepticism as Banting reportedly gave a halting and rambling presentation of his research and discovery. The physicians knew that Banting was a newcomer to diabetes research, and most of the attendees knew little or nothing about either him or his colleague.

The first impression of many people apparently was, who is this interloper that we've never heard of before? However, the mood changed, by some accounts, when Dr. MacLeod, who was also present and was well-known by the diabetes researchers, warmly embraced the discovery. The audience, mostly physicians, quickly realized that they were hearing about a remarkable and historic scientific breakthrough.

Joseph Barach wrote, in his 1928 article on the history of diabetes for *Annals of Medical History*, "It must have come as a great awakening to the savants in medicine, when the wished for remedy came so suddenly and so unexpectedly from such a quiet spot in the medical world. Today, millions of diabetics may eat and live because they have insulin to meet their metabolic requirement."

Also present at that momentous meeting in Connecticut was George Clowes, the director of research for Eli Lilly & Company, a pharmaceutical company. Perceiving the potential value of the discovery, Clowes offered Banting and Best the assistance of Lilly in developing a pure product that could be distributed on a large scale. They were interested; however, Banting did not patent his discovery but instead assigned the rights (for one dollar) to the University of Toronto.

Banting's course was not a smooth one and it was often only by sheer determination that he succeeded at all. For example, he visited the Lilly plant in Indianapolis, Indiana, in July 1922 to find out how they made drugs because he wanted to produce insulin in Canada. He learned that Lilly used a much more sophisticated process than he had available to him and that he would need vacuum stills to make insulin efficiently in Canada. This equipment was expensive and Banting would need $10,000 to buy it. In 1922, this was no small sum.

Undaunted, Banting went to see the chairman of the Board of Governors at the University of Toronto and asked him for the money to buy the vacuum stills. He was told he would have to wait until the entire Board was in session in September. Although September was only a few months away, that was still too long for Banting, who knew that every day that passed counted against the patients who were dying of diabetes, and for them, insulin meant the difference between life and death. The frustrated Banting asked the board chairman if the university would take the money if Banting could get it himself, somehow, and the startled chairman agreed.

Banting's next stop was New York, where he went to see Dr. H. Rowle Geyelin, a doctor treating children who were sick and dying from diabetes. On a previous visit, Geyelin had told Banting that he was going to keep his sickest patients in bed so they could stay alive until they could receive insulin. He had also told Banting that if he ever needed help, to let him know. Banting now asked Geyelin if he would help him obtain the money for the equipment he needed.

Geyelin called up a wealthy man whose daughter was dying of diabetes. The man's only question was who to make the check out to. Banting immediately wired ahead to Toronto to go ahead and buy the equipment and he also wired that Dr. Geyelin should be among the first to receive the insulin when it was ready. Geyelin received advance supplies of insulin in 1922. He used them on his patients, to dramatic effect. (Two of Geyelin's patients are depicted in the before and after photos in this section.)

In the summer of 1923, Eli Lilly & Company made an agreement with the University of Toronto to begin producing insulin in large quantities for North Americans and others with diabetes. At long last, there was true hope for the emaciated, ravaged, and dying victims of Type 1 diabetes.

Despite the lack of popular communications at the time—when very few people had a telephone—word rapidly spread throughout North America that there was a new "cure" for diabetes. Although insulin was not actually a cure of the disease but was instead a treatment (as it still is in modern times), in the eyes of the people who had diabetes and their families, insulin meant continued life. Lack of insulin meant certain death. Thus, it is no wonder that they perceived insulin as curative rather than merely therapeutic.

The clamor for the new drug was very great and it astonished physicians. Dr. Joseph H. Barach wrote in 1928,

> After insulin was announced and given to a number of internists in America for clinical trial, the appeal to these clinics by diabetic patients was tremendous. In my service at the Presbyterian Hospital the demand for treatment was far greater than we could possibly meet. Hundreds of letters from patients and their families, coming from all over the country, reflected the actual plight of the diabetic. These patients wrote that they had had the disease for periods of from one to twenty years, that they had had all kind of treatment by numerous doctors, and that in spite of many efforts to regain health, they were growing progressively worse. They invariably asked this one question, 'Was there really something that could be done to relieve them of their suffering?' Here were evidences of something very different from the complacent picture of the diabetic patient as described in books. The preceding medical treatment of these patients had been a failure, and they craved a return to health and to their occupations. These letters also made it clear that diabetes was not a disease of the rich, an idea which first appeared in the literature of the Hindus and writings of Avicenna, and apparently accepted by many writers even up to the 20th century.

Insulin transformed the lives of many people. For example, Robin Lawrence was a young British doctor who had developed diabetes and was dedicating what he thought were his remaining one or two years of life to treating patients in Florence, Italy. A biochemist friend sent him a

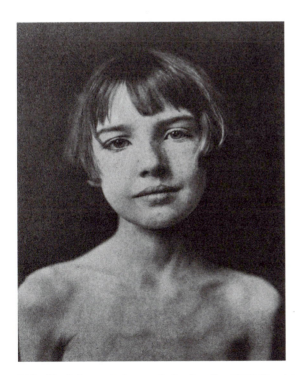
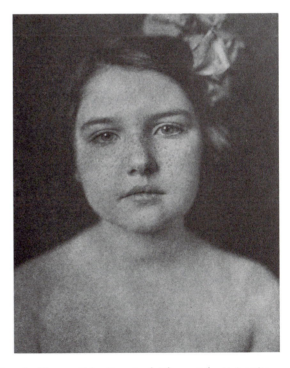

Girl with diabetes, before and after insulin, 1922 *(Reprinted courtesy the Thomas Fisher Rare Book Library at the University of Toronto.)*

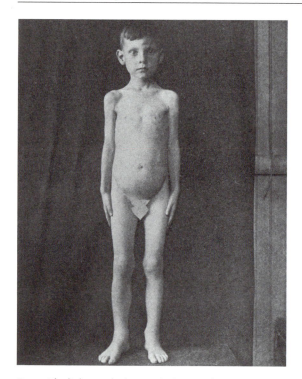 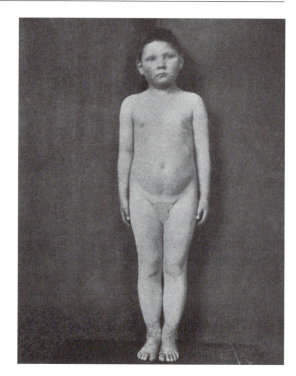

Boy with diabetes, before and after insulin, 1922 *(Reprinted courtesy the Thomas Fisher Rare Book Library at the University of Toronto.)*

telegram that said, "I have got insulin. It works. Come back immediately." Dr. Lawrence returned to England and he received insulin treatment. He subsequently became an eminent diabetologist who treated thousands of patients, educated many doctors, and lived to the age of 76 years, reportedly suffering no complications of diabetes.

Physicians also quickly perceived the potential lifesaving capabilities of insulin for their child patients with diabetes. In 1922, in a paper for the *Journal for Metabolic Research,* Dr. Geyelin (the physician who helped Banting locate the money for his equipment) and his colleagues at the Presbyterian Hospital in New York described the impact of insulin on nine children with diabetes. This article included both "before" and "after" photos of the children, taken before the administration of insulin and afterwards.

Most of the children in the "before" photographs looked very emaciated, even skeletal. After the insulin therapy, the photographs clearly revealed children who looked thin but normal. In fact, the children in the "after" pictures were barely recognizable as the same children in the "before" photographs.

The authors wrote,

One of the most striking and constantly observed effects of insulin in this group of diabetic children has been the rapid and complete disappearance of ketone bodies from the urine. When the initial ketosis was moderate in degree and accompanied by little or no evidence of an acidosis, the urine was occasionally found to be free from diabetic acid within 48 hours after the initiation of insulin therapy. In every case, the amount of diabetic acid in the urine was markedly diminished after the first week of insulin therapy, and in one case . . . did it persist for more than two weeks.

The doctors concluded, "In a series of nine children suffering from severe diabetes, treatment with insulin has been followed by certain definite results: (1) arrest of the downward course of the disease; (2) achievement of a total food intake approximating the normal age requirement in calories; (3) steady gain in weight and growth, with increase in mental and physical vigor; (4) absence of severe or permanent ill effects."

Noted physicians such as Dr. Elliott P. Joslin in Boston actively adopted and promoted the use of insulin. In one case, Joslin brought a five-year-old child before a spellbound audience of physicians, who listened to the child accurately describe a test for sugar in the urine and then expound about the meaning and importance of carbohydrates, proteins, and fats.

Doctors Banting and MacLeod were awarded the Nobel Prize for the discovery of insulin in 1923. Dr. Banting shared his prize with Dr. Best and Dr. MacLeod shared his prize with Dr. Collip. Banting was knighted in 1934 for his discovery, becoming Sir Frederick Banting, and he also received many other much-deserved honors.

There was considerable animosity for years between Banting and MacLeod because Banting made it clear that he felt that Best should have been the other recipient of the Nobel Prize and not Doctor MacLeod. MacLeod contended that he had provided the facilities for the work to be done and that he had also offered important advice and support and thus, his contributions were valuable. Banting's view has been largely vindicated in the judgment of history, which credits the discovery of insulin to Banting and Best.

Through the years, the ingredients and forms of insulin have been changed and improved upon. Insulin was made from beef and pork until the late 20th century, when synthetic forms of insulin were created. There are also different types of insulin in terms of their timeliness. For example, today there are long-acting, intermediate, and short-acting forms of insulin.

There are also various ways to introduce insulin into the body and the insulin pen or the implantable insulin pump are the most recent methods of insulin delivery, and inhaled insulin is another vehicle for introducing the drug into the body. It is easy to forget it but all these drugs and their different forms were predicated on the initial discovery of Doctors Banting and Best.

The American Diabetes Association

No book about diabetes or one that mentions the history of diabetes would be complete without a discussion of the American Diabetes Association (ADA), a powerful and important research and advocacy organization.

In 1940, the ADA was formed by physicians who had become concerned about the complications of diabetes and who wanted to learn more about treatment. The founder and first president was Cecil Striker, a clinician and medical professor at the University of Cincinnati.

In 1950, in concert with the American Dietetic Association and the U.S. Public Health Service, the ADA created the concept of meal exchanges. Foods were divided into six different groups with equivalent portions so that a diabetes patient could choose one food from one group one day and an equivalent food from that group (or another group) on another day.

Today the ADA publishes internationally acclaimed peer-reviewed journals on diabetes, including *Diabetes* and *Diabetes Care*. The ADA also publishes magazines and books for consumers with diabetes and their families.

The ADA has also been active in litigation, most notably in cases where children were barred from daycare centers because of their diabetes, as well as in cases where adults with diabetes have been unfairly denied employment.

The role of the ADA has evolved from an organization centering on treatment to one of research and advocacy as well as information-provider for doctors, patients, and their families. Today the ADA is one of the most powerful and effective nonprofit organizations in the United States.

Dr. Joslin and the Joslin Clinics

Elliott P. Joslin, a Boston physician, was a towering figure in diabetes until his death in 1962, leaving behind the Joslin Diabetes Center, which today is a large organization with affiliates at 23 locations in 12 states, serving more than 40,000 patients with diabetes.

Dr. Joslin's book *The Treatment of Diabetes Mellitus,* was published in 1916. He was globally regarded as one of the most influential and knowledgeable individuals in the field of diabetes. Joslin was one of the six doctors on the "Insulin Committee" that provided patients with the purified form of insulin that was first developed by Eli Lilly & Company in the early 1920s. Joslin also assisted with clinical trials.

Joslin's own mother, who was obese, had suffered from Type 2 diabetes. She died before the development of oral medications for people with diabetes. Perhaps in mind of his mother's weight problem, Joslin himself was said to be a man whose weight never varied more than a pound or so.

Joslin wrote about diabetes prior to the discovery of insulin by Banting and Best and after its introduction he was an immediate and very strong proponent of insulin. Dr. Joslin was also an ardent believer in the importance of careful diet as well as the need to educate patients on how they could best manage their diabetes.

Dr. Joslin's concern for his patients was evident in his work and writing. According to his biographer, Donald M. Barnett, MD, Dr. Joslin wrote in 1921,

Although six of the seven persons, all head of families . . living in [three] adjoining houses . . . on [a] peaceful, elm-lined . . . street . . . in a

country town in New England . . . succumbed to diabetes . . . no one spoke of an epidemic. . . . Consider the measure which would have been adopted to discover the source of the outbreak to prevent a recurrence . . . [as it would] . . . if these deaths had occurred from scarlet fever, typhoid fever or tuberculosis. . . . Because the disease was diabetes, and because the deaths occurred over a considerable interval of time, the fatalities passed unnoticed.

Dr. Joslin founded the Joslin Diabetes Center in Boston in 1898 and the Joslin Clinics actively continue today throughout the United States, treating patients and performing pioneering research. Joslin pioneered the still-important concept of using a team of specialists to treat people with diabetes and he also favored the use of long and short-acting insulins. In addition, Joslin was a strong proponent of frequent testing of glucose levels.

Diabetes Treatment in Modern Times

A variety of important changes occurred in the second half of the 20th century. Insulins were improved upon and people with Type 1 diabetes could use long, intermediate, or short-acting insulins. Humalog, an analog of a human-based insulin, replaced pork and beef insulin. Syringes were improved to be sharper and less painful. Special meters were developed, enabling people with diabetes to test their own blood from the comfort of their homes.

The Evolution of Insulin and Better Devices for People with Diabetes

If Drs. Banting and Best could see the changes to the original insulin that they developed, they would be very proud of how their brainchild has grown and matured. For example, Novo Nordisk Pharmaceuticals, Inc. developed the first slower-acting insulins, in 1936. In 1949, Becton Dickinson and Company produced a standardized syringe for insulin, approved by the American Diabetes Association. This standardization made life much easier for people with diabetes.

In the 1970s, portable glucose meters were introduced, enabling people with both Type 1 and Type 2 diabetes to easily test their blood glucose levels. Before this time, glucose monitoring was primarily managed only in the doctor's office, making daily monitoring difficult or impossible. The 1970s was also when the implantable insulin pump was first introduced, which was perfected further into the 21st century.

In 1986, the first insulin pen delivery system was developed, which ultimately led to the more convenient prefilled insulin pen. This device made injection easier and far less painful for people with diabetes.

Advances in DNA knowledge enabled researchers to create recombinant DNA insulin. The first human insulin analogue, Humalog (lispro) was developed by Eli Lilly & Company and approved by the Food and Drug Administration (FDA) in the United States in 1996. In 1998, studies began to show that inhaled insulin could work as effectively as insulin that was injected.

Development of Better Oral Medications

The 20th century, particularly the latter part of the century, was a time when many more cases of Type 2 diabetes were diagnosed. One disadvantage of an affluent lifestyle was that people had plenty/too much to eat and little need or incentive for physical labor. Rather than laboring in the fields, some people purchased memberships in health clubs.

Of course, not all people with Type 2 diabetes were or are affluent and many are individuals from lower socioeconomic strata. The middle to the end of the 20th century brought new and better oral medications for people with Type 2 diabetes. For example, in 1955, the first drugs in the sulfonylurea class were approved. These drugs induced the pancreas to produce more insulin. In 1961, Eli Lilly & Company developed glucagon for people with severe hypoglycemia.

In 1988, approval was given for angiotensin converting enzyme (ACE) inhibitor medications.

These drugs decreased proteinuria (protein in the urine) and delayed the further development of kidney disease, which was and still is, a major problem faced by many people with diabetes.

In 1995, two major drugs were introduced for people with diabetes. The Bayer Corporation introduced acarbose (Precose). It was an alpha-glucosidase inhibitor that delayed the digestion of carbohydrates.

Bristol-Myers Squibb Company introduced metformin, or Glucophage, in 1995. This was a biguanide drug that prevented the liver from releasing excessive amounts of glucose. Subsequent studies have revealed that people with both Type 2 diabetes and coronary artery disease (CAD) who take metformin have a lower death rate than their peers who take other medications.

In 1997, troglitazone, or Rezulin, was introduced by Parke-Davis for patients with Type 2 diabetes. This drug was subsequently pulled from the market by the Food and Drug Administration (FDA) in 2000 after it appeared to cause serious medical problems in some users.

In 1997, Novo Nordisk Pharmaceuticals, Inc. introduced Prandin (repaglinide). This is an oral medication that is fast acting and is taken by people with Type 2 diabetes before meals.

Another major change came with the home-based management of diabetes. Although people with diabetes still needed to see their physicians in the latter part of the 20th century, blood glucose meters enabled patients to check their own blood levels rather than having to go to a clinic for a blood check. Blood checks were given on a periodic basis in the doctor's clinic. Medicare and most other health insurance companies now provide medical coverage for these devices, making them affordable to the average person.

A Global Look at Diabetes Today and into the Future

After millennia of suffering and death from diabetes, today we can see ahead of us not only better and painless treatments for this disease, but we can also observe that actual cures lie within our grasp. Cures for diabetes encompass transplantations of beta cells as well as transplants of organs such as the pancreas or a pancreas/kidney combination transplant. The "Edmonton Protocol" developed by Dr. Shapiro and his colleagues at the University of Toronto was a breakthrough. Eight very ill patients with Type 1 diabetes received transplanted beta cells from the pancreases of deceased individuals. These transplants enabled them to remain off insulin for longer than one year.

Genetic manipulations may also offer hope for people with diabetes in the near future. In another path of major research, Dr. Aaron Vinik at the East Virginia School of Medicine and his colleagues are performing research with Islets Neogenesis Associated Protein (INGAP). This is a recently discovered, naturally occurring peptide that has been synthesized in the laboratory and that stimulates the growth of insulin-producing cells in the pancreas. It has been tested successfully on animals with diabetes and may mean a cure for humans with Type 1 diabetes in the future. As of this writing 62 human subjects are being tested.

If INGAP is successful in remitting diabetes among human subjects, this will mean a major breakthrough in treatment. It will not require organ transplants or islet cells from donated organs, nor will there be a problem of rejection, since the person's own pancreas will be producing new beta cells that make insulin. It is unknown as of this writing how long it will take to complete trials and, if they are successful, to begin treating the general public. However, it is likely that such treatment is years down the road.

Advances in diabetes are very important and very needed because diabetes is on the rise worldwide and is considered by some experts already to be at an epidemic level, according to reports from the World Health Organization. In a 1998 article published in *Diabetes Care,* Dr. Hilary King and colleagues described the antici-

pated global impact of diabetes, based on World Health Organization data over the period 1995–2025.

According to their findings, the worldwide prevalence of diabetes was about 4 percent in 1995 and was projected to increase to 5.4 percent by 2025. Although an increase of 1.4 percent might seem tiny or insignificant, it is rather a formidable increase when considering the entire population of the world. Another factor that should be considered is that the world population is growing, so that a 1.4 percent increase in today's population is different from a projected 1.4 percent increase in the population that the world faces in 2025.

Even more conservative estimates, released by British diabetologists in *Diabetic Medicine* in 2000, predict at least a 1 percent increase in worldwide diabetes.

One intriguing prediction is that most of the increases in cases of diabetes will be found in developing countries; for example, some experts anticipate a 170 percent increase of cases, from 84 million to 228 million, in the developing countries. Some predict that the number of cases in Asia alone will more than double, from 66 million in 1997 to over 132 million by 2010.

This does not, however, mean that diabetes will stabilize in developed countries such as North America or Europe. Rather, it means that it will go up less precipitously. The authors project an increase from 51 million to 72 million in the developed countries over the 1995–2025 period.

According to the authors, in the developed countries, most people with diabetes are 65 years old or over. In contrast, the majority of people with diabetes in developing countries are 45–64 years old.

It is anticipated that the countries that will have the greatest population of people with diabetes will continue to be as follows: China, India, and the United States.

Globally, more women than men have diabetes. There were 73 million women versus 62 million men with diabetes in 1995. This means that in 1995, about 54 percent of all people in the world with diabetes were women. By 2025, the female excess ratio is expected to decrease worldwide slightly to about 159 women versus 141 men who have diabetes. This means that 53 percent of all people in the world who have diabetes will be female.

In the developed countries, there were 31 million women and 20 million men with diabetes. In the developing countries, the numbers were virtually equal, at about 42 million women and 42 million men.

Many people with diabetes will live in urban (city) areas by 2025. The urban/rural ratio is expected to increase dramatically by more than double, from the 1.6 of 1995 to 3.3 by 2025.

The authors said, "The results of this study suggest that for the world as a whole, between the years 1995 and 2025, the adult population will increase by 64 percent, the prevalence of diabetes in adults will increase by 35 per-cent, and the number of people with diabetes will increase by 122 percent. For the developed countries, there will be an 11 percent increase in the adult population, a 27 percent increase in the prevalence of adult diabetes, and a 42 percent increase in the number of people with diabetes. For the developing countries, there will be an 82 percent increase in the adult population, a 48 percent increase in the prevalence of adult diabetes, and a 170 percent increase in the number of people with diabetes."

Bibliography for the History of Diabetes

Allan, Frank N. "Diabetes Before and After Insulin." *Medical History* 16, no. 3 (July 1972): 66–73.

Allen, Frederick M., M.D. "Blueberry Leaf Extract: Physiologic and Clinical Properties in Relation to Carbohydrate Metabolism." *Journal of the American Medical Association* 89 (November 5, 1927): 1577–1580.

Allen, Frederick M., M.D. "Present Results and Outlook of Diabetic Treatment." *Annals of Internal Medicine* 2, no. 2 (August 1928): 203–215.

American Diabetes Association. "Milestones in Diabetes Treatment." *Diabetes Forecast* (November 1998): 76–82.

Banting, F. G., M.D. "Early Work on Insulin." *Science* 85, no. 2217 (June 25, 1937): 594–596.

———. "Insulin in the Treatment of Diabetes Mellitus." *The Journal of Metabolic Research* (November 1922): 547–604.

Banting, F.G., M.B., and Best, C. H., B.A. "The Internal Secretion of the Pancreas." *The Journal of Laboratory and Clinical Medicine* 8, no. 5 (February 1922): 251–266.

Barach, J., M.D. "Historical Facts in Diabetes." *Annals of Medical History* 10 (1928): 387–386.

Barnett, Donald M., M.D. *Elliott P. Joslin, M.D.: A Centennial Portrait.* (Boston, Mass.: Joslin Diabetes Center, 1998).

Best, Charles H., M.D. "The First Clinical Use of Insulin." *Diabetes* 5, no. 1 (January–February 1956): 65–67.

Bliss, Michael. *Banting: A Biography.* (Toronto, Canada: McClelland and Stewart, 1984).

———. *The Discovery of Insulin.* (Chicago, Ill.: University of Chicago Press, 1982).

Foster, Nellis B., M.D. *Diabetes Mellitus: Designed for the Use of Practitioners of Medicine.* (Philadelphia, Pa.: J. B. Lippincott Company, 1915).

Fulton, John F., M.D. "Reminiscences of the Discovery of Insulin." *Diabetes* 5, no. 1 (January–February 1956): 65–67.

Geyelin, H. Rawle, M.D., et al. "The Use of Insulin in Juvenile Diabetes." *Journal of Metabolic Research* 2, nos. 5 and 6 (1922): 767–791.

Joslin, Elliott, M.D., M.A. *The Treatment of Diabetes Mellitus with Observations upon the Disease Based upon Thirteen Hundred Cases.* (Philadelphia, Pa.: Lea & Febiger, 1917).

Karlsen, Marie, Dorrine Khakpour, and Leslie Lobeda Thomson. "Efficacy of Medical Nutrition Therapy: Are Your Patients Getting What They Need?" *Clinical Diabetes* 14, no. 3 (May–June 1996): 54–61.

Leibowitz, J.O. "The Concept of Diabetes in Historical Perspective." *Israel Journal of Medical Sciences* 8, no. 3 (March 1972): 469–475.

MacCracken, Joan, M.D., guest editor with Donna Hotel. "From Ants to Analogues: Puzzles and Promises in Diabetes Management." *Postgraduate Medicine* 101, no. 4 (April 1997).

MacLeod, J. J. R. "History of the Researches Leading to the Discovery of Insulin." *Bulletin of the History of Medicine* 52, no. 3 (Fall 1978): 295–312.

Myers, Victor C., and Cameron V. Bailey. "The Lewis and Benedict Method for the Estimation of Blood Sugar, with Some Observations Obtained in Disease." *The Journal of Biological Chemistry* 2 (1916): 147–161.

Papaspryos, N. S., M.D. *The History of Diabetes Mellitus.* (Stuttgart, Germany: Georg Thieme Verlag, 1964).

Pyke, D. A. "Preamble: the History of Diabetes." *The International Textbook of Diabetes.* (London, England: John Wiley & Sons, 1997).

Rennie, John, D.Sc., and Thomas Fraser, M.B., M.A. "The Islets of Langerhans in Relation to Diabetes." *The Biochemical Journal* 2, no. 1 (1907): 17–19.

Striker, Cecil, M.D., comp. *Famous Faces in Diabetes.* (Boston, Mass.: G. K. Hall & Co., 1961).

Wallace, George B., M.D. "Recent Advances in the Treatment of Diabetes Mellitus." *Journal of the American Medical Association* 55, no. 25 (December 17, 1910): 2107–2109.

abuse/neglect Causing harm or failing to provide needed care to a person who cannot provide that care to himself or herself. Individuals with diabetes need the ability/capability to check their glucose levels at least several times daily to be able to adjust their diet and activities accordingly. They also need to be able to take oral medication or insulin, or both, if necessary.

If a person is unable to check his or her own levels of blood glucose or administer medication appropriately, because he or she is a child or has a disabling condition that makes it impossible, then it is up to family members or others to ensure that the person with diabetes receives such care. A failure to provide such assistance could be considered abuse or neglect under a state's law, particularly if the individual has Type 1 diabetes and must receive insulin in order to live. If the individual is a child under the age of 18, the parents or guardians could be charged with neglect or, more specifically, "medical neglect." (See also RELIGION/SPIRITUALITY.)

acanthosis nigricans A skin condition that is characterized by many papillomas (benign skin tumors) and also by thickening of the skin (hyperkeratosis). The skin is often described as having a velvety texture. Acanthosis nigricans is primarily found on the neck of the patient, although it may also appear in other areas such as the elbows, knees, groin, underarms, and knuckles. The acanthosis itself only causes cosmetic problems.

This condition may be a risk factor for the development of Type 2 diabetes. It is also found in patients with severe INSULIN RESISTANCE. In addition, it is also found in many patients with lesser degrees of insulin resistance, obesity, acromegaly, and Cushing's syndrome.

James Burke and his colleagues developed a scale to measure acanthosis nigricans, and this scale was published in a 1999 issue of *Diabetes Care*. The scale offers conditions to consider in various parts of the body, as well as their severity, including the neck, axilla (underarm area), knuckles, elbows, and knees. For example, in considering "neck texture," the authors offer four levels, from 0 to 3. A "0" is defined as a neck texture that is "smooth to touch; no differentiation from normal skin to palpation." In contrast, a "3" level is "extremely coarse; 'hills and valleys' observable on visual examination."

As of this writing, there is no treatment for this disease.

James P. Burke, Ph.D., et al., "A Quantitative Scale of Acanthosis Nigricans," *Diabetes Care* 22, no. 10 (October 1999): 2655–2659.

C. A. Stuart et al., "Acanthosis Nigricans As a Risk Factor for Non-Insulin Dependent Diabetes," *Clinical Pediatrics* 37, no. 2 (1998): 73.

acarbose (Precose) An alpha-glucosidase inhibitor that slows the absorption of carbohydrates from the small intestine and thus diminishes the increase in glucose after a meal. It is a medication that is occasionally used for people with Type 2 diabetes and occasionally for patients with Type 1 diabetes. It decreases hyperglycemia (high blood glucose levels) by affecting the absorption of carbohydrates within the intestines.

ACE inhibitors/ACE drugs Angiotensin-converting enzyme (ACE) inhibitors are a class of medications used to reduce high blood pressure (HYPERTENSION), to reverse left ventricular hypertrophy (thickening of the main wall of the heart) and to improve quality of life and increase the survival rate among patients with congestive heart failure. They are also used to slow the progression of renal (kidney) disease, especially among patients who have DIABETIC NEPHROPATHY.

ACE medications were used in the HOPE STUDY among patients with a high risk of developing CARDIOVASCULAR DISEASE. Among the subjects, including patients with diabetes, the researchers found that the medication effectively decreased the risk of serious cardiovascular problems.

The effect of ACE inhibitors in slowing the progression of nephropathy is independent of their effect on blood pressure. This has been clearly demonstrated in patients with both Type 1 and Type 2 diabetes and patients with and without hypertension.

When patients with diabetes use ACE inhibitors, physicians order kidney tests such as BUN, CREATININE, urinary microalbumin/creatinine ratios and potassium to monitor patients, because in rare cases, this class of medication may cause changes that require adjustment of the dosage.

The use of nonsteroidal antiinflammatory (NSAID) medications, often used to reduce pain and inflammation in diseases such as arthritis, may slightly decrease the effectiveness of ACE drugs. Pregnant women should avoid ACE medications completely. The most common side effect found with an ACE medication is cough, and it is often mild and generally well tolerated.

Some examples of commonly prescribed ACE inhibitor medications as of this writing are: captopril (Capoten), enalapril (Vasotec), quinapril (Accupril), fosinopril (Monopril), and benazepril (Lotensin). (See also CORONARY HEART DISEASE, MYOCARDIAL INFARCTION, STROKE.)

acetoacetate One of the two major KETONES (or ketoacids) that the body makes. The other is ß-HYDROXYBUTYRATE. Acetoacetate is the ketone that can be typically measured and monitored by home use urine dipsticks. (See also ACETONE, DIABETIC KETOACIDOSIS [DKA].)

acetone A ketone body or ketoacid. Acetone appears when the body has inadequate insulin effect present or the person is starving. The body then begins to metabolize fat and forms ketoacids. These ketoacids can cause nausea, vomiting, and abdominal pain and can also decrease blood pressure. This is part of what occurs during the process of DIABETIC KETOACIDOSIS (DKA). The two major KETONES are ACETOACETATE and B-HYDROXYBUTYRATE.

acidosis An excess of acid in the body, that may stem from a variety of causes. If the person has diabetes, this excess may escalate and can lead to a dangerous and life-threatening condition that is known as DIABETIC KETOACIDOSIS (DKA). Excess acid in the system can affect blood pressure, the ability of the heart to pump effectively, and its ability to pump regularly (i.e., acidosis may induce an irregular heart rhythm.)

acquired immune deficiency syndrome (AIDS) A chronic viral and severe degenerative illness, for which there is no cure as of this writing, although there are many medications that may help. AIDS results from the human immunodeficiency virus (HIV). Individuals who have both diabetes and AIDS need very careful monitoring.

In 2000, some researchers demonstrated that nondiabetic individuals with AIDS gained benefit from taking very small doses of INSULIN, improving their overall health status and enabling them to gain weight and strength. Further research is needed to determine the full implications of this finding.

Patients with AIDS can develop forms of lipodystrophy, which are abnormal deposits of fat that are usually seen in patients with Cushing's disease/syndrome. Cushing's disease is due to excess steroid effect (produced by the body or taken by the patient for medical reasons). Lipodystrophy is also found among patients with diabetes who inject insulin repetitively into one area of the body. Interestingly, researchers have been using diabetes drugs such as metformin, rosiglitazone, and pioglitazone to try to treat this problem.

acromegaly/gigantism Very rare endocrine disorders of the pituitary gland due to an excessive output of growth hormone. The disease is called "acromegaly" if it occurs after puberty and it is denoted as "gigantism" if it occurs before puberty. Diabetes may also be a consequence of this disease.

The prepubescent individual will attain unusually tall heights because of accelerated bone growth, while the adult who develops acromegaly will develop tissue deformities, such as swelling of the hands and feet, and eventually bony and cartilaginous facial changes that alter the individual's appearance. People who develop the disease after puberty will not grow any taller because the bones have already formed and the growth plates have fused.

About 20 to 30 percent of those with acromegaly/gigantism have diabetes and about 30 to 45 percent have impaired glucose tolerance. This disease is very rare and only about 40 to 60 people per million have it.

Diagnosis of Acromegaly/Gigantism

Diagnosis of acromegaly is often delayed by 15 to 20 years because the onset is very insidious. As a result, diagnosis may not occur until the individual is 35 to 50 years old, when the signs and symptoms have become much more prominent and obvious.

If the disease occurs during childhood, it is more apparent, although it still may go undiagnosed and untreated. The late actor Andre the Giant had gigantism. Some experts speculate that in the Biblical story of David and Goliath, Goliath was a victim of this syndrome.

If the physician suspects acromegaly/gigantism, the doctor can order a fasting blood test of growth hormone. This test alone is not sufficient and should be combined with an ORAL GLUCOSE TOLERANCE TEST because when patients' bodies are overproducing growth hormone, the ingestion of the sugar glucose will not appropriately lower blood growth hormone levels.

Other blood tests, such as for IGF-1 levels, may be ordered. These levels are increased in people with acromegaly/gigantism. Confirming tests such as magnetic resonance imaging (MRI) scans of the pituitary may be ordered.

Causes of the Disorder

In many cases, the excess of growth hormone is caused by a noncancerous tumor in the pituitary gland. Rarely, it may also be caused by secretion of growth hormone–releasing hormone that is made by a tumor in another part of the body.

Resulting Medical Problems

In addition to causing diabetes, other medical problems that stem from acromegaly are hypertension (about 25 percent of acromegaly patients are hypertensive), arthritis, hypothyroidism, and kidney stones. There is also an increased risk for heart disease and the disease may also cause vision problems. In addition, individuals with acromegaly are also at a greater risk for developing polyps in the colon and for colorectal cancer. As a result, experts recommend that a colonoscopy be performed every two to four years, depending on the recommendation of the treating physician.

Key Symptoms

Some signs and symptoms of this disorder are as follows:

- Oily skin
- Achy joints
- Extreme sweating (hyperhidrosis)
- Weakness

- Skin tags (acrochordons)
- Hypertension
- Excess enlargement of the mouth, nose, and tongue (acral growth)
- Deepening voice
- Deformities of teeth and facial bones
- Carpal tunnel syndrome (compressed median nerve, accompanied by numbness, tingling, and weakness in the wrist, thumb, index, or middle finger)

Treating the Disease

Acromegaly is often treated with pituitary surgery (usually transsphenoidal through the sinuses), which is successful in about 80 to 90 percent of cases. Remission of many symptoms generally occurs after surgery.

Medications are also a common form of treatment. Bromocriptine has been found to be successful in improving the quality of life of many patients. In addition, an injectable hormone, such as somatostatin, is also effective in some cases.

A study reported in a 2000 issue of *Drug Week* reported on the success of Somavert, an investigational drug, in effectively blocking the excessive growth hormone secreted by a pituitary tumor. The majority of patients (89 percent) who were at the highest doses of Somavert achieved normal blood levels within 12 weeks, versus the 10 percent of patients on placebo who received normal results over the same timeframe.

Radiation therapy may be used when other treatments have failed, although it is generally considered a last resort for treatment. Doctors may use radioisotope implantation with protein beam and alpha particles. Focused radiation may be performed with a gamma knife. (See also GROWTH HORMONE.)

"Acromegaly," (February 1995) NIDDK, NIH Publication No. 95-3924.

"Acromegaly: Genetically Modified Growth Hormone May Offer Hope for Treatment," *Drug Week* (May 1, 2000).

S. Ezzat et al., "Acromegaly: Clinical and Biochemical Features in 500 Patients," *Medicine* 73, no. 5 (1994): 233–240.

"Giant Leap," *Chemist & Druggist* (October 16, 1999).

Williams Textbook of Endocrinology, (New York, N.Y.: W. B. Saunders, 2001).

adolescents with diabetes Most adolescents with diabetes suffer from Type 1 diabetes but some adolescents have Type 2 diabetes, particularly if they are obese and sedentary. In fact, increasing numbers of children and teenagers in the United States are being diagnosed with Type 2 diabetes. Native American adolescents who have diabetes are more likely to have Type 2 diabetes than Type 1 diabetes, according to the CENTERS FOR DISEASE CONTROL AND PREVENTION (CDC).

There are also a very small number, primarily African American adolescents, who suffer from MATURITY-ONSET DIABETES IN THE YOUNG (MODY). This is a very rare genetic form of Type 2 diabetes that can develop in nonobese teenagers. It may account for 2 percent to 5 percent of all Type 2 diabetes cases in people under age 25, but it is often unrecognized and undiagnosed. MODY is rarely found in white adolescents.

Adolescents with Type 1 Diabetes

Formerly called "juvenile diabetes," "juvenile onset diabetes," or "insulin-dependent diabetes mellitus (IDDM)," the illness was renamed because it may be diagnosed in young adults or even older individuals. Type 1 diabetes is caused by the body's failed ability to make insulin. For this reason, people with Type 1 diabetes must take exogenous insulin to live.

According to the CDC, the prevalence of Type 1 diabetes in the United States among people ages 0 to 19 years is 1.7 per 1,000. In general, Caucasians are more likely to have Type 1 diabetes than are blacks, Asians, or American Indians.

Some adolescents are at risk for developing EATING DISORDERS, particularly females in their early teens. Some girls manipulate their insulin by taking a lower dose or not taking insulin at all, in order to lose weight. One indicator of this behavior is weight loss in the face of an adolescent who is eating normally. The child may also have another form of eating disorder, called "bulimia," in which the person eats, sometimes to excess, and then induces vomiting.

Adolescents with Type 2 Diabetes

Formerly called "adult onset diabetes" or "non-insulin-dependent diabetes mellitus" (NIDDM), Type 2 diabetes is a disease of insulin resistance and the inability to make enough insulin to normalize the blood glucose. This means that the body makes insulin, but for some reason, it is not used properly. Individuals with Type 2 diabetes must also test their blood glucose and follow appropriate nutrition and exercise plans. They may need to take oral medications or insulin to control the disease.

In the late 1990s, researchers discovered that an increasing number of adolescents in the United States were developing classic Type 2 diabetes. According to a 2001 issue of the *British Medical Journal,* Type 2 diabetes is also on the rise among teenagers in other countries as well, and has been reported in children in Canada, Japan, New Zealand, Australia, and other countries.

Native American teenagers have a high risk of developing Type 2 diabetes, especially those who are in tribes such as the PIMA INDIANS. According to the CDC, among 15- to 19-year-old Pima tribe members, 50.9 of every 1,000 people have Type 2 diabetes. This is much higher than the rate of 4.1 per 1,000 for teenagers ages 12–19 in the United States. Researchers have been studying the Pima Indians for years to determine why their rate of Type 2 diabetes is so much higher than for all other racial groups.

Teens with Type 2 diabetes are usually diagnosed between the ages of 12 and 14. Few of the oral medications for treating adult Type 2 diabetes have been tested on adolescents and doctors must rely on these medications to treat children. Adolescents with Type 2 diabetes rarely need insulin, although insulin is an approved drug for children.

Diagnosing Teenagers

Adolescents are diagnosed for diabetes in the same manner as adults are, based on symptoms and the results of blood tests. Often it may not be clear at the start whether the child has Type 1 or Type 2 diabetes, and special blood tests are needed to measure islet cell antibodies, anti-GAD antibodies, and C-peptide levels.

Risk of Diabetic Ketoacidosis

One of the biggest risks that adolescents with Type 1 diabetes face is that of DIABETIC KETOACIDOSIS (DKA). This is a dangerous result of diabetes out of control and can result in COMA and even death. DKA may occur in an adolescent who has not yet been diagnosed. It may also occur in adolescents who know they have diabetes but they are purposely withholding insulin, possibly as a consequence of an eating disorder and an attempt to lose weight.

The other reason for DKA may be that the adolescent has another illness. This is why it is so important to establish SICK DAY RULES. Many people mistakenly believe that when a person with diabetes is sick, they do not have to be careful about their diet or take their medications. Glycemic control may be especially important at this time, however, because of the severe stress that the body is undergoing when another illness is present. If the teenager is so ill that he or she cannot eat or drink (and thus, is susceptible to DEHYDRATION), the risk for DKA increases further.

In several small studies of teenagers with diabetes who died, the majority of deaths were attributed to DKA (about 85 percent) and a small percentage were attributed to HYPOGLYCEMIA. Since hypoglycemia is another indicator of glucose levels that are out of control, this further underlines the importance of monitoring glucose levels at home, especially when the person with diabetes is ill.

General Coping Difficulties

Because teenagers are often self-conscious about their bodies and their behaviors, it can be difficult for them to deal with their diabetes or even admit that they have the illness at all. They may resent the questions of their parents or others about their diet and blood testing regimens, even when those questions are reasonable.

According to a 2000 article by Barbara Schreiner, et al. in *Diabetes Spectrum,* the impact of diabetes on the adolescent varies with age. For example, younger adolescents ages 11–14 years are very self-conscious, and as a result, they may not want anyone to observe them doing a finger stick. Adolescents with diabetes may also worry that others could notice their injection sites. They may also refuse to wear an emergency medical identification. Another concern may be that they will have an attack of hypoglycemia when they are out with their friends.

Possible management solutions that the authors offer are alternative options to traditional medical emergency IDs, such as shoe tags. Parents may use the teen's own self-consciousness to encourage the adolescent to rotate the site of the injection. By pointing out that rotating a site is less likely to make it noticeable, this should encourage site rotation. Pointing out that good glycemic control can avert hypoglycemia may encourage the adolescent to pay more attention to glucose management, especially monitoring.

Teens of this age may have mood swings because of the hormonal changes they are experiencing, and this can affect their glucose levels as well. During the pubertal changes and growth spurts of adolescence, tight glycemic control is difficult because of the counterregulatory hormones that are elevated.

Adolescents in the early years may be defiant and uncooperative, refusing to adhere to meal plans and becoming angry at reminders to test their blood. Experts say that it may be helpful to have the teenager see her diabetes team by herself. Counseling may also be helpful, because the counselor may be able to help the teenager cope with her anger. Some experts say that some teenagers have a fatalistic view about their illness and mistakenly believe that they are doomed to die young. This may also be an excuse to avoid testing their blood and injecting insulin.

Teens who are 15 to 16 years old have other issues, such as an increased demand for independence and more instances of boundary testing. Teens of this age may experiment with tobacco, alcohol, or drugs. They may also become sexually active.

To help teens of this age, experts recommend involving them more in decision making and using negotiation to affect behavior. Teens with diabetes should also be educated on substance abuse and how drugs, alcohol, and tobacco could affect them in relation to their disease. Teens also need to be educated about sexuality.

Older teens (ages 17–18) are often idealistic and they may be interested in becoming involved at the local level with organizations such as the AMERICAN DIABETES ASSOCIATION. Teens of this age are also beginning to think about their future and seek greater independence. Adolescents of this age may wish to see the doctor on their own. They also continue to need education about their diabetes. Adults may think teenagers already know what they need to know about diabetes but sometimes important issues that were discussed earlier may not have made an impression or were not understood at the time.

Problems with adherence It can be difficult for adolescents to self-monitor their glucose levels and their diabetes symptoms for several reasons. One reason is that they are emotionally immature and often very distractible. Another reason is that most adolescents seek to be like everyone else, but everyone else does not have diabetes, nor do they have to test their blood, inject medication, watch their diet, and so forth. As a result, adolescents with diabetes may agree to eat foods that are inadvisable, fail to check their blood glucose levels regularly, and not take their medicine in the proper dose (or at all). They may also ignore symptoms of hypoglycemia and other indicators of problems. In some cases, adolescents with diabetes (especially younger teenagers) may develop eating disorders.

Attitude Is Key

Adolescents and children who believe they can manage their diabetes have measurably better glucose levels than teenagers who believe their disease controls them and there is little they can do about it. There is an apparent self-fulfilling prophecy at work: those teenagers who think they can control their diabetes are successful at controlling it. Those who believe that there is little or nothing they can do about their illness often do not bother to take appropriate actions to manage their illness. As a result, they have poor control and they are at greater risk for consequences.

A study reported in a 2001 issue of *Diabetes Care* demonstrated adolescents' beliefs toward their illness affected the outcome of their blood levels. The researchers studied 144 adolescents and children with diabetes from the United Kingdom. They found that girls had worse levels of glycemic control than boys did and higher rates of depression and anxiety. Females were also more likely to report that diabetes impaired their lives.

The authors said, "These results indicate that the more adolescents believe that their treatment regimen will control their diabetes, the better their subsequent dietary self-management will be. Better dietary self-care and gender [male] were associated with better glycemic control of diabetes. The greater impact a young person perceives diabetes to have on his or her life, the more anxiety he or she subsequently experiences."

E. Boland et al., "A Primer on the Use of Insulin Pumps in Adolescents," *The Diabetes Educator* 24, no. 1 (1998): 78–86.

Kathryn S. Bryden, R.N., "Eating Habits, Body Weight, and Insulin Misuse," *Diabetes Care* 22, no. 12 (December 1999): 1956–1960.

Denis Daneman, M.B., B.Ch., F.R.C.P.C., "Diabetes-Related Mortality: A Pediatrician's View," *Diabetes Care* 24, no. 5 (2001): 801–802.

The Diabetes Control and Complications Trial Research Group, "Effect of Intensive Diabetes Treatment on the Development and Progression of Long-Term Complications in Adolescents with Insulin-Dependent Diabetes Mellitus: Diabetes Control and Complications Trial," *The Journal of Pediatrics* 125, no. 2 (August 1994): 177–188.

Anne Fagot-Campagna, K. M. Venkat Narayan, and Giuseppina Imperatore, "Type 2 Diabetes in Children," *British Medical Journal* 322 (2001): 377–378.

Damian McNamara, "Overcoming Juvenile Diabetes with a Little Planning and High Tech," *FDA Consumer* 34, no. 4 (July 2000): 28.

Stephen W. Ponder, M.D., C.D.E., et al., "Type 2 Diabetes Mellitus in Teens," *Diabetes Spectrum* 13, no. 2 (2000): 95.

Rosenbloom et al., "Emerging Epidemic of Type 2 Diabetes in Youth," *Diabetes Care* 22, no. 2 (1999): 345–354.

Barb Schreiner, R.N., M.N., C.D.E., et al., "Management Strategies for the Adolescent Lifestyle," *Diabetes Spectrum* 13, no. 2 (2000): 83.

T. Chas Skinner, Ph.D., and Sarah E. Hampson, Ph.D., "Personal Models of Diabetes in Relation to Self-Care, Well-Being, and Glycemic Control: A Prospective Study in Adolescence," *Diabetes Care* 24, no. 5 (May 2001): 828–833.

(See also CHILDREN, EATING DISORDERS.)

adult onset diabetes One of the former names for Type 2 diabetes, also formerly known as noninsulin diabetes mellitus or NIDDM. The name was changed because it is possible for the "onset" to occur in childhood or adolescence. In fact, increasing numbers of children in North America are being diagnosed with the disease, particularly if they are obese, sedentary, and have a family history of diabetes. Type 2 diabetes is as serious an illness as is Type 1 diabetes and should be treated as aggressively.

By definition, patients with this illness still make some insulin and may be treated with diet, exercise, and pills. In some cases, they may also require insulin. Patients with Type 2 diabetes both make insufficient insulin and are unable to properly use it.

If people with Type 2 diabetes are ill or stressed enough, they can develop DIABETIC KETOACIDOSIS (DKA), although this occurs much less commonly than among patients who have

Type 1 diabetes. With very high glucose levels, these patients can also develop HYPEROSMOLAR COMA, a life-threatening condition. (See also TYPE 2 DIABETES.)

advanced glycosylation end products (AGEs)
Tissue chemicals that can be measured in the skin and the urine. Elevated levels indicate the presence of DIABETIC RETINOPATHY or DIABETIC NEPHROPATHY.

These elevated levels occur when glucose binds to proteins that are both inside and outside the cells. AGEs affect protein and its cellular and organic structure and function. They are also associated with complications such as diabetic retinopathy and diabetic nephropathy. Researchers are now exploring ways to inhibit the formation of AGEs, in order to slow or altogether prevent such complications.

African Americans with diabetes African Americans who suffer from either Type 1 or Type 2 diabetes, although Type 1 diabetes is far less frequent among African Americans. About 90 to 95 percent of African Americans with diabetes have Type 2 diabetes. According to the National Diabetes Education Program, there are more than 2.3 million African Americans with diabetes in the US, including 1.5 million who have been diagnosed and 730,000 who have not yet been diagnosed. Black women are at particular risk.

African Americans with diabetes have a higher prevalence of complications linked to diabetes for several basic reasons. Some of the key factors that are involved include:

- Genetic predisposition to diabetes
- High blood pressure
- High glucose levels
- Lower education (less knowledge about risks and complications)

A growing problem The numbers of African Americans with diabetes has greatly increased over the course of a generation: compared to 1968, there are four times as many African Americans in 2000 who were diagnosed with diabetes.

Blacks in United States Have Higher Risk for Diabetes than Whites
African Americans with diabetes are overrepresented in the U.S. population. Although African Americans represent only about 11 percent of the total population in the United States, their numbers account for 17 percent of all Americans with diabetes. Another grim statistic: the death rate among blacks with diabetes is 27 percent higher than among whites with the illness.

Individuals who are of African-American descent have twice the risk of developing Type 2 diabetes than do whites in North America. African-American children and adolescents, particularly when obese, are also at high risk for developing Type 2 diabetes. However, African American children in the United States are less likely to have Type 1 diabetes than white children.

Age is another factor in the incidence of diabetes. Middle-aged and older African Americans are more likely to have diabetes than are their younger same-race counterparts, just as the rates of diabetes increase with age in other racial and ethnic groups. However, black women are at greater risk for the disease than WOMEN WITH DIABETES in other races.

In an article reported in a 2000 issue of the *Journal of the American Medical Association (JAMA)*, researchers Frederick Brancati and colleagues reported on their Atherosclerosis Risk in Communities (ARIC) study of 2,646 African Americans and 9,461 Caucasians ages 45–64, drawn from various parts of the United States and followed up over nine years.

None of the subjects were diagnosed with diabetes when the study began. At the conclusion of the study, researchers reported their findings of a greater incidence of Type 2 diabetes among African-Americans, particularly African-American women. Black women were 2.4 times more likely to have diabetes than white women. Black men were 1.5 times more likely to have diabetes than white men.

According to the researchers, black women and men both had higher systolic and diastolic blood pressures (HYPERTENSION) than white women or men. In addition, black women had a significantly higher BODY MASS INDEX than white women, although black men and white men were similar in this measure. OBESITY is a major risk factor for the development of Type 2 diabetes.

Experts believe that at least half of the risk factors contributing to the development of diabetes in African-American men and women could be modified with lifestyle changes, such as diet, exercise, weight loss, controlling blood pressure, smoking cessation, and taking other actions.

High Risk of Diabetes Among Black Women

As mentioned, African-American women are particularly at risk for developing Type 2 diabetes. An estimated 28 percent of all African-American women over age 50 have diabetes, as do about 19 percent of African-American males who are over 50 years. About one of every three African-American women between the ages of 65–74 have diabetes, an extremely high rate.

Complications of Diabetes Are More Frequent and More Severe Among African Americans

Diabetes is also associated with other diseases and with more severe complications. According to a study released in 2000 and published in the *Journal of Clinical Epidemiology*, African-American women with diabetes have a higher rate of coronary heart disease, cardiovascular disease, and death when compared to other racial groups. (See DEATH.)

African Americans with diabetes are twice as likely to suffer from blindness and three to five times as likely to experience END-STAGE RENAL DISEASE as whites. Their risk of suffering from AMPUTATION is also twice as high as that for whites.

DIABETIC RETINOPATHY is another common problem among African Americans with diabetes. Blacks with diabetes face a 40–50 percent greater risk of developing diabetic retinopathy over that experienced by whites. In a study reported in a January 2000 issue of *Archives of Ophthalmology,* researchers included 725 black patients with Type 1 diabetes and evaluated their risk for diabetic retinopathy. The key risk factors that they found leading to the development of diabetic retinopathy were the existence of renal (kidney) disease, poor glycemic control, long-term diabetes, and a high systolic blood pressure.

As a result of the frequency and severity of complications that African Americans with diabetes can incur, particularly females, African Americans need to be very vigilant about the prospect of diabetes and educated about associated risks and complications. Screening should begin in early adulthood if there is a family history of diabetes as well as other risk factors.

Study after study has shown that EARLY DETECTION can prevent or diminish the impact of the severe complications that can result when diabetes has gone untreated for many years.

High rates of hypertension HYPERTENSION may be another factor contributing to or associated with the high rate of diabetes among blacks. In a study of 342 American adults with Type 2 diabetes, including 142 African Americans (reported in a 1999 issue of *Ethnicity and Health*), researchers found that blacks had an average higher diastolic blood pressure than whites. They also had worse glycemic control. The African-American females in the study were most likely to experience hypertension.

The researchers also found that insufficient glycemic control was *more* associated with the appearance of diabetic symptoms in black subjects than in white subjects. Thus, good glycemic control is even more essential for African Americans who have diabetes.

Quality of Care

Some question whether African Americans are receiving sufficient care, since blacks with diabetes are so overrepresented among those with diabetes and its severe complications. It appears to some researchers that some blacks with diabetes are shortchanged in healthcare, although the cause for this is unknown. It may be a combination of genetic, socioeconomic, cultural, and other factors that are yet to be discovered.

Researchers analyzed the care received by elderly African Americans with diabetes and who were on Medicare, reporting on their findings in a 1998 issue of *Diabetes Care*.

They found that African Americans visited their physicians fewer times per year and were much less likely to have had appropriate measurements of their blood glucose levels recorded by medical staff. They were also more likely to use the Emergency Room of the hospital when they were ill rather than see a physician in an office or clinic. The black subjects were also far less likely to have obtained an influenza vaccination (16 percent) than their white counterparts (57 percent). The authors said,

> African-Americans were less likely to receive several recommended services. These discrepancies may reflect a preference by African-Americans to avoid medical testing and procedures, but they could also result from a less aggressive treatment style by physicians for African-Americans or difficulties by African-Americans in gaining access to the health care system.

Hopefully, the reasons for the discrepancy will be identified and overcome so that African Americans receive adequate health care.

Impact of Diet

Although it is generally assumed that a poor diet is responsible for a higher rate of diabetes among African Americans than among individuals of other races, one study seemed to indicate the reverse. Researchers studied black and white children in Birmingham, Alabama, reporting on their findings in a 2000 issue of *Patient Care*.

The researchers found that the African-American children consumed 25 percent more vegetables and double the number of fruits as the white children did. Their consumption of dairy products was about 40 percent of that reported by the white children. (The information on food intake was self-reported and not verified.) Total cholesterol levels were higher in the African-American children and acute insulin responses were about double that of levels that were seen in the white children (indicating possible early insulin resistance). Thus, a genetic predisposition to increased insulin resistance may be the factor explaining this difference.

Black Children and Glycemic Control

Numerous studies have documented the essential importance of good glycemic control in adults with diabetes. This finding holds true for adolescents and children as well.

A study reported in a 2000 issue of the *Journal of Diabetes and Its Complications* revealed that black children diagnosed with diabetes had far worse records of glycemic control than did their white counterparts. Researchers studied children in Baltimore and New Orleans. The African-American children had a mean glycosylated hemoglobin level of 12.5 versus the more improved level of 10.7 in the Caucasian children in the area. Clearly, good glycemic control is another area the medical community needs to emphasize to blacks of all ages who have diabetes. (See also PREGNANCY; RACE/ETHNICITY.)

Cynthia L. Arfken, Ph.D., et al., "Development of Proliferative Diabetic Retinopathy in African-Americans and Whites with Type 1 Diabetes," *Diabetes Care* 21, no. 5 (May 1998): 792–795.

Frederick L. Brancati, M.D., M.H.S., et al., "Incident Type 2 Diabetes Mellitus in African American and White Adults: The Atherosclerosis Risk in Communities Study," *Journal of the American Medical Association* 283, no. 17 (May 3, 2000): 2253–2259.

Marshall H. Chin, M.D., M.P.H., "Diabetes in the African-American Medicare Population: Morbidity, Quality of Care, and Resource Utilization," *Diabetes Care* 21, no. 7 (July 1998): 1090–1095.

Maureen I. Harris, Ph.D., M.P.H., "Racial and Ethnic Differences in Health Insurance Coverage for

Adults with Diabetes," *Diabetes Care* 22, no. 10 (October 1999): 1679–1682.

Joseph C. Konen, M.D., P.S.P.H., et al., "Racial Differences in Symptoms and Complications in Adults with Type 2 Diabetes," *Ethnicity and Health* 4, no. 1–2 (February–May 1999): 39–49.

Mary Desmond Pinkowish, "Diabetes and CVD Risks in African American Children: The Role of Insulin Metabolism," *Patient Care* 34, no. 9 (May 15, 2000): 23.

Monique S. Roy, M.D., "Diabetic Retinopathy in African Americans with Type 1 Diabetes: The New Jersey 725," *Archives of Ophthalmology* 118, no. 1 (January 2000): 105–115.

Leonard M. Thaler, M.D., et al., "Diabetes in Urban African-Americans: XIX. Prediction of the Need for Pharmacological Therapy," *Diabetes Care* 23, no. 6 (June 2000): 820–825.

age/aging and diabetes The impact of growing older on the incidence of diabetes as well as how older people are affected by diabetes. In general, diabetes is an increasing risk with aging, rising with middle age and reaching its peak in individuals who are over age 60. However, people of any age, including children, may develop diabetes.

Aging also presents a risk factor for people with diabetes to develop COMPLICATIONS that can occur from diabetes. For example, the risks for CARDIOVASCULAR DISEASE, DIABETIC NEPHROPATHY, and DIABETIC RETINOPATHY all increase with age, as do risks for many other illnesses that are directly and indirectly associated with diabetes.

In the past, diabetes was primarily perceived as either a problem for children and adolescents, hence "juvenile onset diabetes" or for middle-aged or older adults, hence "adult onset diabetes." However, researchers have learned that adults may have the disease diagnosed primarily in children—and children may have the form of diabetes found in older adults.

As a result, rather than defining diabetes in terms of age alone, it is defined in terms of its primary symptoms. Type 1 diabetes is an illness in which the individual's body stops producing insulin and, as a result, he or she needs supplemental insulin in order to live. This condition is usually diagnosed in children or adolescents but it may also be found in adults of any age.

Type 2 diabetes is a disease in which the person's body produces some insulin but the body fails to use it properly (INSULIN RESISTANCE) and the amount of insulin is inadequate to normalize

SIX LEADING CAUSES OF DEATH AMONG MEN AGE 65 OR OLDER (1997)				
White	**Black**	**Asian/Pacific Islander**	**American Indian/Alaska Native**	**Hispanic**
1. Heart disease	Heart	Heart	Heart	Heart
2. Cancer	Cancer	Cancer	Cancer	Cancer
3. Stroke	Stroke	Stroke	**Diabetes**	Stroke
4. COPD*	COPD	Flu/pneumonia	Stroke	**Diabetes**
5. Flu/Pneumonia	Flu/pneumonia	COPD	COPD	Flu/pneumonia
6. **Diabetes**	**Diabetes**	**Diabetes**	Flu/pneumonia	COPD

SIX LEADING CAUSES OF DEATH AMONG WOMEN AGE 65 OR OLDER (1997)				
White	**Black**	**Asian/Pacific Islander**	**American Indian/Alaska Native**	**Hispanic**
1. Heart disease	Heart	Heart	Heart	Heart
2. Cancer	Cancer	Cancer	Cancer	Cancer
3. Stroke	Stroke	Stroke	**Diabetes**	Stroke
4. COPD	**Diabetes**	Flu/pneumonia	Stroke	**Diabetes**
5. Flu/pneumonia	Flu/pneumonia	**Diabetes**	Flu/pneumonia	Flu/pneumonia
6. **Diabetes**	COPD	COPD	COPD	COPD

*chronic obstructive pulmonary disease

the blood glucose (BETA CELL DYSFUNCTION). Both abnormalities worsen with age and are also modified by environmental factors, such as weight and activity levels, as well as medications and intercurrent illnesses. Type 2 diabetes is primarily diagnosed in middle-aged and older adults but is also on the rise among children and adolescents.

The incidence of Type 2 diabetes has increased and a study of nearly 150,000 individuals in the US, published in a 2000 issue of *Diabetes Care,* revealed an increase in the overall prevalence of 33 percent. The greatest increase was among people ages 30–39 years, where the prevalence increased dramatically by 76 percent. Researchers believe that most of this increase could be attributed to an increased incidence of obesity among the afflicted individuals. (See also ADOLESCENTS WITH DIABETES, CHILDREN WITH DIABETES, SCHOOL-AGE; ELDERLY.)

Ali H. Mokdad, Ph.D., et al., "Diabetes Trends in the U.S.: 1990–1998," *Diabetes Care* 23, no. 9 (September 2000): 1278–1283.

Alaska Natives and diabetes   Native Americans/American Indians residing in or from Alaska in general are at high risk for developing diabetes. A 2000 study in *Diabetes Care* revealed that the risk in recent years has increased. Looking at diagnoses over the years from 1990–97, researchers found that the prevalence of diagnosed cases of diabetes had increased by 29 percent. The increased prevalence varied according to region and ranged from a 16 percent increase in the Northern Plains Indians to a 76 percent increase among Alaska Natives.

A further disturbing finding is that the increased prevalence falls largely among middle-aged rather than elderly individuals. Although about half the people with diabetes in the United States are age 65 and over, among Alaskan natives and Native Americans, only 24 percent of the diabetic population is 65 and over. Authors of the study say, "This greatest percentage of diabetic cases in the Native American and

Alaskan diabetic population (49 percent) is among those aged 45–64 years." This data is similar to that from developing countries in which there are more middle-aged individuals with diabetes than elderly individuals with diabetes.

Alaska Natives also have a greater proportion of their members who are dying from diabetes. According to the report, "Older Americans 2000: Key Indicators of Well Being," released by the Federal Interagency Forum on Aging-Related Statistics in 2000, diabetes is the third leading cause of death among American Indian and Alaska Natives age 65 or older. Diabetes is the fourth leading cause of death among Hispanics and the fifth or sixth leading cause among other ethnic groups.

In contrast, although diabetes is a problem for other racial and ethnic groups, it is not as severe a problem as it is for American Indians and Alaska Natives. The charts on the preceding page compare the key causes of death among older people from various racial and ethnic groups. There are two charts because the death risks from diseases vary by gender.

As can be seen from the charts, there are no ethnic or gender differences when it comes to the top two causes of death. The number one killer is heart disease for all races, ethnicities, and genders. The number two killer for all groups is cancer. But although the third biggest killer for most groups was stroke, this pattern did not hold for American Indians and Alaska Natives. Instead, in their cases, diabetes was their third leading cause of death among elderly individuals.

(See also AMERICAN INDIANS.)

"Prevalence of Diabetes among Native Americans and Alaska Natives, 1990–1997," *Diabetes Care* 23, no. 12 (December 2000): 1786–1790.

albuminuria   Albumin is a protein that is sometimes found in the urine and that may be noted in the urine of people who have had diabetes for many years. The presence of albumin in the urine can be a sign of HYPERTENSION (high blood pressure), and may also be an indicator or a possible precursor of kidney problems. It is very important to determine whether the person has hypertension, because when uncontrolled hypertension is combined with diabetes, it can lead to a rapid decline in kidney function. Yet if hypertension is identified, it is eminently treatable.

People with diabetes should have an examination for macroalbuminuria (large amounts of albumin in the urine) at least once a year. This can be done at the time of an office visit by dipping a REAGENT STRIP into a small amount of the patient's urine, to check for protein. If that examination is negative, then an examination for microalbuminuria (small amounts of albumin in the urine) should be performed. This can be done in the doctor's office with a different type of test or it can be sent to the laboratory for evaluation. Often the doctor may repeat this test on several occasions because there are several confounding variables such as fever, exercise, uncontrolled blood glucose, and other factors that may temporarily increase the amount of protein or albumin in the urine. (See also PROTEINURIA.)

alcohol   Wine, beer, or distilled spirits. According to the U.S. Department of Agriculture, the moderate use of alcohol is safe and without significant negative effect in patients with well-managed diabetes. Moderate consumption is defined as no more than one drink per day for women and no more than two drinks per day for men. A "drink" is defined as 12 ounces of beer or 5 ounces of wine or 1.5 ounces of 80 proof spirit.

An estimated 75 percent of the population in the United States drink alcohol and individuals in many other countries also imbibe alcoholic beverages. Alcohol affects people with diabetes beyond the intoxicating effects that alcohol can have on everyone. For example, alcohol has little or no nutritional value (although it does have calories), while at the same time, it decreases the liver's ability to produce glucose.

It should also be noted that calories from alcohol increase the risk of OBESITY, yet another factor that is strongly linked to Type 2 diabetes.

As a result, if a person with diabetes who is drinking alcohol does not also consume food, then he or she risks developing HYPOGLYCEMIA. A further complication is the fact that often the effects of hypoglycemia are misinterpreted as intoxication, by the individual or by other people, and thus treatment does not ensue. This can be very dangerous for the person with diabetes. Note: if children with diabetes accidentally or purposely ingest alcohol, they may also suffer a severe bout of hypoglycemia.

Hypoglycemia and Chronic Alcoholism
Severe hypoglycemia is one consequence of chronic ALCOHOL ABUSE by patients who have diabetes. A large study, reported in a 2000 issue of *Diabetes Care,* indicated that a regular high level of alcohol intake is associated with the later development of Type 2 diabetes in men. (A high alcohol intake may also have the same effect on women, but such a study has not yet been reported, as of this writing.)

In this study, 8,663 nondiabetic men ages 30–79 were evaluated according to alcohol intake and other factors. The men were followed for six years and 149 of them developed Type 2 diabetes. The men were divided into five groups, including nondrinkers and four quartiles of drinkers.

The quartiles of drinkers were as follows: Quartile 1 drank between 1.0 to 61.8 grams per week. Those in Quartile 2 drank from 61.9 to 122.7 grams per week. Those in Quartile 3 drank 122.8 to 276.6 grams per week. Lastly, those in Quartile 4 drank any amount over 276.6 grams weekly.

The researchers found a statistical link between alcohol consumption at the higher quartiles and the subsequent development of Type 2 diabetes. The men in the third and fourth quartiles had a 2.2 to 2.4 greater risk of developing diabetes than the other groups, with the highest risk faced by heavy drinkers.

Interestingly, the nondrinkers had a 1.8 greater risk of developing diabetes, which the researchers could not explain, although they hypothesized that perhaps the nondrinkers were recovering alcoholics or were ill. The risk for the moderate drinkers of developing diabetes was actually lower than for the nondrinkers. Based on this study, it appears that excessive consumption of alcohol is a risk factor for the development of Type 2 diabetes among males.

In this study, heavy drinkers were more likely to also be heavy smokers. Smoking is yet another risk factor for the development of Type 2 diabetes.

Other studies have shown that moderate drinkers face an increased risk for developing Type 2 diabetes over nondrinkers. It is also known that excessive alcohol consumption can contribute to OBESITY.

Expert Advice

According to British authors Williams and Pickup, in their book, *Handbook of Diabetes,* alcohol should be "forbidden completely in those with hyperlipidaemia [hyperlipidemia], hypertension, pancreatic disease, or recurrent, severe hypoglycaemia [hypoglycemia]." They also note that alcohol consumption is associated with an increase in ERECTILE DYSFUNCTION (impotence).

If people with diabetes do choose to consume alcoholic beverages, experts offer the following basic tips:

- Do not drink more than one or two drinks per evening

- Mix your own drinks so that you know exactly what is in them

- Understand that some beers have a high alcohol content, as do liqueurs

- Wear an emergency medical identification bracelet, necklace, or anklet, so that you are identified as a person with diabetes

- Bring a fast-acting carbohydrate source such as juice or specially prepared items for people with diabetes, should you develop hypoglycemia

- Consume food to avoid the risk of hypoglycemia as well as decrease the risk for intoxication

- Check glucose levels every few hours

- Learn what medications can have bad or even dangerous interactions when mixed with alcohol since many common medications for diabetes should not be mixed with alcohol

(See also ALCOHOL ABUSE.)

Ming Wei. M.D., et al., "Alcohol Intake and Incidence of Type 2 Diabetes in Men," *Diabetes Care* 23, no. 1 (January 2000): 18–22.

Gareth Williams and John C. Pickup, *Handbook of Diabetes* (London, England: Blackwell, 1999).

J. Zielke, "Alcohol: A Primer: How Does Alcohol Affect Diabetes?" *Diabetes Forecast* 52, no. 3 (1999): 64–66.

alcohol abuse/alcoholism   Excessive consumption of alcohol or addiction to alcohol. Heavy drinking is very risky for a person with diabetes. An abuser of alcohol may develop alcoholism if the abuse occurs on a regular basis and meets other criteria for alcoholism.

According to the Substance Abuse and Mental Health Services Administration in the United States, about 5.6 million people in the United States abuse alcohol. In addition, there are another 8 million people who meet the diagnostic criteria for alcoholism. Alcohol abuse/alcoholism is a serious problem in many other countries as well. It is unknown how many people who have diabetes also have problems related to alcohol.

According to the National Institute on Alcohol Abuse and Alcoholism (NIAAA) in the United States, alcohol abuse is characterized by a drinking pattern that includes at least one of the following aspects over a 12-month period:

- Failure to perform responsibilities at work, home, or school

- Consumption of alcohol while driving a car or operating equipment

- Arrest for driving under the influence of alcohol or for assaulting someone while under the influence of alcohol

- Consumption of alcohol despite relationship problems that are caused or made worse by alcohol

As mentioned, alcohol abuse may escalate into alcoholism, which is a disease characterized by an urgent craving and dependency on alcohol and a need for greater amounts to achieve the same level of intoxication. It is also characterized by symptoms of withdrawal when the person abstains from alcohol. Alcoholism is a serious disease and one that is very dangerous for people with diabetes. It affects and can damage virtually every organ in the body, including the PANCREAS, the brain, the stomach, the heart, and other vital organs.

Chronic Risks of Alcohol Abuse/Alcoholism for People with Diabetes

One reason why heavy drinking is particularly perilous for people with diabetes is that those who are heavy alcohol consumers may not consume any or enough food. As a result, in addition to the impaired judgment that all people who abuse alcohol experience, the person with diabetes also risks the development of HYPO-GLYCEMIA, which may be severe.

In addition, chronic alcohol abuse increases the risk of HYPOGLYCEMIC UNAWARENESS, when the intoxicated person does not recognize the classic signs of hypoglycemia, such as a racing heart, sweatiness, and other symptoms. Because he is unaware of these signs, he will not take appropriate actions such as drinking fruit juice or consuming special foods designed to combat hypoglycemia. As a result, the problem can escalate further and develop into a medical emergency.

It is also possible for a person with diabetes to become both severely intoxicated and also hypoglycemic, and yet not receive treatment from others in the environment who don't know about the person's diabetes or who may be unfamiliar with hypoglycemia. They may mistake hypoglycemic symptoms or even unconsciousness as a common result of excessive drinking. Thus, they fail to recognize a hypoglycemic crisis. (This could also be a mistake made by law enforcement people or even paramedics.) This is yet another reason why all persons with diabetes should wear a medical emergency identification in the form of a bracelet, necklace, anklet, or other easily visible item.

Among those who *do* eat normally, chronic alcohol consumption may result in HYPER-GLYCEMIA, although researchers are not sure if one specific mechanism is to blame. The hyperglycemia may be the result of biochemical interactions in the liver or pancreas, or it could be attributed to the failure of heavy drinkers to take their prescribed medications. Probably the hyperglycemia results from a combination of causes.

Other Risks of Alcohol Abuse

According to Emanuele et al. in their 1998 article for *Alcohol Health & Research World*, heavy alcohol consumption by people with diabetes can cause or exacerbate DIABETIC KETOACIDOSIS (DKA), DYSLIPIDEMIA, CARDIOVASCULAR DISEASE, ERECTILE DYSFUNCTION, DIABETIC RETINOPATHY, and PERIPHERAL NEUROPATHY. It is clearly best for people with diabetes to either abstain from alcohol altogether or to drink only very limited amounts on an occasional basis.

Alcohol abuse causes disease Some studies have indicated that heavy alcohol consumption may lead to the development of Type 2 diabetes. Chronic and excessive alcohol consumption may also cause a variety of other diseases, most notably pancreatitis or cirrhosis of the liver. Alcoholism is also linked to the development of HYPERTENSION, heart disease, and other illnesses. There is some evidence that alcohol abuse may also lead to the development of breast cancer in women, although further research is needed.

Studies also have revealed that heavy drinkers are much more likely to be heavy smokers, thus increasing their risk for the development of a variety of smoking-related ailments, such as lung cancer, cardiovascular disease, heart disease, bronchitis, and asthma. In addition, SMOKING has been proven to accentuate the complications caused by diabetes.

Ethnic risks Studies indicate that alcohol use is more prevalent among whites in the United States than among Hispanics or other ethnic groups (with the exception of Native Americans). According to the 1999 National Household Survey on Drug Abuse, more than half (51 percent) of all whites in the United States use alcohol versus 42 percent of Hispanics. However, when it comes to heavy alcohol use, whites and Hispanics are roughly equivalent, at 5.8 percent of whites and 6.2 percent of Hispanics. About 5 percent of blacks are heavy drinkers.

As for binge drinking (five or more drinks on the same occasion at least 1 day in the past month), the percentage of whites reporting such behavior was 16.0 percent in 1998 (reported to be the same in 1999), and the percentage of Hispanics was 15.0 percent. The percentage of blacks was much lower, at 10.9 percent. Binge drinking is especially dangerous for people who have diabetes, because it accelerates the risk of hypoglycemia.

Adolescents who drink When a teenager has diabetes and then complicates her illness with alcohol abuse, very severe complications, up to and including death may be the end result. The most common complications of alcohol abuse among teenagers with diabetes are either diabetic ketoacidosis (DKA) or hypoglycemia.

Peer pressure is a major problem for many teenagers and it is also a driving force leading adolescents to drink alcohol, smoke, and use illegal drugs. Adolescents with diabetes may already feel out of the mainstream because of their disease, and thus, it may be hard for them to resist social pressure to abuse alcohol and drugs. Parents who think their children may be abusing alcohol need to consult with physicians and counselors immediately, particularly when that child also has diabetes. Even if parents are cer-

tain that their children do not drink, they should still educate them about the risks of alcohol abuse.

Medication interactions Many people who take medication on a regular basis don't realize that when they consume alcohol, the combination of the drug and the alcohol can sometimes cause very serious side effects. The medication and alcohol interact with each other even when they are not consumed at the same time, because many medications stay in the system for hours.

According to Weathermon and Crabb in their 1999 article for *Alcohol Research & Health,* people who take the following medications for diabetes risk suffering from severe nausea, vomiting, sweating, and other serious reactions after consuming alcohol:

- Diabinese (chlorpropamide)
- Glynase, Micronase and DiaBeta (glyburide)
- Tolazamide (generic drug)

Other medications taken by people with diabetes will cause problematic interactions with alcohol, even for those who are not heavy drinkers. For example, Diabinese can cause hypoglycemia when taken with alcohol. Excessive alcohol intake with or without liver disease can lead to an increased risk of lactic acidosis in patients on METFORMIN (Glucophage).

People with diabetes may take other medications for illnesses such as hypertension, arthritis, or other medical problems they may have. These medications may also interact negatively with alcohol. Even a medication as seemingly harmless as acetaminophen (Tylenol) can result in a harmful reaction when combined with excessive amounts of alcohol.

Treatment for Alcohol Abuse

People with diabetes who have a problem with alcohol abuse or full-blown alcoholism should inform their physicians. Many people are embarrassed or afraid to report this behavior to their doctors, but most doctors can provide suggestions to help. The doctor may recommend a therapist who is an expert at treating people with alcohol-related problems. He may also advise that the individual attend support group meetings or self-help groups such as Alcoholics Anonymous.

Some people need intensive outpatient or inpatient care for their alcoholism. People with diabetes who enter such facilities should be sure that the facility is made aware of the diabetes and the medications that the person takes, as well as their complete medical history.

Note: it is important that whatever group is recommended is one that is *not* opposed to all medications, because the person with diabetes should not go off drugs unless or until his or her own doctor advises that course of action. The doctor should not be working at cross-purposes with the self-help organization.

Some doctors believe that people with alcohol abuse problems are "self-medicating" because of an underlying problem with DEPRESSION. If so, the doctor may believe that a course of an anti-depressant or another medication would be helpful. A self-help group that decries the use of such medications would be inadvisable.

There are also some medications that have shown success in decreasing the desire for drinking in some people who have problems with alcoholism, including such medications as nal-trexone and ondansetron. Johnson and Ait-Daoud described such medications in their 1999 article for *Alcohol Research & Health.* Of course, it is essential that the person with diabetes verifies with the prescribing physician (as well as with the pharmacist) that such medications will not interfere with medicine taken for diabetes.

For further research on alcohol and health, one comprehensive source is the *10th Special Report to the U.S. Congress on Alcohol and Health: Highlights from Current Research,* published by the National Institute on Alcohol Abuse and Alcoholism in 2000.

For further information, contact the National Institute on Alcohol Abuse and Alcoholism (NIAAA) at:

Willco Building, Suite 409
6000 Executive Boulevard
MSC 7003
Bethesda, MD 20892-7003
(301) 443-3860
www.niaaa.nih.gov

(See also ALCOHOL.)

Nicholas V. Emanuele, M.D., et al., "Consequences of Alcohol Use in Diabetics," *Alcohol Health & Research World* 22, no. 3 (1998): 211–219.

Bankole A. Johnson, M.D., Ph.D. and Nassima Ait-Daoud, M.D., "Medications to Treat Alcoholism," *Alcohol Research & Health* 23, no. 2 (1999): 99–106.

Office of Applied Studies, Substance Abuse and Mental Health Services Administration, Department of Health and Human Services, "Summary of Findings from the 1999 National Household Survey on Drug Abuse," 2001.

Ron Weathermon, Pharm.D., and David W. Crabb, M.D., "Alcohol and Medication Interactions," *Alcohol Research & Health* 23, no. 1 (1999): 40–54.

alpha cell   A cell from within the islets of the pancreas (also called the islets of Lagerhans). It produces and releases glucagon, a hormone that increases the blood sugar (glucose) level of an individual by breaking down stored GLYCOGEN in the liver.

alpha-glucosidase inhibitors   A class of drugs used mainly to treat people with Type 2 diabetes. They slow down the digestion of carbohydrates after meals and are often used to treat elderly individuals who have diabetes. By slowing the absorption of glucose after a meal, these medications also decrease the rise in glucose subsequent to eating a meal.

Precose (ACARBOSE) and Glycet (miglitol) are two drugs in this class, as of this writing. These medications are taken with food. Alpha-glucosidase inhibitors may cause gastrointestinal disturbances such as gas and loose stools.

alternative medicine/complementary medicine
Nontraditional, nonprescribed medications,

remedies, and treatments. Such treatments are extremely popular among the general population, both with and without diabetes, as evidenced by the billions of dollars spent on alternative medications by consumers. A 2001 study reported in *Diabetes Medicine* found that 31 percent of 502 Canadian patients with diabetes were using alternative medicines and remedies, most commonly using garlic, echinacea, vitamin E, vitamin C, and calcium supplements.

Alternative remedies may be very helpful to many people; however, some drugs may also be very dangerous, particularly if they purport to "cure" diabetes, cancer, and other serious ailments. (Some drugs may claim to cure all major diseases. They are to be especially avoided.)

According to an article in a 1998 issue of *The Diabetes Educator,*

> Patients who believe that a natural product will lower their glucose level may stop taking their oral medications or insulin, with the result being an increase in blood glucose levels. Such an increase could be very dangerous, especially when it is sustained.

Alternative medications are offered in health food stores throughout the United States as well as in supermarkets and pharmacies. A proliferation of alternative medicines and remedies are offered to consumers worldwide over the Internet.

In general, alternative medication encompasses such categories as:

- herbal remedies
- supplemental vitamin or mineral therapy
- homeopathic remedies

Herbal Remedies

There are a wide variety of roots, teas, berries, and other items sold as herbal remedies. The market for herbal remedies is estimated at about $5 billion in the United States alone. (Not including the market for vitamin supplements and minerals or homeopathic remedies. The estimated total market was about $14 billion in 2000.)

The key impetus to this growth in the United States was the passage of the Dietary Supplement Health and Education Act of 1994. Based on this legislation, herbal remedies and vitamin supplements were thereafter regulated differently from both over-the-counter and prescribed medications.

The key difference: most pharmaceutical companies must offer considerable proof in the form of clinical studies to the Food and Drug Administration (FDA) before a new medication may be offered to the public. These studies must indicate not only that a new drug is safe but also that it is efficacious and that it improves the condition that it treats.

In contrast, the Dietary Supplement Health and Education Act of 1994 in the United States made the situation quite different for the sale of herbs and supplemental vitamins and minerals. In this case, it is the federal government, rather than the drug company that must provide proof. Also, rather than prove that the drug is safe and efficacious, the government must instead prove that the herbal remedy is dangerous before it can be removed from the market. This is a much more difficult burden of proof. Of course, the FDA can and does issue press releases when it believes an alternative remedy may be harmful.

As a result, if the herbal remedy or mineral is harmless, even if it has as little value as a sugar pill ("placebo"), the FDA cannot pull it off the market. It is true that manufacturers are supposed to limit their medical claims under the law, but as of this writing, there seems to be little or no investigation or enforcement of this requirement, possibly because of the sheer volume of the thousands of products on the market.

Most medical experts believe that individuals with diabetes should not take any herbal remedies unless specifically advised to take them by their medical doctor. Breastfeeding mothers, with or without diabetes, should also avoid *all* supplemental herbs, minerals, and other alternative remedies, unless their physician specifically recommends them.

Another issue is that the purity of herbal remedies has been questioned in some cases, as have their contents. Some random studies have indicated that some herbal remedies have been adulterated with substances not described on the packaging while others have revealed that there is little or none of the substance that is purported to be included.

Sometimes herbal remedies contain high doses of substances that may be harmful, such as ephedra (*ma huang*). In a person who already has hypertension, cardiac ailments, or other medical complications caused by or related to diabetes, taking ephedra and similar drugs can be very dangerous.

Some particularly dangerous herbs are:

- lobelia
- poke root
- those used in teas for dieters
- pennyroyal
- willow bark
- wormwood
- mistletoe
- skullcap

Supplemental Vitamins and Minerals

In some cases, alternative remedies have proven very useful in helping those with diabetes; however, individuals should always check with their physicians first before instituting any new medication regimen, including vitamin or mineral therapy.

Controlled studies have indicated that supplemental Vitamin E may improve the health of individuals with diabetes; however, Vitamin E in high doses may also result in bleeding disorders, as may some herbal remedies such as ginkgo biloba.

Some experts have also recommended that individuals with diabetes suffering from ulcers should use supplemental ZINC to aid in healing.

Some German studies of alpha-lipoic acid (ALA) have indicated that ALA can be effective in treating DIABETIC NEUROPATHY. Studies on ALA are currently under way in the United States. ALA is an accepted treatment in Germany.

A July 2000 issue of *Alternative Medicine Alert Archives* included an article which provided an overview on studies of ALA in treating diabetic neuropathy. Most of the studies have concentrated on positive results from injected ALA, a treatment not available in the United States as of this writing. Study results on the effects of orally administered ALA were mixed or inconclusive.

ALA is also found in red meat, although many people in the United States with and without diabetes have cut back on their consumption of red meat.

Scientists have also been studying the impact of minerals such as chromium and others on people with diabetes, but to date, they have not yet found any clear indications for recommending supplementation to patients with diabetes. Some experts believe that a magnesium deficiency can worsen complications of diabetes, but further research is needed.

One common supplement that may be *harmful* to people with diabetes is chromium picolinate, a supplement used by some people with arthritis based on best-selling books recommending the supplement. Some studies have indicated that this supplement may cause HYPO-GLYCEMIA; however, contradictory findings have also been made in other studies. As of this writing, individuals with diabetes should not take chromium picolinate unless a physician expert in the treatment of diabetes recommends this supplement.

Homeopathic Remedies

Homeopathy is a system that was developed by German physician Samuel Hahnemann in the early 19th century. This physician had stopped practicing medicine but he continued experimenting on herbs. Hahnemann noted that large quantities of the drug quinine made healthy individuals feverish and shaky, with malaria-like symptoms. Much smaller doses, however, helped people who actually had malaria.

Many physicians in the United States discount the value of homeopathic remedies although doctors in Germany and other European countries accept them.

Hahnemann devised his concept of the "law of similars," which was based on his belief that large quantities of substances may cause illness, but very tiny quantities of the same substance may provide relief. For example, belladonna, a deadly drug for most people, is used by homeopaths in tiny quantities to cure migraine headaches. Hahnemann's experiments are compiled in an 1811 reference guide called *Materia Medica.*

Other Alternative Treatments

Some practitioners recommend relaxation therapy, hypnosis, massage, chiropractic therapy, Ayurveda, yoga, aromatherapy, tai chi, and a very broad array of other options to improve health and overall wellness; however, it's important to understand that although such treatments may decrease a person's stress level, they cannot take the place of insulin or other prescribed medications for diabetes.

To obtain more information on alternative remedies and complementary medicine, contact the National Institutes of Health's Office of Alternative Medicines Clearinghouse. The telephone number is toll-free: (888) 644-6226.

"Alternative Therapies Gain Popularity Among Patients," *Diabetes Management Archives* (November 1, 1999).

Nancy Cooper, R.D., C.D.E., "Using Herbal Therapies Safely," *Diabetes Self-Management* 16, no. 3: 6–8, 10–13.

Missalee Gori, Pharm.D. candidate, and R. Keith Campbell, R.Ph., Fa.Pha., FASHP, "Natural Products and Diabetes Treatment," *The Diabetes Educator* 24, no. 2: 201–202, 205–206, 208.

Vincent Morelli and Roger J. Zoorob, "Alternative Therapies: Part I. Depression, Diabetes, Obesity," *American Family Physician* 62, no. 5 (September 2000): 1051–1060.

Robert J. Nardino, M.D., "Alpha-Lipoic Acid for the Prevention and Treatment of Diabetic Neuropathy," *Alternative Medicine Alert Archives* 3 (July 2000): 73–77.

E.A. Ryan, M.E. Pick, and C. Marceau, "Use of Alternative Medicines in Diabetes Mellitus," *Diabetes Medicine* 18, no. 3 (March 2001): 242–245.

Alzheimer's disease A brain disease and the most common form of DEMENTIA, or an illness in which the individual loses the ability to think rationally. Cognitive abilities continue to decline, eventually causing death. The rate of deterioration may be rapid or slow, depending on many factors, but it generally occurs over a period of from two to 20 years. Some studies have indicated that people with diabetes are at much greater risk for developing Alzheimer's disease or other forms of dementia than are nondiabetics, although the cause for this is unknown.

In the United States, there were an estimated 4 million people who had Alzheimer's in 2000 and also about 317,000 Canadians who were diagnosed with the disease. Globally, it was estimated that 12 million people had Alzheimer's disease in 2000 and this number was anticipated to rise with the increasingly older global population.

Gender plays a role in Alzheimer's disease: over 2/3 (68 percent) of those afflicted with Alzheimer's in the United States are women. Most people with Alzheimer's (85 percent) in the United States are white. Many are unhealthy, and an estimated 66 percent of elderly individuals with Alzheimer's are in fair to poor health versus the 27 percent who don't have Alzheimer's and are in poor to fair health.

According to Medicare data, 22 percent of Medicare beneficiaries who have Alzheimer's disease also have diabetes. Other health problems among Medicare beneficiaries who have Alzheimer's include stroke (24 percent), osteoarthritis (26 percent), and coronary artery disease (33 percent). In addition, 20 percent of Medicare beneficiaries who have Alzheimer's also have cancer.

Note: "Dementia" is a broad term that refers to a brain dysfunction that directly affects the intellect. Dementia may have other causes, such as stroke, end stage Parkinson's disease, head trauma, chronic alcohol or drug abuse and other illnesses, or even may result from taking some medications.

The disease is degenerative and as of this writing, it is not curable although there are effective medications and treatments to delay the memory loss of afflicted individuals. However, extensive ongoing medical research is expected to result in dramatic improvements in treatment and possibly, even a cure, within the next decade.

The Discovery of Alzheimer's Disease

The disease was first diagnosed by German physician Alois Alzheimer in 1906, after an autopsy on Auguste D., who had reportedly said poignantly at some point before her death, "I have lost myself." Auguste D. had experienced increasingly difficult and severe problems with her memory and behavior, and she died at age 51.

The autopsy on Auguste D. startled Dr. Alzheimer, who discovered brain cells that were shaped differently from the norm for the cerebral cortex of the brain. This is the area of the brain that is responsible for memory and reasoning. He also found tangles of a plaque substance, which are not seen in a normal brain. These lesions are still found in the brains of Alzheimer's victims after their deaths. Currently, they cannot be identified in brain tests on living individuals, such as magnetic resonance imaging (MRI) or other radiologic tests.

Alzheimer's disease is usually found among individuals who are over age 65 but it can occur in someone who is age 50 or younger. However, neither is it "normal" for most older people to have Alzheimer's disease and, in fact, only a minority of older people do have this illness. However, the percentage of people affected by Alzheimer's does increase with age. About 10 percent of North Americans over age 65 have Alzheimer's disease but the percentage of those afflicted increases to 30–50 percent of people who are older than age 85.

Early and Late Onset of Alzheimer's

Medical experts differentiate between "early" and "late" onsets of Alzheimer's disease. A person who has early-onset Alzheimer's disease is under age 65. In these cases, there appears to be a much stronger genetic link than for the late-

onset group. To fit the criterion of late-onset Alzheimer's disease, the individual must be over age 65, and this group represents 90 percent of all cases.

Baby Boomers and Alzheimer's

One key impetus that continues to propel research on Alzheimer's disease is that scientists, politicians, and others are concerned about the massive scale of the potential problems that could come from the aging Baby Boomer cohort of people born in the years 1946–64 as well as from the aging global population. Under today's paradigm, these particular individuals would seem to be increasingly at risk for Alzheimer's disease as they age, given today's conditions. However, scientists are very hopeful that they will succeed at averting or limiting these problems with medications and treatments that are under development at this time.

Alzheimer's and Diabetes

Some research has indicated that people with both Type 1 and Type 2 diabetes may be at greater risk for developing Alzheimer's disease than are nondiabetics. One study performed in the Netherlands (the Rotterdam study) and reported in 1999, looked at 6,370 older people who were screened for both diabetes and dementia. The researchers reported that the individuals with diabetes had twice the risk for dementia, in general, and for Alzheimer's disease, in specific, than the risk experienced by nondiabetics. The dementia risk was highest among diabetics receiving insulin and it was lowest among those with mild cases of diabetes or people who had just been diagnosed.

When a person who has diabetes also has Alzheimer's disease, there is definitely an increasing impact from both of these illnesses. For example, as cognitive abilities decline, others must take over the caregiving and make sure that the individual takes his or her medication and performs the necessary blood testing. Insulin injections must eventually be performed for the person because he or she cannot manage them. This may be difficult for family members and may require that the individual be placed in a SKILLED NURSING FACILITY (SNF).

Experts also report that the physician's goals for a patient with Alzheimer's disease may become less stringent. The reason for this is that tight control of glucose levels may lead to hypoglycemia and it may become very difficult or even impossible for a person with dementia to recognize the symptoms of hypoglycemia or hyperglycemia. It may also be very difficult for the caregiver assisting the person with Alzheimer's to maintain more than standard levels of glucose control.

A Careful Diagnosis Is Important

As of this writing, Alzheimer's disease can only be diagnosed with certainty after a person has died and an autopsy has been conducted on the deceased person's brain. Instead, physicians ask the individual a series of predetermined questions to assess the likelihood of the illness, and they also observe the behavior of the person. Doctors use such tests as the Mini-Mental State Examination (MMSE) to determine both short- and long-term memory capabilities, as well as the patient's abilities in writing and speaking.

Physicians should be sure to perform a very careful evaluation of older individuals who seem confused. Alzheimer's may be misdiagnosed in a person who suffers from undiagnosed diabetes or who may be more properly diagnosed with a variety of other ailments including depression, Vitamin B_{12} deficiency, syphilis, Parkinson's disease, heart disease, and other medical problems. Alzheimer's disease may also be misdiagnosed in a person whose primary problem is that he or she is abusing drugs or alcohol.

Diagnostic breakthroughs appear imminent

In 2000, researchers developed a test that appears to be sensitive to the early stages of Alzheimer's disease, and thus, may be able to detect the illness. The test looks for a special protein that is present in high concentrations in the brains of people with Alzheimer's but is found in unusually low concentrations in their blood. The advantage of early identification is that physicians can treat individuals in the early stages of the disease, so that brain function can be preserved for a longer period.

Symptoms of Alzheimer's

Many middle-aged and older individuals may fear that they are showing signs of Alzheimer's disease merely because they misplace their car keys or forget someone's name. These are common memory errors and they are not indicative of Alzheimer's disease. Some possible indicators of Alzheimer's disease (although other medical causes should be ruled out first) are:

- Refusal to bathe
- Failure to recognize people who have been known for a long time
- Extreme suspiciousness of others or paranoia
- Rages and combativeness
- Trouble with tying shoes or dressing, unrelated to any physical disabilities
- Wandering around the house (or outside) at night
- Aphasia (difficulty in speaking or understanding the meaning of words used by others)

Possible Causes of Alzheimer's

Medical researchers actively dispute among themselves what causes Alzheimer's disease; however, there appear to be several major camps of theorists. One group believes that the disease is caused by an amyloid protein, which causes the sticky plaque formations characteristic of the brain of a person with Alzheimer's disease.

Other groups say these plaque formations are only the results of the "true" cause. Some of these individuals believe the real culprit is another brain substance called "tau," a substance they believe is responsible for killing brain cells.

There are also genetic susceptibilities to Alzheimer's disease, although much of the disease cannot as yet be attributed to heredity. Consequently, having a parent or even parents with dementia does not condemn their children to developing the illness when they are older. The key susceptibility gene for Alzheimer's disease is APOE4, as of this writing.

A 1996 study of thousands of families that include a relative with Alzheimer's disease found that the risks are as follows:

11 percent if neither parent has Alzheimer's
36 percent if one parent has the disease
54 percent if both parents have the disease
40–50 percent if an identical twin has
    Alzheimer's disease

Another factor, which may be causal, is an individual's neurochemical (brain chemical) composition and interaction with other neurochemicals. There are neurochemical changes to the brains of people with Alzheimer's disease. For example, the level of acetylcholine is greatly reduced in the brains of people who have Alzheimer's disease.

Delaying the Degeneration

Although Alzheimer's disease is not curable as of this writing, physicians are working to delay the severity of the deterioration with medications. Physician Serge Gauthier, director of the Alzheimer's disease research unit at the Montreal, Canada–based McGill Centre for Studies in Aging told *Macleans* magazine in 2000,

> If we can delay the onset of symptoms by five years, we will decrease the number of persons with Alzheimer's by half. If we can delay the onset of symptoms by 10 years, we will reduce the number affected by Alzheimer's in one generation by 75 per cent.

As of this writing, there are three primary medications used to slow the memory loss experienced by patients diagnosed with Alzheimer's disease, including Aricept, Exelon, and Reminyl. Other medications are under development.

Looking Ahead

In one exciting apparent breakthrough reported in 2000, medical researchers at Elan Pharmaceuticals in San Francisco described their experiments with mice who had been bred to have brain plaques. The mice were then injected with beta-amyloid. This substance appeared to stimulate the immune system of the mice and the plaques then began to disappear. A year later, seven of the nine mice were free of all brain plaque. More mice were injected in subsequent experiments and again, the plaque disappeared. In some cases, the performance of the mice on maze experiments improved after receiving the vaccine.

However, mice are very different from people, and human clinical trials are needed to determine if the vaccine could be effective in helping humans who are suffering from Alzheimer's disease. As of this writing, a small number of people (24) with mild to moderate Alzheimer's disease in the United States have received the nasal beta-amyloid vaccine, although it is too soon to tell if the vaccine will be successful in improving the cognitive abilities of humans. As of this writing, no side effects have been identified in the administration of the vaccine. Another clinical trial using the vaccine on 80 Alzheimer's patients in the United Kingdom was launched in 2000, and further trials will be conducted.

Recruitment of humans in the United States with mild to moderate Alzheimer's disease to participate in clinical trials of the AN-1792 vaccine that was developed by Elan began in 2001. If it is as effective as it appears to be in mice, the vaccine may not only help people who already have Alzheimer's but may also prevent Alzheimer's in people who are at risk for developing it. (See also DEPRESSION, ELDERLY, EMOTIONAL PROBLEMS.)

For further information about Alzheimer's disease, contact the Alzheimer's Association, a nationwide organization with local chapters, at:
Alzheimer's Association
919 North Michigan Avenue
Suite 1100
Chicago, IL 60611-1676
(Toll-free) 800-272-3900 or (312) 335-8700
www.alz.org

"Diabetes, Head Trauma, Marriage and Dementia," *Psychiatric Medicine in Primary Care Archives* (March 1, 2000).

E. W. Gregg et al., "Is Diabetes Associated with Cognitive Impairment and Cognitive Decline Among Older Women?" *Archives of Internal Medicine* 60, no. 2 (2000): 174–180.

Meena Kumari et al., "Minireview: Mechanisms by Which the Metabolic Syndrome and Diabetes Impair Memory," *Journals of Gerontology* 55, no. 5 (May 1, 2000): B228–B232.

A. Ott et al., "Diabetes Mellitus and the Risk of Dementia: The Rotterdam Study," *Neurology* 53 (1999): 1937–1942.

Lee Shirey et al., "Alzheimer's Disease and Dementia: A Growing Challenge," *Challenges for the 21st Century: Chronic and Disabling Conditions* 1, no. 11 (September 2000): 1–6.

John Travis, "Possible Alzheimer's Vaccine Seems Safe," *Science News* 158, no. 3 (July 15, 2000): 38.

American Academy of Family Physicians (AAFP) Nationwide professional organization of family doctors who are interested in a broad array of ailments, including diabetes. In 1999, the group published "The Benefits and Risks of Controlling Blood Glucose Levels in Patients with Type 2 Diabetes Mellitus."

AAFP
11400 Tomahawk Creek Parkway
Leawood, KS 66211-2672
(913) 906-6000
www.aafp.org

American Academy of Pediatrics (AAP) Professional organization of pediatricians nationwide in the United States. Because children and adolescents can suffer from both Type 1 and Type 2 diabetes, these are issues of concern to Academy members. The AAP publishes *Pediatrics,* which includes peer-reviewed journal articles on a variety of topics including diabetes.

American Academy of Pediatrics
601 13th Street, NW
Suite 400 North
Washington, DC 20005

(202)347-8600
www.aap.org/

American Association of Clinical Endocrinologists (AACE) A professional and international organization of physicians who specialize in endocrinological diseases such as diabetes and thyroid disease. AACE publishes a peer-reviewed journal, *Endocrine Practice.*

In 2000, the group released "The American Association of Clinical Endocrinologists Medical Guidelines for the Management of Diabetes Mellitus: The AACE System of Intensive Diabetes Self-Management—2000 Update," published by the Diabetes Medical Guidelines Task Force, which was chaired by Stanley Feld, M.D., M.A.C.E.

AACE
1000 Riverside Avenue
Suite 205
Jacksonville, FL 32304
(904) 353-7878
www.aace.com

American Association of Diabetes Educators (AADE) An organization of more than 10,000 health care professionals involved in diabetes care and education. The mission of the AADE is to advance the role of the diabetes educator and to improve the quality of diabetes education and care. Most certified diabetes educators (CDEs) are members of AADE and their state chapters. Publishes *The Diabetes Educator,* a bimonthly journal.

AADE
100 West Monroe
4th floor
Chicago, IL 50503
(312) 424-2426
www.aadenet.org

American Diabetes Association (ADA) Formed in 1940 by physicians concerned about diabetes treatment and research, this vitally important and very influential health organization supports clinical research on both Type 1 and Type 2 diabetes and provides information to a broad array of physicians, nurses, and patients with diabetes and others. The ADA has offices in each state as well as the District of Columbia. According to information provided by the American Diabetes Association, their mission is to prevent and cure diabetes, and improve the lives of everyone affected by diabetes.

The ADA is also an active advocacy organization, providing support and information on discrimination and violations of the AMERICANS WITH DISABILITIES ACT in the school and the workplace. It has also provided court briefs in several successful lawsuits on behalf of children and adults with diabetes. In addition, the ADA lobbies Congress and other groups on issues of importance to those who have diabetes.

The ADA has been a cosponsor with major federal agencies on very large clinical trials of patients with diabetes, such as the DIABETES CONTROL AND COMPLICATIONS TRIAL (DCCT) as well as many other vitally important studies. In fact, the ADA supports about 250 medical researchers at 100 institutions in the United States today.

The American Diabetes Association provides information to diabetes professionals and consumers with diabetes. The ADA also produces the four most widely read professional peer-reviewed journals, including *Diabetes, Clinical Diabetes, Diabetes Care,* and *Diabetes Spectrum.*

In 1994, the American Diabetes Association Research Foundation was formed to raise funds for diabetes research. In fiscal year 2000, the fundraising done by this arm of the ADA led to the funding of $22.4 million in diabetes research.

American Diabetes Association (ADA)
1701 North Beauregard Street
Alexandria, VA 22311
(800) 232-3472 or (703) 549-1500
www.diabetes.org

American Indians/Native Americans Individuals who are descendants of tribal groups in the United States. Many are at very high risk for developing Type 2 diabetes. It is estimated that the risk for Native Americans developing diabetes is about 2.7 times the risk for the general population.

At particular risk are the PIMA INDIANS of Arizona, a group that has been studied by the National Institutes of Health since 1965. Over half of this group over the age of 35 years have Type 2 diabetes. They also experience a death rate from diabetes that is 10 times greater than the rate for Caucasians. However, the high rate appears to be largely influenced by diet and inactivity because very few of the Pima Indians who

NUMBER AND INCIDENCE* OF AMERICAN INDIANS/ALASKA NATIVES WITH DIABETES WHO INITIATED TREATMENT FOR DIABETES-RELATED END-STAGE RENAL DISEASE, BY YEAR AND SEX—UNITED STATES, 1990–1996

Year	Men		Women		Total	
	No.	Incidence	No.	Incidence	No.	Incidence
1990	182	516.9	212	439.0	394	472.4
1991	190	549.9	249	489.9	439	514.7
1992	229	601.2	294	533.0	523	561.1
1993	207	515.5	298	527.3	505	524.3
1994	260	571.6	356	569.7	616	573.0
1995	286	611.9	402	608.1	688	610.9
1996	309	589.0	410	577.5	719	584.3

* Per 100,000 persons with diabetes. Incidence of treatment was age-adjusted based on the 1980 U.S. population with diabetes.

live in Mexico have Type 2 diabetes. The children of Pima Indians who have diabetic nephropathy appear to inherit their parents' risk for this complication of diabetes.

The Indian Health Service (IHS) offers a program to document diabetes problems and provide prevention and control programs to American Indian and Alaska Native communities.

Organizations that provide assistance to American Indians are:

Association of American Indian Physicians
1235 Sovereign Row
Suite C-9
Oklahoma City, OK 73108
(405) 946-7651

Indian Health Service Headquarters
Diabetes Program
5300 Homestead Road NE
Albuquerque, NM 87110
(505) 248-4544
www.his.gov/MedicalPrograms/Diabetes

Diabetes Control Program HIS
3200 Canyon Lake Drive
Rapid City, SD 57702
(605) 355-2378

Society of American Indian Dentists
P.O. Box 15107
Phoenix, AZ 85060
(602) 954-5160

(See also ALASKA NATIVES, RACE/ETHNICITY.)

"End-Stage Renal Disease Attributed to Diabetes Among American Indians/Alaska Natives with Diabetes—United States, 1990–1999," *Morbidity and Mortality Weekly Report* 49, no. 42 (October 27, 2000): 959–962.

D. J. Pettitt et al., "Familial Predisposition to Renal Disease in Two Generations of Pima Indians with Type 2 Non-Insulin Dependent Diabetes Mellitus," *Diabetologia* 33, 7, no. 7 (1990): 438–443.

Americans with Disabilities Act (ADA)

Signed into law in 1990, the Americans with Disabilities Act prohibits discrimination against disabled individuals in the workplace, schools, and in other areas used by disabled individuals.

Work and the ADA

In the workplace, the ADA applies when employers have 15 or more workers. There are many provisions in the ADA but several are key to keep in mind. For example, according to the Equal Employment Opportunity Commission, one provision is that employers who are interviewing job applicants may not question the prospective employee about his or her disability, even if it may be related to the job.

If the interviewer decides to make a conditional offer of employment at that point, he or she may inquire about disabilities and may also request medical examinations, if such inquiries would be made for others applying for the same type of job. After the person is hired, questions about a disability can be made only if they are related to the job. The same holds true about requiring a medical examination after the person has been hired: under the ADA, a medical examination can only be mandated if it is job-related. The specific wording is as follows:

> A covered entity shall not require a medical examination and shall not make inquiries of an employee as to whether such employee is an individual with a disability or as to the nature and severity of the disability, unless such examination or inquiry is shown to be job-related and consistent with business necessity.

Impact of the Americans with Disabilities Act

According to attorney Michael A. Greene, in his 1999 article for *Diabetes Spectrum*, the enactment of the ADA was "the sunrise of legal advocacy for diabetes." Greene also stated that the efforts of the American Diabetes Association that preceded its passage resulted in a "legislative history replete with medical and scientific references to diabetes."

Prior to the passage of the ADA, disabled individuals fell under a broad range of state statutes that varied greatly from state to state. The ADA, a federal law, provided one prevailing standard for all children and adults with disabilities, although many lawsuits have tested the law since its passage.

Lawsuits under the ADA

The American Diabetes Association has appeared as a plaintiff in some lawsuits filed under the provisions of the Americans with Disabilities Act. For example, in the case of *Stuthard and the American Diabetes Association v. KinderCare Learning Centers,* an Ohio daycare center refused to accept a child with Type 1 diabetes because he needed insulin injections. The daycare provider would not allow any staff members to give the injections even though the child was a toddler and was too young to perform self-glucose testing or to self-inject.

The case was resolved in favor of the family and the American Diabetes Association. Attorney General Janet Reno said, "Children with diabetes shouldn't be left on the sidelines. We hope that other child care facilities will do the right thing and follow KinderCare's lead." (See also FAMILY AND MEDICAL LEAVE ACT, LAWSUITS.)

Michael A. Greene, J.D., "The Age of Legal Advocacy for Diabetes," *Diabetes Spectrum* 12, no. 4 (1999).

amino acid　The primary material that is found in the cells of the body and that is also the "building block" of proteins. Insulin is comprised of two chains of 51 amino acids.

amputation　The surgical removal of a body part such as an arm, leg, finger, or toe. Diabetes is the number one cause of nontraumatic amputations in the United States and people with diabetes have about 40 times the risk of experiencing an amputation than nondiabetics. There are about 86,000 lower limb amputations performed on people with diabetes in the United States each year, at a cost of over $860 million annually. These amputations represent 60 per-

cent of all lower extremity amputations that are performed for any reason in a year.

Experts believe that as many as half of all the amputations that are experienced by people with diabetes could have been prevented with appropriate examinations and patient education.

According to the CENTERS FOR DISEASE CONTROL AND PREVENTION (CDC), about 60 percent of all diabetes-related amputations occur to patients over age 65. The rate goes up with aging: amputation rates for those over age 75 are more than twice as high as those aged 65–74 years.

Rates of amputation were higher among men than women and also higher among blacks than whites.

Reason for Amputation

If an injury progresses to the point of GANGRENE or tissue death, which is subsequently followed by bacterial infestation, then the gangrenous part must be amputated to avoid further spreading of the gangrene and infection and subsequent certain death.

Amputations are more common among individuals with Type 1 diabetes, although those who have had Type 2 diabetes for many years may also be at risk for amputations.

The main reason why people with diabetes are at greater risk than nondiabetics is that they lose feeling in their feet and may not feel or notice an injury. This nerve damage is also called DIABETIC NEUROPATHY. The injury becomes progressively worse and may deteriorate to the point of gangrene before it is noticed by the individual or by doctors.

Other risk factors　It is also important to minimize or eliminate other risk factors that can contribute to future amputations, such as OBESITY, SMOKING, and uncontrolled HYPERTENSION. The following patients should see a podiatrist for prevention every eight to 12 weeks. Patients who:

- Cannot see or assess their own feet for injuries, because of obesity or another reason
- Have diabetic neuropathy

- Have diabetic retinopathy or other causes of visual loss
- Are on anticoagulants
- Have known peripheral vascular disease (intermittent claudication)

Medicare and many other health plans will cover an annual payment for therapeutic shoes for patients with diabetes. Patients need to obtain a prescription for the shoes from their medical doctor.

Long-term Studies on Amputation Patients

In a large study based on 906 patients who were taking insulin and had an onset of diabetes before age 30 (drawn from the Wisconsin Epidemiologic Study of Diabetic Retinopathy [WESDR]), researchers reviewed the outcome of these patients 14 years later. They found a higher incidence of amputations among men (11.4 percent) than women (2.9 percent). Individuals who experienced amputation were also more likely to have the following risk factors:

- Hypertension/high blood pressure
- High pulse rate
- High consumption of alcohol (more than 30 mL/day)
- Proteinuria (protein in the urine, a precursor of kidney disease)
- History of prior ulcers of the feet or ankles
- Proliferative diabetic retinopathy or moderate retinopathy
- Current or former smoker
- Non-aspirin-user (daily ASPIRIN use apparently has a mitigating effect against amputation)

In another large study of 776 veterans in Seattle, Washington, reported in *Diabetes Care* in 1999, researchers looked for incidence and risk factors in individuals who had lower extremity amputations. The former military patients were mostly male (98 percent) and

white (78 percent) and their median age was 65 years, although the age range was 28–91 years. The large majority, or 93 percent of the patients, had Type 1 diabetes.

Thirty of the patients required an amputation. These patients were more likely to have had a history of heart disease and past problems with foot ulcers, blisters, and sores. They were also more likely to have had diabetes for more than 14 years. In addition, they were more likely to have had a previous amputation. The researchers said,

"Short of preventing diabetes itself, this study implies that prevention of foot lesions and even neuropathy in individuals with diabetes may markedly reduce the incidence of LEA [lower extremity amputation]."

Heel ulcers preceding amputation   In another study on lower extremity amputations, researchers described the results of 86 patients with severe heel ulcers, including 38 diabetic and 48 nondiabetic patients in *Wounds* in 2000. The researchers reported that 97 percent of the diabetic patients with severe heel ulcers required limb amputation while a lower percentage of 85 percent of the nondiabetic patients required amputation.

The common factors among all patients requiring amputation were smoking, hypertension, and heart disease. One difference between the patients with diabetes and those without diabetes (all of whom had amputations) was that obesity was a more prominent feature among the diabetic patients: 74 percent of the patients with diabetes were obese versus 40 percent of the nondiabetic patients. Clearly, OBESITY is a very high-risk amputation factor for individuals with diabetes.

The authors concluded,

The increased morbidity [illness] seen in diabetic patients with heel ulcers often results in above-the-knee or below-the-knee amputations. Currently, with the advent of microvascular surgery and free-tissue transfers, the chronic heel ulcer is no longer associated with definitive amputation. However, prevention remains the best treatment for heel ulcers in all settings. Working with a team of endocrinologists, podiatrists, nurses, and vascular surgeons, diagnosis and screening tests in high-risk patients should increase the limb-salvage rate.

Foot Care Is Essential

To greatly reduce the risk of amputation, physicians emphasize the importance of good FOOT CARE, including daily examination of the entire foot by the patient, particularly the bottoms of feet, but also including the heel and between the toes. Because it can be hard to study the soles of one's own feet, mirrors may help with this task, or family members may be taught to examine the individual's foot for injuries.

Experts say that when a person with diabetes visits the doctor, an examination of the foot should be as routine as a blood pressure or weight check. Yet many physicians still do not perform regular foot examinations of diabetic patients. To help their doctors, people with diabetes should remove their shoes and socks at doctor visits, before the physician even enters the room.

Economic Issues

Some researchers created a model to evaluate the economic savings of preventing lower extremity amputation in individuals with diabetes, reporting on their findings in a 1998 issue of *Diabetes Care.*

Looking at a population of 10,000 adults with diabetes and who would avoid amputations, the researchers found an annual savings of $3,000–$4,000 per individual with foot ulcer. The researchers extrapolated these results to a savings of about $3 million per year. The greatest benefits were found in educating patients who were 70 years old or younger. The researchers said,

> Given the significant cost, morbidity, and mortality associated with lower-extremity amputation, we advocate the formation of a partnership between government, private payers, health care service providers and producers,

and individuals with diabetes to establish amputation prevention strategies as standard components of routine diabetes care.

Emotional Impact of Amputation

Clearly, the emotional impact of losing one or more limbs is a devastating one for patients as well as their families. The patient may develop problems with feelings of hopelessness and DEPRESSION and may require psychiatric intervention. Some patients are so depressed that they are suicidal.

A psychiatrist or therapist cannot bring back the missing limb but may be able to provide assistance in developing ways to help the patient cope with the problem or help the patient connect with others who have dealt with their amputations. The patient may also benefit from taking antidepressant medication, although this option should be discussed between the patient and physician.

Amanda I. Adler, M.D., Ph.D., "Lower-Extremity Amputation in Diabetes," *Diabetes Care* 22, no. 7 (July 1999): 1029–1035.

Tikva S. Jacobs, M.D., and Morris D. Kerstein, M.D., "Is There a Difference in Outcome of Heel Ulcers in Diabetic and Non-Diabetic Patients?" *Wounds* 12, no. 4 (2000): 96–101.

Daniel A. Ollendorf, M.P.H., "Potential Economic Benefits of Lower-Extremity Amputation Prevention Strategies in Diabetes," *Diabetes Care* 21, no. 8 (1998): 1240–1245.

E. Moss Scot, M.A., "The 14-Year Incidence of Lower-Extremity Amputations in a Diabetic Population," *Diabetes Care* 22, no. 6 (1999): 951–959.

angiopathy   A general term for damage to blood vessels. Some individuals who have had diabetes for many years have this condition.

angiotensin receptor blockers (ARBs)   A category of blood pressure medications that are given to people who suffer from HYPERTENSION. Many people who have diabetes also have hypertension. ARB drugs work to reduce protein in the urine (PROTEINURIA) as well as delay kidney damage. Some examples of ARBs are: losartan, valsartan, candesartan, and irbesartan. ARBS differ from the angiotensin-converting enzyme (ACE) inhibitor drugs in that they block the effects of angiotensin by preventing it from binding to its receptor. The effect is to prevent the angiotensin in the system from increasing blood pressure.

ACE drugs work by blocking the conversion of angiotensinogen to angiotension I, and thus, they cause lower levels of angiotensin II to be available. Angiotensin II is one of the most potent constrictors of blood vessels known. Therefore, if there are lower levels, there is also less constriction of the arteries, and thus the vessels are more relaxed and blood pressure decreases. In addition, if there is less angiotensin II, there is also less stimulation of the adrenal to make aldosterone, which would cause the retention of some salt and water and raise blood pressure. Aldosterone also causes loss of potassium by the kidney. If the formation of angiotensin I and II is blocked, then blood pressure will be lower and potassium levels will be increased.

Similar to the ACE drugs, ARBs are very well tolerated, with as few side effects as a placebo. They do not cause cough, which is one of the most common side effects of ACE drugs, albeit a side effect that is often minor and tolerated by many people.

ACE drugs have been available for nearly 20 years in the United States and are still considered first-line therapy for hypertension and for the prevention of development or progression of DIABETIC NEPHROPATHY; however an ARB medication is often used as a second choice if the patient is unable to tolerate the ACE drug. Multiple studies are underway to determine whether or not ARBs are as effective as ACE drugs in protecting the diabetic kidney.

animals and diabetes   Nonhuman species, particularly dogs, cats, rats, and mice that have played a large role in the research and treatment of diabetes in humans as well as animals. Animals can also develop diabetes in their later years, and they are usually treated with insulin.

The first successful experiments on injected insulin, performed by Drs. Banting and Best in 1921 in Canada, were performed on a dog. Many subsequent experiments have been performed on other animals as well as mice and rats, some of which have been specially inbred so that they would develop diabetes. Experiments have been done on animals to determine the effects of diabetes, to find underlying genetic causes of OBESITY, and for many other purposes. Some people are opposed to experimentation on animals.

Animals may also develop diabetes, particularly as they age, and they may require oral medication or insulin injections in order to survive. According to *Diabetes Mellitus* by Porte and Sherwin, Type 1 diabetes occurs in about 1 in every 200 dogs and occurs in 1 of 800 cats. Other animals may also develop diabetes. The authors say,

> Diabetes has been reported in horses, ferrets, and ground squirrels. In zoological gardens, in which animals are liberally fed as compared to the nutrition available in their native habitat, diabetes has been reported in dolphins, foxes, and a hippopotamus.

Veterinarians are very familiar with diabetes among animals and have researched many ways to help animals. Some researchers seeking to help animals have made findings that could also benefit humans; for example, an article in a 2000 issue of *Veterinary Medicine* revealed that chromium and vanadium, trace elements needed by both humans and animals, may be useful as a supplemental treatment for both cats and people with Type 2 diabetes. Further research is needed on this topic.

Daniel Porte, Jr., M.D., and Robert S. Sherwin, M.D., *Ellenberg & Rifkin's Diabetes Mellitus* (Stamford, Conn.: Appleton & Lange, 1997).
"Two Transition Metals Show Promise in Treating Diabetic Cats," *Veterinary Medicine* 95, no. 3 (March 1, 2000): 190–193.

antibodies to insulin Proteins made by B-lymphocytes that can bind to and neutralize insulin that it mistakenly considers as an intruder to the body.

Anyone who takes insulin will develop antibodies against insulin. These antibodies are generally in low levels that do not cause clinical effects.

In fact, patients who have Type 1 diabetes develop antibodies to insulin *before* the diagnosis of diabetes and before insulin therapy has begun. Part of their disease was the destruction of the beta cells that produced natural insulin.

Modern insulin is much purer than past formulations, and thus, antibody levels (titers) are less.

Stopping and starting insulin can increase a person's antibody levels to insulin, and consequently, is not recommended.

The Controversy over Insulin Antibodies

The effects of insulin antibodies are under debate. Theoretically, they can bind to insulin and worsen GLYCEMIC CONTROL, thus preventing insulin from working. They can also buffer large amounts of free insulin that is released from the body's subcutaneous (fat) stores and help with smoothing out insulin levels and improving glycemic control.

Insulin antibodies apparently may exacerbate complications of diabetes. They have been found in the eyes and kidneys of animals that experienced diabetic complications. But no one has yet proven a direct cause and effect link between insulin antibodies and complications of diabetes.

anti-GAD antibody A substance produced by the body (antibody) that attacks glutamic acid decarboxylase (GAD), an enzyme that is necessary to the production of insulin in the pancreas. Anti-GAD antibodies are found in the majority (85–90 percent) of people newly diagnosed with Type 1 diabetes.

Patients with anti-GAD antibodies may also have other autoimmune diseases in addition to diabetes, such as Graves' disease (a form of hyperthyroidism) or Addison's disease.

Appropriate Blood Pressure Control in Diabetes Trial (ABCD Trial) A clinical study of 470 patients who had both diabetes and HYPERTENSION. Patients were assigned to two groups, one treated with enalapril (an ACE drug) and the other group treated with nisoldipine (a calcium channel blocker not available in the United States but similar to amlodipine and felodipine). Patients averaged 57–58 years old and had had diabetes for eight and a half years.

The initial blood pressure for patients was 155/98 in both groups. After five years of follow up, there were 25 heart attacks in the nisoldipine group versus five in the enalapril group. There were also 43 strokes in the nisoldipine group and seven in the enalapril group. The blood pressure decline was the same in both groups. The use of the ACE drug enalapril clearly conferred an advantage to the patients who took it, and it had effects other than just lowering blood pressure. The nisoldipine did not make the patients worse: they just did not do as well as the ACE group.

artificial pancreas Previously a hospital-based machine that provided a constant reading of blood glucose levels and was usually used for clinical research studies. Today, with fingerstick bedside monitoring, most people with diabetes who are hospitalized are placed on an intravenous insulin drip with frequent glucose checks.

The term "artificial pancreas" also refers to the concept of combining the still experimental implantable insulin pump with a device to continually measure glucose levels and feed back that information to the insulin pump. In contrast, the external pump requires the patients to check their own glucose levels and to then adjust the rate of insulin delivery.

Asians/Pacific Islander Americans (APIA) People of Chinese, Filipino, Japanese, Asian

Indian, Korean, Hawaiian, Samoan, and Vietnamese origin as well as people from an additional 28 Asian and 19 Pacific Islander ethnic groups. (See table.) Members from some of these groups have a high risk of developing diabetes.

Some researchers study Pacific Islanders alone. These are people who are ethnic descendants of individuals from Hawaii, Samoa, or the South Seas. Although they do not have a high rate of Type 1 diabetes, many Pacific Islanders have a high risk of Type 2 diabetes, which is greater than the risk for Caucasians and people of other races. This risk is believed to stem from genetics as well as lifestyle factors such as obesity and a sedentary lifestyle. As a result, they are prone to the COMPLICATIONS that stem from diabetes.

Studies indicate that people of APIA origin have four times the risk of developing Type 2 diabetes as do Caucasians in the United States. The risk is particularly high among Native Hawaiians, where some studies indicate over 22 percent of those over age 30 have Type 2 diabetes and the incidence increases to 40 percent for Native Hawaiians over age 60. Native Hawaiians as a group have at least double the risk of having Type 2 diabetes over that found among Caucasians in the United States. According to the National Institutes of Health, an estimated 73 percent of all APIA live in the following states: California, Hawaii, Illinois, New Jersey, New York, Texas, and Washington State.

The key factors leading to diabetes among this ethnic group, in addition to possible genetic risk factors are the same as for other groups: obesity, sedentary lifestyle, and high caloric diet. Interestingly, in some communities, the rate of diabetes varies depending on whether people live in rural or urban settings. For example, in Western Samoa, the rate of diabetes among rural residents was only 3.4 percent, compared to the more than double rate of 7.8 percent found among city dwellers.

In addition, a study that compared Japanese people who remained in Japan to Japanese people who relocated to Hawaii found that the Japanese people who relocated to Hawaii were more obese and they had over twice the risk of developing Type 2 diabetes. In general, Asians living in the United States have a greater risk of developing Type 2 diabetes: their risk is two to four times greater than the risk for people of the same race but who live in China, the Philippines, and other Asian countries. Clearly, environmental impacts are profound. Much of the high risk of Type 2 diabetes is attributed to obesity, poor diet, and a sedentary lifestyle. Interestingly, Asian and Pacific Islander children are less likely to have Type 1 diabetes than white children.

ASIANS AND PACIFIC ISLANDER ETHNICITIES IN THE UNITED STATES

Asian	Pacific Islander
Asian Indian	Carolinian
Bangladeshi	Fijian
Bhutanese	Guamanian
Bornean	Hawaiian
Cambodian	Korean
Celebesian	Melanesian
Ceram	Micronesian
Chinese	Northern Mariana Islander
Filipino	Palauan
Hmong	Papua New Guinean
Indochinese	Ponapean
Iwo Jiman	Polynesian
Japanese	Samoan
Javanese	Solomon Islander
Korean	Tahitian
Laotian	Tarawa Islander
Malayan	Tongan
Maldivian	Trukese (Chuukese)
Nepali	Yapese
Okinawan	
Pakistani	
Sikkimese	
Singaporean	
Sri Lankan	
Sumatran	
Thai	
Vietnamese	

Source: "Diabetes in Asian and Pacific Islander Americans," National Institute of Diabetes and Digestive and Kidney Diseases (NIDDK), NIH Publication No. 00–4667, November 1999

Organizations that provide assistance to Asians and Pacific Islanders with diabetes are:

Asian Health Services
Walk for Health Program
818 Webster Street
Oakland, CA 94607
(510) 986-6800
www.ahschc.org/walk.htm

Association of Asian Pacific Community Health
   Organizations
1440 Broadway, #510
Oakland, CA 94612
(510) 272-9536
www.aapcho.org

aspartame   An artificial sweetener that is derived from amino acids which is 180–200 times sweeter than sucrose (table sugar). Aspartame was first approved in 1981 under the brand name NutraSweet. It is used in diet drinks and foods and has 0 calories per gram.

Aspartame does not alter glucose levels in patients with diabetes and has been found to be safe.

Council on Scientific Affairs, "Aspartame: Review of Safety Issues," *Journal of the American Medical Association* 254 (1985): 400–402.

aspirin therapy   Aspirin taken on a daily basis as a preventive measure against heart disease or stroke. People who have diabetes face between double to quadruple the risk of death from cardiovascular disease (CVD) as nondiabetics. However, a regular dose use of aspirin, taken under the advice and care of a physician, has been found to be effective in decreasing deaths after heart attacks by about 23 percent. It has also been shown to cut the risk of a repeat heart attack by about 50 percent.

According to the American Diabetes Association, those who benefit the most from aspirin therapy are people with diabetes who are over age 65 and have HYPERTENSION or CARDIOVASCULAR DISEASE.

Patients with diabetes have very reactive or "sticky" platelets in their blood, and thus, these platelets are more likely to clot than the platelets of patients without diabetes. Thus, taking aspirin may particularly help patients with diabetes by blocking or decreasing this excessive clotting action.

According to a position statement from the American Diabetes Association in 2001, analyses of studies of cardiovascular diseases reveal that

> low dose aspirin therapy should be prescribed as a secondary prevention strategy, if no contraindications exist. Substantial evidence suggests that low-dose aspirin therapy should also be used as a primary prevention strategy in men and women with diabetes who are at high risk for cardiovascular events.

Aspirin is particularly recommended to reduce the risk of heart disease in patients who:

- have a family history of coronary heart disease
- continue to smoke cigarettes (although it is always best to cease all smoking)
- have hypertension
- have protein in their urine
- have an obesity problem
- have low density lipids (LDL) under 130 ("bad" cholesterol)
- have high density lipids (HDL) over 40 ("good" cholesterol)
- have triglycerides over 250

Aspirin has also been shown to be effective in decreasing risks for patients with the following medical problems:

- heart attack
- stroke
- transient ischemic attack ("mini-stroke")
- peripheral vascular disease
- angina (chest pains related to heart disease)

A clinical study that was comparing the results of low-dose aspirin therapy to Vitamin E in decreasing cardiovascular problems was actually halted prematurely when the researchers found clear evidence that aspirin had major benefits to patients. According to a 2001 article in *Lancet,* the researchers found that cardiovascular deaths were reduced from 1.4 percent to 0.8 percent and total cardiovascular events dropped from 8.2 percent to 6.3 percent in the aspirin group. In this study, Vitamin E did *not* confer these benefits.

Since the researchers did not wish to deny these benefits to the non-aspirin group, they ended the study earlier than they had planned so they could advise the patients to begin aspirin therapy.

The authors said the results should give doctors "the confidence to recommend low doses of aspirin (80–100 mg daily) for primary prevention in individuals who have one or more risk factors but whose blood pressure is contained within the normal range."

Despite the advantages of aspirin therapy, many people with diabetes who have CVD are not taking aspirin. According to a 2001 study in *Diabetes Care,* about 27 percent of people with diabetes have CVD, but only about one third (37 percent) use aspirin on a regular basis.

African Americans and Mexican Americans are less likely to use aspirin than whites.

Side Effects

Side effects of aspirin therapy may be allergy as well as minor or major gastrointestinal bleeding. Coated and lower-dose aspirin may decrease this problem. For this reason, it's important for patients using aspirin therapy to report any problems to their physicians. Aspirin therapy is not recommended for those who are under age 21, or those receiving anticoagulant medication, or who have had recent problems with gastrointestinal bleeding, or have problems with easy bleeding.

American Diabetes Association, "Aspirin Therapy in Diabetes," *Diabetes Care* 24, suppl. 1 (2001): S62–S63.

Collaborative Group of the Primary Prevention Project, "Low Dose Aspirin and Vitamin E in People at Cardiovascular Risk: A Randomised Trial in General Practice," *Lancet* 357 (2001): 89–95.

Samuel K. Kajubi, M.D., "Aspirin in the Treatment of Type 2 Diabetes," *Archives of Internal Medicine* 160, no. 3 (2000): 394.

D. B. Rolka, et al., "Aspirin Use Among Adults with Diabetes: Estimates from the Third National Health Nutrition Examination Survey," *Diabetes Care* 24, no. 2 (2001): 197–201.

assisted living facilities (ALF)   Refers to rooms or apartments for older and/or disabled individuals in a facility where the staff provides assistance to residents. These facilities usually don't provide as much care as a person would receive in a SKILLED NURSING FACILITY (nursing home), but they do offer more care than the individual would receive if he or she were living at a private home. For example, most assisted living facilities provide meals, social events, and a nurse available on the premises as well as a physician on call.

Many assisted living facilities also offer special care to residents with diabetes, cognitive impairments such as ALZHEIMER'S DISEASE, and who suffer from other medical problems. In addition, the staff in an ALF often assists residents in making sure that needed medication is taken. Most staff members also offer or arrange for transportation for residents to get to their doctor appointments and shopping facilities.

Demographics of Assisted Living Residents

According to a summary of a report in a 2000 issue of *Contemporary Longterm Care,* most residents (75 percent) of assisted living facilities are female. The average age of residents is about 84 years for women and 83 years for men. An estimated 41 percent of residents are wheelchair users. About 10 percent of ALF residents receive special assistance with managing their diabetes and about 29 percent of residents receive help with managing their medications.

Advantages of Assisted Living Facilities

Older individuals with diabetes may find it difficult to live completely independently and yet they may also be fairly self-sustaining. As a result, they don't need or want the high level of care and the more limited freedom of a skilled nursing environment. Instead, the mid-level care offered in an assisted living facility may be sufficient for their needs. Study after study has demonstrated that many people intensely dislike the idea of moving to a skilled nursing facility; consequently, the interim step of an assisted living facility may provide residents with the convenience and the care that they need.

Disadvantages of Assisted Living

Most assisted living facilities are "private pay," and thus Medicare or Medicaid will not cover the cost of residence fees. Residents must use their own income and savings or must liquidate assets or find some other means to afford fees.

It should not be assumed that assisted living facilities follow the same state and federal regulations as skilled nursing facilities. Instead, state laws vary greatly on requirements that ALFs must meet; however, in general, the requirements are not as strict as they are for skilled nursing facilities. Of course, new ALFs must meet state and local building code requirements.

In 2000, the average rate for a private studio apartment in an ALF was estimated at about $2,000 per month, although fees vary greatly from area to area. The cost also depends heavily on the type of facility that is chosen and the services provided; for example, some ALFs advertise that they offer gourmet meals to residents. As one might expect, fees at such facilities are higher than where facilities provide nutritious but nongourmet fare.

Medicaid Waivers
May Cover ALF Fees

It should be noted that in many states, and in assisted living facilities that wish to participate and are approved, a limited number of units are set aside in a special program for Medicaid recipients. In this "Medicaid waiver" program, requested by the state to the federal govern-ment, individuals who are receiving Medicaid benefits may have all or part of their rent paid for out of Medicaid funds. This program may be expanded in the future; however, as of this writing, it represents only a tiny portion of all assisted living units.

"ALF Overview Preview," *Contemporary Longterm Care* 23, no. 6 (June 2000): 9.

atherosclerosis/arteriosclerosis A complex condition in which the surface of the blood vessel (endothelium) is remodeled as the result of various processes. Atherosclerosis is a medical problem faced by many people with diabetes. It is an active process involving lipids (fats), white blood cells, antibodies, platelets, and other hormones and proteins that are all participants.

If the process continues long enough, it may block a blood vessel. More frequently, the plaque that builds up in the vessel ruptures and exposes lipids and other proteins to the circulation, setting off an acute clot (thrombus). This results in the blocking of blood flow and oxygen to the affected organ. Depending on the severity of the blood flow blockage, atherosclerosis may lead to MYOCARDIAL INFARCTION (heart attack), STROKE, or other serious medical problems. (See also CARDIOVASCULAR DISEASE, HS-CRP TEST, STROKE.)

Australia An estimated 800,000 Australians have diabetes, and half of them have not yet been diagnosed with the disease, according to Diabetes Australia, an organization that provides information on diabetes. The Diabetes Australia Research Trust (DART) provides grants to support research on diabetes.

For further information, contact

Diabetes Australia
1st Floor Churchill House
218 Northbourne Avenue
Braddon ACT 261
Australia
www.diabetesaustralia.com.au

autoimmune disease   A disease in which the body's own immune system destroys essential body tissue because it has mistakenly identified it as a foreign invader of the body. Type 1 diabetes is believed by most experts to be an autoimmune disease because the immune system attacks and destroys the beta cells that lie within the pancreas and that make insulin.

Examples of other autoimmune diseases are rheumatoid arthritis, pernicious anemia, vitiligo, Graves' hyperthyroidism, and Hashimoto's thyroiditis. Having any one autoimmune disease often makes a person more prone to having another such disease.

autonomic neuropathy   Refers to nerve problems involving the automatic functions of the body, such as the emptying of the stomach, colon, and bladder, as well as nerve problems with sexual function (erectile dysfunction in men and vaginal dryness and arousal failure in women).

If the stomach does not empty well, the condition is called GASTROPARESIS DIABETICORUM. When the bladder is affected, it can cause NEUROGENIC BLADDER. When the colon is affected, it can cause diabetic diarrhea. It may also cause colonic dysmotility, a malfunction of the colon that may result in severe constipation, sometimes to the point of requiring the surgical removal of part of the colon.

Autonomic neuropathy can also affect heart function and lead to cardiac arrhythmias and sudden death. The blood pressure can also be affected. ORTHOSTATIC HYPOTENSION is a condition in which the systolic blood pressure of the person falls by more than 20 mm Hg when the person moves from lying to standing and has symptoms of lightheadedness and faintness. The person may actually faint. (See also DIABETIC NEUROPATHY.)

babies See INFANTS.

balanitis A YEAST infection of the foreskin of the penis, typically due to *Candida albicans*. It is much more common among men with diabetes. If a man has such an infection, he should also be screened for diabetes. Recurrent infections of balanitis can lead to scarring and serious medical conditions that may ultimately necessitate circumcision in an uncircumcised male. (If a man has already been circumcised, this condition is rare.)

behavioral modification A purposeful changing and shaping of behavior. For example, psychologists may use behavioral modification techniques to help patients with diabetes exhibit better medication adherence and improve their diet, lose weight, and quit smoking, among some of the available choices. In their 1998 article for *Clinical Diabetes,* authors Harris and Lustman note that the psychologist or social worker can help the patient improve his or her health. They also state that,

> The bulk of the psychological services in diabetes care are provided to patients who do not have diagnosable psychological problems. For example, nonadherence to the diabetes regimen is the most common reason for psychological referral, although in a statistical sense, it represents the norm and not the exception. Nonadherence to treatment is not itself evidence of a psychological problem.

Common psychological goals are:

- to improve adherence to diet and insulin/medication
- to promote exercise and a healthy lifestyle
- to aid the patient in eliminating harmful behavior such as smoking
- to evaluate psychological problems that may exist and make appropriate referral

Of course, sometimes patients with diabetes do have serious psychological problems, such as DEPRESSION, and it's estimated that at least one third of all patients with diabetes will experience depression or anxiety at some point in their lives. Sometimes antidepressants or other medications are prescribed. The psychiatrist or treating physician should carefully coordinate any medication that is prescribed for a patient with diabetes with the patient's primary physician. The patient should also be sure to tell his or her physician about the psychiatrist or any other medical doctor being seen, so that any risks of medication interactions are minimal. (See also MEDICATION NONADHERENCE/NONCOMPLIANCE.)

Maryanne Davidson et al., "Teaching Teens to Cope: Coping Skills Training for Adolescents with Adolescent-Dependent Diabetes Mellitus," *Journal of the Society of Pediatric Nurses* 2, no. 2 (April–June 1997): 65–73.

Sarah E. Hampson, Ph.D., et al., "Behavioral Interventions for Adolescents with Type 1 Diabetes," *Diabetes Care* 23, no. 9 (September 2000): 1416-1422.

Michael A. Harris, and Patrick J. Lustman, "The Psychologist in Diabetes Care," *Clinical Diabetes* 16, no. 2 (April 1998): 91–94.

beta cell   Specialized cell found in the islets of Langerhans along with alpha cells (glucagon) and delta cells. It is this cell that produces insulin and that may become defective and stop producing insulin.

People with Type 1 diabetes have pancreases that produce no insulin because their immune system has destroyed the beta cells. In contrast, people with Type 2 diabetes usually have a pancreas with beta cells that produce some insulin; however, their bodies have developed a resistance to the effects of insulin.

Current research is focused on attempts to infuse/transplant beta cells to cure diabetes. The limiting issue, however, is the availability of pancreases from which to harvest the beta cells. Intense efforts are ongoing to grow beta cells in the laboratory in order to create a dependable and renewable supply. (See also ISLET CELL TRANSPLANTATION.)

B-hydroxybutyrate   One of the two major KETONES that the body makes. The other is ACETOACETATE. B-hydroxybutyrate cannot be measured in the urine by commercially available urine dipsticks, as can acetoacetate. (See also ACETONE, DIABETIC KETOACIDOSIS [DKA].)

biguanides   A class of drugs used to treat people with Type 2 diabetes. As of this writing, the only drug in the class is Glucophage (METFORMIN). Drugs in this class work to boost or improve the use of glucose in the body and lower the amount of insulin in the body. Glucophage does not cause HYPOGLYCEMIA as do some other diabetes medications, nor does it cause weight gain. Since many people with Type 2 diabetes have a problem with OBESITY, this is an important asset.

Glucophage may cause nausea and can initially lead to changes in bowel habits, especially loose stools. Taking the pill with a meal and slowly titrating the dose up to 2,000 to 2,550 milligrams per day often diminishes these side effects. Glucophage should not be used in patients with renal insufficiency or moderate-to-severe liver dysfunction. Nor should it be used in patients with congestive heart failure.

birth control   Devices used to prevent conception from occurring, such as birth control pills, intrauterine devices, condoms, diaphragms with spermicides, sponges, and "natural" methods, such as charting when conception is most likely to occur and avoiding intercourse at that time. (Also known as the "rhythm" method.) Women with diabetes can, in general, use most of the same methods and devices for birth control as women with normal glucose levels. Caution must be taken, however, in using oral birth control contraceptives.

Experts caution women with diabetes against using progesterone-containing intrauterine devices (IUDs) for contraception because of the risk of infection. However, it is felt that women with diabetes may safely use copper-containing IUDs.

Contraception Enables Preconception Care

Contraception is also important for the woman with diabetes because before conception, experts strongly advise that extra care should be taken to avoid later harm to both mother and baby. Preconception care has proven to provide significant health benefits to both mother and child. (See also PREGNANCY.)

Birth Control Pills

If women with diabetes use birth control pills for contraception, they need to realize that the female hormone in the pills may affect their blood glucose levels. Birth control pills may increase insulin resistance. This is especially true for progesterone-only contraceptives. Women with diabetes who use birth control pills may require an adjustment in their therapy to continue to maintain their usual level of glycemic control. Monophasic pills (pills with a steady level of hormone on each day, with no variation) supply a steady level of hormone and thus may cause fewer ups and downs in glucose levels. If a woman has diabetes, is over 30, is a smoker, or has high blood pressure, oral contraceptives may not be the safest option.

Women who are also at risk for diabetes, because of close family members with diabetes or whose doctors say they are at risk for another reason, should also be cautious in taking birth control pills. Women with normal glucose tolerance who have risk factors for diabetes and take birth control pills may develop IMPAIRED GLUCOSE TOLERANCE (IGT). In addition, women who already have IGT and who then take birth control pills may then progress to overt diabetes.

Birth Control for Women Who Had Gestational Diabetes

Birth control is also important for the mother who has had a previous experience with GESTATIONAL DIABETES MELLITUS (GDM) and who does not wish an active involvement in diabetes self-care. The rate for recurrent GDM is about 50 percent. To avoid unplanned pregnancies, contraception is important.

Tubal ligation, a form of surgical sterilization, is another option for women who do not wish to have any more children. It's important to realize, however, that it is usually difficult and may be impossible to reverse this procedure.

Male Contraception

There are fewer contraceptive options available for men, although condoms are about 90 percent effective when used correctly. Vasectomy is an excellent choice for couples who do not wish to have more children, and it is a much less invasive procedure than tubal ligation for women. As with tubal ligation, this decision needs to be taken very carefully, as reversal is very difficult and may prove to be impossible.

bladder diseases Medical problems related to the bladder and urinary tract. Individuals with diabetes may suffer from a variety of bladder problems, such as incontinence, NEUROGENIC BLADDER, spastic bladder, bladder inflammation, (CYSTITIS), URINARY TRACT INFECTIONS and other urological problems. Most bladder problems experienced by people with diabetes are likely to stem from nerve damage, or DIABETIC NEUROPATHY. In the case of bladder problems stemming from AUTONOMIC NEUROPATHY, patients should urinate on a regular basis and should also exert pressure in the lower pelvic area, just above the pubic bone (suprapubic pressure), when they urinate. This will facilitate a more complete emptying of the bladder and decrease the risk of a urinary tract infection.

blindness The inability to see or loss of vision. Diabetes is the main cause of blindness in individuals ages 20–74 in the United States, and the disease accounts for up to 24,000 of new cases of blindness each year. People with diabetes have about 20 times the risk of nondiabetics of developing blindness. In many cases, an eye examination and treatment could have prevented the loss of vision.

According to the CENTERS FOR DISEASE CONTROL AND PREVENTION (CDC), about 1.6 million people, or 25 percent of those with diabetes, have some form of visual impairment up to and including blindness. Experts emphasize that early detection and treatment could prevent up to 90 percent of cases of blindness that are related to diabetes, or about 18,000 cases per year. In addition to saving the eyes of these patients, the annual savings to the federal budget would be over $470 million.

Although good medical treatment is available, many people with diabetes do not obtain such treatment and they lose their eyesight; for example, the CDC estimates that 60 percent of individuals with diabetes fail to have their eyes checked annually with a dilated eye examination. This is a crucial eye examination, which can reveal early signs of eye problems that may eventually lead to blindness.

As a result of concern over this serious problem on the part of government officials in the United States and OPHTHALMOLOGISTS, individuals who are over age 65 and who cannot afford eye examinations may now obtain free examinations and treatment, as a part of the NATIONAL DIABETES EYE EXAMINATION PROGRAM.

Another reason for having an annual examination is that often serious eye diseases may have no noticeable symptoms until it is very difficult or too late to repair the damage. An ophthalmologist or an optometrist trained in diabetic eye diseases can detect such diseases in the early stages when treatment will still be effective.

In most cases, DIABETIC RETINOPATHY is the cause of blindness among people with diabetes. Other diseases that may lead to blindness if not treated are CATARACTS, GLAUCOMA, and MACULAR EDEMA.

blood glucose meters Special hand-held devices that test the blood glucose levels, thus helping a person with diabetes determine if the glucose level is normal or not. Many devices require the person to prick a finger with a LANCET, so that a drop of blood may be tested. Some devices incorporate the blood extraction with the testing, enabling a person to extract the drop of blood from the forearm, where there are fewer nerve endings, and thus, less pain and to then obtain readout results in 8–30 seconds.

Many meters have memories, and an individual can make comparisons to previous readings. The patient may also be able to download the information to a computer for later use.

Many devices offer prompts to alert the patient to the presence of ketones or to advise the person to get a snack or adjust his or her insulin. Blood glucose meters may be small or very large and prices for them vary greatly. Insurance companies may provide payment for such devices. MEDICARE covers blood glucose meters for individuals with diabetes, although as of this writing, actual diabetes medications such as insulin and others are not covered.

Most meters now automatically convert the whole blood glucose reading to a plasma level so that it would be comparable to a venous (vein) reading taken in a laboratory. *Diabetes Forecast*, a publication of the AMERICAN DIABETES ASSOCIATION, includes a "Resource Guide" supplement at the end of each year that is devoted to reviewing blood glucose meters and other devices that are needed by or that are helpful to people with diabetes.

The major blood glucose meter manufacturers are as follows:

Abbott Laboratories/MediSense Products
(800) 527-3339
www.Medisense.com

Bayer Corporation Diagnostics Division
(800) 348-8100
www.glucometer.com

LifeScan, Inc.
(800) 227-8862
www.lifescan.com

Roche Diagnostics
(800) 858-8072
www.accu-chek.com

TheraSense, Inc.
(888) 522-5226
www.TheraSense.com

blood glucose monitoring Periodic testing of blood glucose levels, followed by possible action based on the results of the test. For example, if glucose levels are high, more medication may be needed. If they are very low or the person may be experiencing symptoms of HYPOGLYCEMIA, the individual will consume a glucose gel/tablet or a high carbohydrate food or drink.

One of the major developments in diabetes over the past 80 years is that patients can monitor their own glucose levels with a tiny drop of blood. Noninvasive options (BLOODLESS TESTING) may be available to patients in the early 21st century, thus alleviating the pain of the FINGER PRICK. Self-monitoring is really the cornerstone of care, and enables the person with diabetes to judge the effects of diet, exercise, medications, stress, insulin, and other factors. (See also GLYCEMIC CONTROL, HOME BLOOD GLUCOSE MONITORING.)

bloodless testing Testing of blood glucose levels without the need to draw blood. Because of the discomfort that comes with pricking their fingers for a blood drop to test, many people with diabetes fail to test their blood frequently enough and sometimes do not test their blood at all. As a result, they do not know what changes should be made to their diet and medication. Experts increasingly seek devices that can provide bloodless testing so that people with diabetes would be more likely to perform testing and at the frequency recommended by their physicians.

The Glucowatch, manufactured by Cygnus Therapeutics, has been approved by the FDA and should be available to the public in 2002. This device, worn just like a wristwatch, includes a special highly sensitive pad that is placed on the skin and fits under the "watch." The special pad will measure the wearer's blood glucose every 15–20 minutes after a two- to four-hour warmup period. These measurements will be taken for up to 12 hours. As of this writing, the cost of the pads is estimated at $5 to $10 per day.

The key advantage to the Glucowatch is that it eliminates the need for frequent blood testing. However, it is still a good idea at this time for most people with diabetes to perform a daily finger stick test at least once a day.

blood pressure/hypertension See HYPERTENSION.

blood sugar Blood glucose levels, which are usually high (HYPERGLYCEMIA) in a person with untreated diabetes. If blood sugar drops to a low state, the person with diabetes is having an episode of HYPOGLYCEMIA, which can cause an array of serious problems and medical complications. (See also GLYCEMIC CONTROL.)

blood urea nitrogen (BUN) A waste product produced by the kidneys. Increased levels of BUN may be an early warning sign of kidney disease and should be followed up. It can also indicate DEHYDRATION.

blurred vision Clouded or distorted vision. For a person with diabetes, sudden blurred or clouded vision is a danger sign and means that he or she should see an ophthalmologist (doctor who specializes in eye diseases) immediately. The blurred vision could be a sign of the onset of DIABETIC RETINOPATHY with hemorrhage and impending BLINDNESS. If caught early, it may be possible to avert such severe complications. Blurred vision might also be a warning sign of CATARACTS. Untreated cataracts lead to blindness.

Blurred vision may also be caused by major shifts in glucose levels. Glucose gets into the lens of the eye, where it is converted to sorbitol. Water osmotically follows and the lens changes its shape. As a result, the person's eyes cannot refract properly. For these reasons, physicians recommend no change in eyeglass prescriptions until glucose levels have been stable for about four to six weeks.

Body Mass Index (BMI) A specific formula that is based on height and weight, and which helps to determine whether a person is underweight, of optimal weight, or is overweight or obese. The United States and the World Health Organization rely primarily on the Body Mass Index (BMI) to determine levels of OBESITY and to stratify a patient's risk for a variety of diseases and complications. It should also be noted that a BMI chart for an adult should not be used to determine whether a child is overweight or obese. Instead, physicians should refer to pediatric BMI charts for boys and girls. (See Appendix X.)

In the past, physicians and other experts primarily relied on height/weight charts alone; however, the BMI measure is seen as a better measure of determining excessive weight.

Because OBESITY is a strong predictor of Type 2 diabetes, BMI is an important concept in diabetes.

BODY MASS INDEX CLASSIFICATION

Underweight: Less than 18.5
Normal weight: 18.5–24.9
Overweight: 25–29.9
Obesity (Class 1): 30–34.9
Obesity (Class 2): 35–39.9
Extreme Obesity: 40 or over

BMI is also usually a very effective measure to denote obesity. But it should also be noted that, in a few cases, such as the case of weightlifters or very athletic and heavily muscular people, they might appear to be overweight according to BMI charts, although they are not.

The converse is also true. Some studies indicate that in the case of some Asian individuals, because their bones and body build are smaller than the Western standard, Asians may be overweight or obese at lower weights than indicated by the BMI chart. As a result, some Asians may be at risk for diabetes or actually have diabetes, but because of the BMI chart, doctors think they do not have a weight problem and they do not realize when there is a risk for Type 2 diabetes.

According to a report on obesity in Asia, published in 2000, new criteria for overweight and obesity are needed. The authors say, "While in some Asian populations the prevalence of obesity is lower than that in Europe, the health risks associated with obesity occur at a lower body mass index (BMI) in Asian populations."

This source offered such criteria. For example, the normal range of BMI for an "adult Europid" (person from Europe) was 18.5–24.9. The authors proposed that a normal BMI for adult Asians should be 18.5–22.9. Thus, Asians would be considered overweight at lower levels than non-Asians.

"The Asia-Pacific Perspective: Redefining Obesity and Its Treatment," International Diabetes Institute, a World Health Organization Collaborating Centre for the Epidemiology of Diabetes and Health Pro-

BODY MASS INDEX (BMI) TABLE																	
BMI	19	20	21	22	23	24	25	26	27	28	29	30	31	32	33	34	35
Height	Weight (in pounds)																
4'10" (58")	91	96	100	105	110	115	119	124	129	134	138	143	148	153	158	162	167
4'11" (59")	94	99	104	109	114	119	124	128	133	138	143	148	153	158	163	168	173
5' (60")	97	102	107	112	118	123	128	133	138	143	148	153	158	163	168	174	179
5'1" (61")	100	106	111	116	122	127	132	137	143	148	153	158	164	169	174	180	185
5'2" (62")	104	109	115	120	126	131	136	142	147	153	158	164	169	175	180	186	191
5'3" (63")	107	113	118	124	130	135	141	146	152	158	163	169	175	180	186	191	197
5'4" (64")	110	116	122	128	134	140	145	151	157	163	169	174	180	186	192	197	204
5'5" (65")	114	120	126	132	138	144	150	156	162	168	174	180	186	192	198	204	210
5'6" (66")	118	124	130	136	142	148	155	161	167	173	179	186	192	198	204	210	216
5'7" (67")	121	127	134	140	146	153	159	166	172	178	185	191	198	204	211	217	223
5'8" (68")	125	131	138	144	151	158	164	171	177	184	190	197	203	210	216	223	230
5'9" (69")	128	135	142	149	155	162	169	176	182	189	196	203	209	216	223	230	236
5'10" (70")	132	139	146	153	160	167	174	181	188	195	202	209	216	222	229	236	243
5'11" (71")	136	143	150	157	165	172	179	186	193	200	208	215	222	229	236	243	250
6' (72")	140	147	154	162	169	177	184	191	199	206	213	221	228	235	242	250	258
6'1" (73")	144	151	159	166	174	182	189	197	204	212	219	227	235	242	250	257	265
6'2" (74")	148	155	163	171	179	186	194	202	210	218	225	233	241	249	256	264	272
6'3" (75")	152	160	168	176	184	192	200	208	216	224	232	240	248	256	264	272	279

Source: Evidence Report of Clinical Guidelines on the Identification, Evaluation, and Treatment of Overweight and Obesity in Adults, 1998. NIH/National Heart, Lung, and Blood Institute (NHLBI)

motion for Noncommunicable Disease, February 2000, Australia.

bolus An extra injection of insulin that is taken by a person with diabetes in anticipation of a rise in glucose from eating a meal. (See also BOLUS RATES/BASAL RATES.)

bolus rates/basal rates The speed at which insulin is supplied, whether through an extra injection, or BOLUS, or through a continuous supply (basal) of low levels of insulin, as with an insulin pump.

brain attack See STROKE.

breastfeeding Directly providing breast milk to an infant, and a highly regarded method of nutrition for babies. In past years, women with diabetes were discouraged from having children. If they did have babies, bottle feeding rather than breastfeeding their infants was encouraged by doctors. Today most doctors work with mothers who have diabetes to help them have an optimal pregnancy and a healthy child. Breastfeeding is no longer discouraged by physicians, who are aware of the strong bond that develops between the breastfeeding infant and the mother as well as the nutritional and medical benefits that come with breastfeeding.

According to the Centers for Disease Control and Prevention (CDC) in their 2001 report on women and diabetes, new mothers who have Type 1 diabetes are about as likely to choose breastfeeding for their babies as nondiabetic mothers; however, they are more likely to begin adding supplementary formula within weeks of delivery. A copious milk production can also be delayed among women with Type 1 diabetes. The worse the GLYCEMIC CONTROL of the mother, the longer the delay in sufficient milk production.

There are also some studies that indicate that infants whose mother has Type 1 diabetes and who also receive cow's milk formula may be at risk for developing diabetes based on their increased immune response. Of course, the infants also are at genetic risk as well. More research is needed on this controversial topic.

Some Difficulties to Overcome

WOMEN WITH DIABETES need to be aware that they must continue to be prudent in checking their glucose levels, a task that can become cumbersome among the many duties of a new mother. In addition, many new mothers are tired from lack of sleep and sleep deprivation can upset glucose levels for the diabetic woman. A third risk for breastfeeding mothers who have diabetes is that they are more prone to infections than nondiabetic women, and need to be sure to contact the physician if their breasts become painful or swollen. This may indicate a yeast or bacterial infection.

Women with diabetes who are breastfeeding will often need a small snack prior to breastfeeding a child and should also be sure to test their glucose levels about an hour after breastfeeding to make sure there is no problem with excessively low levels of glucose (HYPOGLYCEMIA), which could lead to a dangerous situation for the mother and child.

Breastfeeding mothers should also be very careful about medications that they take. For example, oral hypoglycemic medications that can be secreted into breast milk should be avoided because they may cause the infant to suffer from hypoglycemia.

One caveat with regard to breastfeeding is that there is some suggestive evidence that if a mother has Type 1 diabetes, her baby may be at risk for developing diabetes because antigens in the breast milk may trigger an autoimmune response in the baby that could eventually lead to diabetes. Women with diabetes should be sure to discuss all the pros and cons of breastfeeding with their own physicians as well as with the baby's pediatrician.

In rare cases, breastfeeding should be avoided altogether. This is true in the case of women with diabetes who have proliferative retinopathy (an eye disease that can lead to blindness), because breastfeeding can further accelerate the retinopathy.

For Further Information

La Leche League International offers assistance to nursing mothers. Breastfeeding mothers should contact La Leche League to find the nearest group in their area. Contact the organization at:

La Leche League International
1400 North Meacham Road
Schaumburg, IL 60173-4840
(847) 519-7730
www.lalecheleague.org

La Leche League International also publishes a pamphlet on breastfeeding for mothers with diabetes, "The Diabetic Mother and Breastfeeding."

Elizabeth Bird, editor and compiler, "The Diabetic Mother and Breastfeeding," La Leche League International, pamphlet 1999.

J. Paronen et al., "Effect of Cow's Milk Exposure and Maternal Type 1 Diabetes on Cellular and Humoral Immunization to Dietary Insulin in Infants at Genetic Risk for Type 1 Diabetes," *Diabetes* 49, no. 10 (2000): 1657–1666.

brittle diabetes A condition in which glucose levels are very variable and very difficult to control. When this type of problem occurs, it is nearly always diagnosed in patients with Type 1 diabetes and no immediate apparent or clear-cut cause is found. Further investigation is required to seek out the cause.

In their chapter on brittle diabetes in *Ellenberg and Rifkin's Diabetes Mellitus,* authors David S. Schade and Mark R. Burge define brittle diabetes as, "Specifically, a brittle diabetic patient is one who is either incapacitated or whose life-style is disrupted more than 3 times per week by repeated episodes of hyperglycemia or hypo-glycemia *after the patient has been educated in the techniques of intensive insulin therapy."* (Italics in original.)

Schade and Burge contend that until it is clear that the patient is fully educated and that the problem does not stem from misunderstanding about self-treatment, brittle diabetes should not be diagnosed.

They also state that in about half of the cases, once the underlying cause of the brittle diabetes is corrected, the patient then becomes "nonbrittle."

In his article on this topic in a 2000 issue of *Diabetes Forecast,* Dr. Michael Pfeiffer agrees that there are always reasons for wide swings in glucose levels. Some reasons that he suggested may be the causes are:

- Insulin that has been improperly stored and as a result, has gone bad
- Errors with insulin measurement or mixing
- Digestive disorders such as GASTROPARESIS, or slow stomach emptying
- Physical and/or psychological stress

Other causes noted by Schade and Burge include:

- narcotic drug addiction
- early morning hyperglycemia (dawn phenomenon)
- endocrine disorders
- insulin resistance
- psychological problems

Michael A. Pfeiffer, M.D., "Brittle Diabetes," *Diabetes Forecast* 53, no. 11 (November 2000): 13.

David S. Schade and Mark R. Burge, "Brittle Diabetes: Pathogenesis and Therapy," in *Ellenberg and Rifkin's Diabetes Mellitus* (Oxford, England: Appleton & Lange, 1999).

calcium channel blockers (CCBs) A class of medications that is prescribed for people with HYPERTENSION (high blood pressure) in order to lower their blood pressure levels. Many people with diabetes also suffer from hypertension. The combination of diabetes and hypertension can cause severe complications including premature death. Some examples of calcium channel blocker medications are, as of this writing: nifedipine, amlodipine, isradipine, diltiazem, and verapamil.

CCBs are further broken down into the dihydropyridine (DHP) class and the non-DHP (NDHP) class. The DHP calcium channel blockers may cause mild headache and swollen ankles when given in large doses. The NDHP calcium channel blockers may cause constipation and may slow the heart rate, and they need to be used carefully with other drugs that could affect heart rate or any aspect of the heart's electrical conduction system. This has been an area of controversy as some studies have shown that although the DHP CCBs are very well tolerated and very effective, at the same time, they may be less effective than the NDHP CCBs at protecting kidney function in patients with diabetes.

Dr. George Bakris has done a number of studies showing that low-dose NDHP CCBs in combination with ANGIOTENSIN-CONVERTING ENZYME (ACE) inhibitor drugs or beta-blocker drugs may be the best choice. The exact combinations that are best will continue to be a source of controversy as newer drugs are developed. At this time, most experts feel that the most important issue is getting the blood pressure as low as the patient will tolerate, at a minimum under 135/85 or,

ideally, as low as 120/70. If an optimal blood pressure can be achieved, then the exact choice of medications has less impact on the overall outcome. (See also CARDIOVASCULAR DISEASES, STROKE.)

G. Bakris et al., "Effects of an ACE inhibitor/calcium antagonist combination on proteinuria in diabetic nephropathy," *Kidney International* 54, no. 4 (1998): 1283–1289.

camps for children and adolescents with diabetes Summer camps for school-age children and adolescents who have diabetes. These camps are specifically oriented to their needs.

Summer camp can be a valuable experience, according to many experts, enabling children to meet new friends and providing an opportunity for children to learn that other children share the same struggles. It can help them feel less alone and more normal, as they discuss problems and solutions they have developed. Some children who have been resistant to self-injecting may overcome their fears when they see other children self-inject in a matter-of-fact manner. Camp counselors may also be adolescents and young adults who have diabetes and can be empathetic with the children about the disease and yet, at the same time, not overly fearful.

Camp can also be a break for parents or others who care for children with diabetes, and who must constantly consider issues such as blood checks, medication, and dealing with problems related to the disease.

According to Joanne D. Moore, R.N., C.D.E., in her article on sending a child to camp for the first time, in a 1996 issue of *Diabetes Self-Management,* parents should take the following steps to ease the way for both parent and child:

• Talk to the child about the camp beforehand and emphasize its assets

• Decide whether to send the child to a day camp or a residential camp. Day camps may be preferable for children under age nine

• Make sure that the camp is accredited by the AMERICAN DIABETES ASSOCIATION

• Read camp brochures

• If the camp offers an open house opportunity to ask questions, attend it

• Learn how the camp copes with medical problems and how they reach a physician if one is needed

The American Diabetes Association (ADA) has created a position statement on the management of diabetes at diabetes camps. According to the ADA, each camper should have a form that provides medical information on the child, as well as immunization information and the child's medication regimen.

While children are in camp, daily records of their blood glucose levels and insulin dosages should be recorded. Some modifications, such as reductions, may need to be made to insulin dosages because many children will be much more active at camp than at home. If the child uses an insulin pump, the camp director and medical staff should be familiar with the device and ensure that extra batteries are available.

American Diabetes Association, "Management of Diabetes at Diabetes Camps," *Diabetes Care* 24, Supp. 1 (January 2001): S113–S115.

Joanne D. Moore, R.N., C.D.E., "Sending Your Kid to Camp for the First Time," *Diabetes Self-Management* (March/April 1996): 23–26.

Canada and diabetes There are more than 2 million Canadians who have diabetes, according to the CANADIAN DIABETES ASSOCIATION. Of these, about 90 percent have Type 2 diabetes. Canadians also suffer from the complications of diabetes; for example, about 28 percent of the cases of severe kidney disease are experienced by Canadians with diabetes. ERECTILE DYSFUNCTION and many other illnesses are also problems.

Canada is comprised of diverse ethnic groups, and, as in the United States, minority groups are generally at a much greater risk for the development of Type 2 diabetes.

Interestingly, it has been Canadian scientists who have made great advances in helping people with diabetes. Most importantly, in 1922, Canadian scientists, Frederick Banting and Charles Best, proved that insulin could mitigate the impact of diabetes. Banting (with laboratory director Dr. MacLeod) later received the Nobel Prize for this work. It was truly an incredible life-saving discovery, responsible for improving quality of life for millions of children and adults with diabetes.

In 2000, Dr. James Shapiro and his colleagues at the University of Alberta in Edmonton reported a breakthrough success with islets of Langerhans transplants, causing 11 patients to remain diabetes-free one year later. Dr. Shapiro attributed at least part of the success to the avoidance of steroid medications, which had apparently inhibited success in past trials. As of this writing, Shapiro's "Edmonton Protocol" is being tested and utilized on patients in the United States, Canada, and the United Kingdom.

Many other clinical studies on diabetes, too numerous to cite in this essay, have been performed by Canadian physicians and researchers. (See also ISLETS OF LANGERHANS, TRANSPLANTATIONS.)

Canadian Diabetes Association (Association Canadienne du Diabète) Formed in 1953, the Canadian Diabetes Association is a nongovernmental advocacy organization for research and education that helps an estimated 2 million Canadians who have diabetes. It has 150 branches throughout the country. The Canadian Diabetes Association estimates that by 2010, the number of Canadians with diabetes will increase to 3 million.

The organization produced "Guidelines for Nutritional Management of Diabetes Mellitus in the New Millennium" in 2000 to assist people with diabetes and others who need helpful information. That same year, the Canadian Diabetes Association produced "Kid with Diabetes in School," a kit created to help teachers and administrators understand the needs of children with diabetes.

The organization also funds research through the Charles H. Best Research Fund.

Canadian Diabetes Association.
National Office
15 Toronto Street
Suite 800
Toronto, Ontario M5C 2E3
Canada
(416) 363-3373 or (800) BANTING (Toll-free in
  Canada)
www.diabetes.ca

Provincial Offices:
British Columbia-Yukon Division
1385 West 8th Avenue
Suite 360
Vancouver, BC V6H 3V
Canada
(604) 732-1331 or (800) 665-6526 (Toll-free in
  Canada)

Alberta/Northwest Territories Division
1010-10117 Jasper Avenue, NW
Edmonton, AB T5J 1W8
Canada
780-423-1232 or (800) 563-0032 (Toll-free in
  Canada)

Saskatchewan Division
104-2301 Avenue C North
Saskatoon, SK S7L 5Z5
Canada
(306) 933-1238 or (800) 996-4446 (Toll-free in
  Canada)

Manitoba Division
102-310 Broadway Avenue
Winnepeg, MB R3C 0S6
Canada
(204) 925-3800 or (800) 226-8464 (Toll-free in
  Canada)

Ontario Division
15 Toronto Street
Suite 800
Toronto, ON M5C 2E3
Canada
(416) 363-3374 or (800) 226-8464 (Toll-free in
  Canada)

New Brunswick Division
165 Regent Street
Suite 3
Fredericton, NB E3B 7B4
Canada
(506) 452-9009 or (800) 884-4232 (Toll-free in
  Canada)

Nova Scotia Division
6080 Young Street
#101 Halifax, NS B3K 5L2
Canada
(902) 453-4232 or (800) 326-7712 (Toll-free in
  Canada)

Prince Edward Island Division
Charlottetown Area Health Centre
1 Rochford Street
Charlottetown, PEI C1A 9L2
Canada
(902) 894-3005

Newfoundland and Labrador Division
354 Water Street
Suite 217
St. John's, NF A1C 1C4
Canada
(709) 754-0953

Affiliate:
Association diabète Québec
5635, rue Sherbrooke est
Montreal, PQ H1N 1A2
Canada

(514) 259-3422
(800) 361-3504 (Numero sans frais)

carbohydrate A source of energy and one of the three main food groups. The other two food groups are fats and proteins. Carbohydrates include sugars and starches. They contain 4 kilocalories per gram. When the body cannot draw on glucose (sugar) levels that are within the blood for energy, then it cannot properly use carbohydrates. In such a situation, the body draws on its fat reserves. If the glucose levels fall too precipitously, the person with diabetes may develop HYPOGLYCEMIA. (See also CARBOHYDRATE COUNTING, OBESITY.)

carbohydrate counting A meal-planning tool that allows for good nutrition as well as glycemic control. People with diabetes who are treated with insulin learn their own carbohydrate-insulin ratios, and thus, they can estimate their insulin dosages more precisely. For example, if a person has a carbohydrate to insulin ratio of 10 to 1, and will consume 50 grams of carbohydrates at breakfast, he or she will then inject 5 units of rapid or short-acting insulin.

There is no evidence that complete restriction of sucrose (sugar) is helpful for people with diabetes. However, this does not mean that it's acceptable or advisable for people with diabetes to eat large amounts of sugar-filled foods. Instead, sugar should be consumed in moderation.

Carbohydrate counting enables people with diabetes to achieve an appropriate level of moderation. Patients with diabetes need to learn, for example, that one slice of bread is equivalent in carbohydrate grams to one small apple or 1 cup of milk. Another example of carbohydrate equivalence: $1/2$ cup of popcorn is equal to 2 tablespoons of raisins or 1 tablespoon of sugar. (See also CARBOHYDRATES.)

Mary A. Johnson, M.S., R.D., C.D.E., "Carbohydrate Counting for People with Type 2 Diabetes," *Diabetes Spectrum* 13, no. 3 (2000): 156–158.

Diane Reader, R.D., L.D., C.D.E., "Carbohydrate Counting for Pregnant Women," *Diabetes Spectrum* 13, no. 3 (2000): 152–153.
Susan Saffel-Shrier, M.S., R.D., C.D., Certified Gerontologist, "Carbohydrate Counting for Older Patients," *Diabetes Spectrum* 13, no. 3 (2000): 158–162.
Hope S. Warshaw, and Karmen Kulkani, *Complete Guide to Carb Counting* (Lincolnshire, Ill.: NTC Publications Group, 2001).

cardiac dysfunctions See CARDIOVASCULAR DISEASES.

cardiologist Physician who is an expert in the treatment of heart disease. Many people with diabetes are at risk for CARDIOVASCULAR DISEASE and CORONARY HEART DISEASE. WOMEN WITH DIABETES have a particularly high risk for death from heart disease.

cardiovascular disease (CVD) Diseases of the heart itself or of the blood vessels of the heart. Primarily includes CORONARY HEART DISEASE, HYPERTENSION, NEPHROPATHY (kidney disease), and STROKE. Cardiovascular diseases are the leading causes of death and disability in the United States, and coronary heart disease is the number one cause of death for both men and women. The American Heart Association estimates that at least 58 million people in the United States have some form of cardiovascular disease. According to the CENTERS FOR DISEASE CONTROL AND PREVENTION (CDC), 960,000 Americans die of CVD each year, or 41 percent of all deaths. There are an estimated 6 million hospitalizations each year due to CVD events.

Cardiovascular Disease and Diabetes
Cardiovascular diseases are very common among people with diabetes, particularly coronary heart disease, kidney disease, and hypertension (high blood pressure).

According to the CDC, almost half (43 percent) of the people who die from diabetes-related deaths have cardiovascular diseases.

WOMEN WITH DIABETES are particularly at risk for dying from cardiovascular disease.

Great progress has been made in limiting the overall number of deaths from cardiovascular diseases. The CDC reported that between 1980 and 1996, age-adjusted death rates from CVD dropped by one third and death rate decreases were seen among all races as well as in both men and women. Unfortunately, people with diabetes have seen fewer improvements and the situation has actually worsened for women with diabetes.

Women with diabetes are at grave risk for CVD As mentioned, WOMEN WITH DIABETES have a higher rate of CVD than nondiabetic women. Studies have shown that although heart disease deaths have dropped by 27 percent among nondiabetic women, they have actually *increased* by 23 percent for women with diabetes. The findings are more favorable for men. Nondiabetic men have seen a 36 percent decline in CVD deaths, versus a 13 percent decline among men with diabetes.

Ethnic risks Some ethnic groups are more likely to suffer from CVD than others. Cardiovascular diseases and the serious complications associated with them are more commonly found among African Americans. In 1996, blacks experienced 40 percent more deaths from cardiovascular diseases than did whites. American Indians are also at high risk for cardiovascular disease and death.

In the Strong Heart Study of cardiovascular risk factors, researchers evaluated 1,846 men and 2,703 women ages 45–74 from 13 American Indian communities over the period 1989–92. The findings of this research were reported by Barbara V. Howard and her colleagues in *Diabetes Care* in 1999. The researchers found a distinct tie between diabetes and cardiovascular disease among the studied subjects.

The researchers found a high prevalence of diabetes that ranged from about 32–71 percent of the group, with the highest rates among American Indians in Arizona. The researchers compared men and women with diabetes to those without diabetes. They found that the subjects with diabetes were significantly more obese than the nondiabetic subjects, had more body fat, and more of the fat was distributed in the abdominal area, as measured by the WAIST-TO-HIP RATIO.

The subjects with diabetes were also much more likely to suffer from hypertension and higher triglyceride levels, and greater numbers of them had ALBUMINURIA.

American Indian women with diabetes were more obese than the men who had diabetes and they also had more fat around the waist (central adiposity). In addition, the women had more cases of DYSLIPIDEMIA than the men, with greater decreases in HDL (good) cholesterol. All of these factors combined made the women with diabetes more at risk for cardiovascular disease than the men with diabetes.

Risk Factors for CVD among Patients with Diabetes

Both Type 1 and Type 2 diabetes are risk factors for the development of CVD. Other risk factors for CVD that are common to many people with diabetes (in addition to the aforementioned risk of hypertension) are OBESITY (usually among those with Type 2 diabetes) and lack of exercise. Cigarette smoking is another known risk factor for the development of CVD.

The Honolulu Heart Program was one of many studies that demonstrated that diabetes brings an increased risk for cardiovascular disease. This ongoing program is a study of Japanese American men who were 45–68 when the study began in 1965. At that time, none of the 8,006 men had cardiovascular disease. The men were followed for over 23 years. The researchers found that the men with glucose intolerance or diabetes had a greater risk for coronary heart disease or death. This risk was present independent of age or other known risk factors for cardiovascular disease. They were also at greater risk of suffering from a stroke.

INSULIN RESISTANCE, or the failure of the body to adequately use the insulin produced (a problem for people with Type 2 diabetes), is also a risk factor for CVD. Insulin resistance is worsened in large part by obesity and lack of physical activity.

In addition, people with diabetes are more likely to experience dyslipidemia. According to Dr. Grundy and his colleagues in a 1999 article in *Circulation,* LDL is a very critical factor in the development of CVD. In fact, it is a more major factor than the other known risks. The authors say,

> In populations having very low LDL cholesterol levels, clinical CHD [coronary heart disease] is relatively rare, even when other risk factors— hypertension, cigarette smoking, and diabetes— are common. In contrast, severe elevations in LDL cholesterol can produce full-blown atherosclerosis and premature CHD in the complete absence of other risk factors.

Some people with diabetes have greater risks than others Among people who have diabetes, some groups have more of a risk for developing cardiovascular disease. Whites who have diabetes have the highest risk for developing cardiovascular disease, followed by blacks, and then Hispanics or Latinos. Also, the risk for cardiovas-

cular disease clearly rises with age for people with diabetes. The rate of cardiovascular disease is 38 per 100,000 people for those under age 45. The rate rises dramatically to 306 per 100,000 for those ages 45 to 64 years and then makes another marked rise to 850 per 100,000 for those ages 65 to 74 years old. The highest risk, a staggering 3,222 per 100,000, is faced by those who are age 75 and older.

Treatment for CVD

In addition to recommending that patients with diabetes attain good GLYCEMIC CONTROL and give up SMOKING, doctors also urge patients who are obese to lose weight and become more physically active. However, these lifestyle changes may not be sufficient to control hypertension or dyslipidemia.

Medications help considerably Studies such as the SCANDINAVIAN SIMVASTATIN SURVIVAL STUDY (4-S) and other major studies have demonstrated that medications in the statin class such as simvastatin and pravastatin can lower lipid levels and reduce the risk for heart attack or, among those who have not yet developed coronary artery disease, reduce the risk of its development.

Patients with diabetes benefited more than nondiabetics in the 4-S study. CVD risk decreased by 32 percent in patients who did *not* have diabetes but decreased 55 percent in those who were diagnosed with diabetes.

Patients may also need medications such as beta-blockers or ANGIOTENSIN-CONVERTING ENZYME (ACE) INHIBITORS. The HOPE STUDY demonstrated that ramipril, an ACE inhibitor, decreased the risk of myocardial infarction, stroke, and death. The findings were so positive that the study was ended early so that those patients on placebo could be given the drug.

Drugs in the thiazolidinediones class can help patients who use insulin improve their glycemic control and may have direct effects on the endothelial layer of the blood vessels to help lower the risk of atherosclerosis. Some examples of drugs in this class are rosiglitazone and pioglitazone.

Persons with Diabetes, 1997	Cardiovascular Disease Deaths
	Rate per 100,000
TOTAL	343
Race and ethnicity	
American Indian or Alaska Native	93
Asian or Pacific Islander	223
Asian	263
Native Hawaiian and other Pacific Islander	113
Black or African American	283
White	359
Hispanic or Latino	270
Select populations	
Age groups (not age adjusted)	
Under age 45 years	38
45 to 64 years	306
65 to 74 years	850
75 years and older	3,222

ASPIRIN THERAPY has also been proven to be a significant help in preventing cardiovascular disease, whether patients have diabetes or not.

In 2001, the AMERICAN DIABETES ASSOCIATION and the National Diabetes Education Program (NDEP) launched initiatives to increase public awareness of the relationship between diabetes and cardiovascular disease. One initiative was the Diabetic Cardiovascular Disease Initiative, a three-year project to increase public awareness of the link between diabetes and cardiovascular disease and to educate diabetes patients on their risks and appropriate self-management. An additional emphasis was to educate health care providers on the proper diagnosis and treatment of cardiovascular disease and its risk factors. (See also MYOCARDIAL INFARCTION, STROKE.)

Scott M. Grundy, M.D., Ph.D., Chairman, et al., "Diabetes and Cardiovascular Disease: A Statement for Healthcare Professionals from the American Heart Association," *Circulation* 100 (1999): 1134–1146.

Barbara V. Howard, Ph.D., et al., "Adverse Effects of Diabetes on Multiple Cardiovascular Disease Risk Factors in Women: The Strong Heart Study," *Diabetes Care* 21, no. 8 (August 1998): 1258–1265.

Beatriz L. Rodriguez, M.D., Ph.D., et al., "Glucose Intolerance and 23-Year Risk of Coronary Heart Disease and Total Mortality," *Diabetes Care* 22, no. 8 (1999): 1262–1265.

Karen Z. Walker, Ph.D., et al., "Effects of Regular Walking on Cardiovascular Risk Factors and Body Composition in Normoglycemic Women and Women with Type 2 Diabetes," *Diabetes Care* 22, no. 4 (April 1999): 555–556.

CARE Trial (Cholesterol and Recurrent Events Trial) A clinical study of heart disease, including subjects with and without diabetes. In this study, subjects were 4,159 patients, ages 21–75 years, who had suffered a MYOCARDIAL INFARCTION and were placed on either pravastatin or a placebo over five years. The study found that the drug lowered LDL cholesterol levels by 28 percent, and that fatal and nonfatal myocardial infarctions dropped by 24 percent. Patients with diabetes had an even more favorable result than

did nondiabetics. Other studies, such as the SCANDINAVIAN SIMVASTATIN SURVIVAL STUDY (4-S), proved that simvastatin, another drug in the statin class, lowered fatality rates among patients at risk for heart attack. (See also CARDIOVASCULAR DISEASE, CORONARY HEART DISEASE.)

Penny Kris-Etherton, and T.A. Pearson, "For Your Information," *American Dietetic Association Journal* 100, no. 10 (October 1, 2000): 1126–1130.

cataract An eye illness that causes an opaqueness of the lens of the eye. Cataracts are common among people with diabetes. A cataract is a clumping up of the protein in the lens of the eye and, once started, it continues to grow. As the disease progresses, it becomes more and more difficult for the individual to see through the cloudy film of the cataract.

People with diabetes have about twice the risk of developing cataracts than nondiabetics, according to the National Institutes of Health (NIH). Cataracts often appear in people with diabetes at a younger age and progress at a faster rate than among nondiabetics. Some studies have indicated that high blood glucose levels may be linked to the development of cataracts. Experts also believe that if glucose levels are kept at lower/near-normal levels, then the probability of cataracts developing will also be reduced.

Cataracts appear more commonly among people who smoke. However, people who neither smoke nor have diabetes may also develop cataracts, usually as an age-related disease among those over age 65. Ultraviolet light from sun exposure is also a risk factor for the development of cataracts.

Symptoms of Cataracts

When cataracts first develop, there may be no symptoms or may be only a slight clouding of a small area of what is seen. Some people experience a few early warning symptoms. For example, the person may find sunlight more glaring than in the past. Oncoming headlights of a car at night may seem far too bright. Colors may also seem duller than in the past. It is very easy to dismiss such symptoms as not important or as a normal part of aging. It is also easy for patients and even doctors not to realize that these can be signs of cataracts. It's better to be diagnosed and treated at an early stage of the disease. This is why experts recommend that people with diabetes have an annual eye examination.

As the cataract grows, it becomes harder to read and perform everyday tasks and the person eventually realizes that there is a serious problem.

Diagnosis and Treatment

An OPHTHALMOLOGIST or OPTOMETRIST can diagnose the existence of cataracts. If surgery is required, the ophthalmologist can perform this procedure. The eye professional may decide on a "wait and see" approach if the cataract is small and does not significantly impair vision. If it begins to grow or is already large when it is diagnosed, the doctor may recommend surgery. The cataract will be removed and often a synthetic clear plastic lens will be implanted in the eye.

The National Eye Institute, a part of the National Institutes of Health, is researching whether some minerals or vitamins may be effective in delaying the growth of cataracts or in preventing them from forming altogether. Results should be available in several years. (See also BLINDNESS, DIABETIC RETINOPATHY, EYE DISEASES, GLYCEMIC CONTROL, GLAUCOMA.)

celebrities with diabetes Well-known people who have diabetes. Famous people, infamous people, and "just regular" people suffer from diabetes and its complications. Some celebrities have publicly spoken out about their diabetes, such as the actress Mary Tyler Moore, chairman of the Juvenile Diabetes International Foundation and the former child star Jerry Mathers of *Leave It to Beaver*. The late Carroll O'Connor, the star of the TV show *All in the Family*, and many movies, also had diabetes and suffered an AMPUTATION of his toe in 2000.

Horror novelist Anne Rice has reportedly suffered from a diabetic COMA, from which she recovered. TV celebrity Delta Burke was reported to have purposely lost considerable weight when she learned that she had developed diabetes.

There are many other celebrities who have diabetes such as Olympic gold medal winner Gary Hall, Jr. According to Hall, when he was diagnosed with Type 1 diabetes, his physician told him he would have to give up swimming. He changed doctors, trained for and, subsequently, won in the Olympics.

Other celebrities include former Miss America Nicole Johnson, the late Jerry Garcia of the Grateful Dead, Chris Dudley of the National Basketball Association, and Michelle McGann of the LPGA. This list only touches the surface of celebrities who have either Type 1 or Type 2 diabetes.

Centers for Disease Control and Prevention (CDC) Primary federal agency over other agencies that provide research and information on diabetes and other diseases. For example, the Diabetes Translation Program interprets research into information that is subsequently used in public health programs. The National Center for Health Statistics compiles data and statistics on diabetic complications, death rates and other statistical data that are related to diabetes, and publishes reports on findings.

Three key agencies that conduct diabetes-related activities within the CDC include the National Center for Chronic Disease Prevention and Health Promotion (NCCDPHP), the National Center for Environmental Health (NCEH), and the National Center for Health Statistics (NCHS). Each of these agencies is further subdivided into organizations.

For example, within the NCCDPHP, the Division of Diabetes Translation provides fact sheets, statistical data, publications, and information about diabetes programs in different states at their website: www.cdc.gov/diabetes.

Contact these organizations at:

National Center for Chronic Disease Prevention
and Health Promotion
Mail Stop K-10
4770 Buford Highway, NE
Atlanta, GA 30341-3717
(877) CDC-DIAB
www.cdc.gov/diabetes

cerebrovascular diseases Diseases that cause damage to the blood vessels in the brain and neck which can lead to STROKE or HEART DISEASE. People with diabetes have a higher risk of developing cerebrovascular diseases than nondiabetics.

Charcot's arthropathy/Charcot's joint A condition that usually results from diabetes and which causes the joints and soft tissue, usually those of the feet, to become malformed and distorted. It can cause an acute painful destruction of the joint. Also called "neuropathic arthropathy" or "Charcot's joint." It occurs when there is abnormal sensation in the feet although the circulation is usually normal.

Repeated minor traumas can lead to a widened foot that is shorter and with a flattened arch. It is most commonly found in the ankle and tarsal joints of the feet.

The patient is treated by an orthopedic or podiatric surgeon familiar with the disease. Treatment is nonweight bearing, which means that the patient can either remain in bed or the affected foot is placed in a special cast so that it is immobilized and has a chance to recover. The person may use crutches to walk. After the foot has recovered and the cast has been removed, the patient may still be considered at risk for future ulcerations. As a result, the physician may recommend a special leg brace and/or custom-molded shoes.

If Charcot's arthropathy is not treated, then ulceration may develop and progress to the point that gangrene develops and AMPUTATION of a limb is the only course of action to save the life of the patient.

Acutely ill patients may experience a warm to hot foot with an increased blood flow and pain.

The bisphosphonate drugs, such as Fosamax (alendronate), Didronel (etidronate), and Actonel (risedronate) may be used to decrease the pain and inflammation, although they are not approved by the FDA for this specific indication. These drugs are used to treat OSTEOPOROSIS, Paget's disease, and other bone problems.

Gregory M. Caputo, M.D., et al., "The Charcot Foot in Diabetes: Six Key Points," *American Family Physician* (June 1998).

children of diabetic mothers The offspring of women who have Type 1 or Type 2 diabetes. Some studies indicate that children of mothers with diabetes are also affected by the illness, whether as a fetus, through genetic transmissions or by other means. The children may develop diabetes, whether they develop Type 1 diabetes as children or at an older age, or they develop Type 2 diabetes, usually later in life. They may not develop diabetes but may instead be more likely to suffer from other health problems than children of nondiabetic mothers.

In a study of the children of African mothers with Type 2 diabetes, published in a 2000 issue of *Diabetes Care*, researchers studied families in Cameroon and found that both diabetes and impaired glucose tolerance were much more common among the children of mothers with diabetes than among the African children who were born to nondiabetic mothers.

The researchers said, "The 4 percent prevalence of diabetes and 18 percent prevalence of IGT in the offspring of type 2 diabetic parents is four and nine times greater, respectively, than that found in the general population, which is estimated to be 1 and 2 percent in urban Cameroon." The researchers speculated that this problem may be driven by impairment of beta cells function. (See also GESTATIONAL DIABETES MELLITUS [GDM].)

Dana Dabelea et al., "Effect of Diabetes in Pregnancy on Offspring: Follow-up Research in the Pima Indians," *Journal of Maternal-Fetal Medicine* 9, no. 1 (January–February, 2000): 83–88.

Jan-Claude N. Mbanya, M.D., Ph.D., M.R.C.P. (UK), et al., "Reduced Insulin Secretion in Offspring of African Type 2 Diabetic Parents," *Diabetes Care* 23, no. 12 (December 2000): 1761–1765.

Peter A. M. Weiss, M.D., et al., "Long-Term Follow-Up of Infants of Mothers with Type 1 Diabetes," *Diabetes Care* 23, no. 7 (July 2000): 905–911.

children with diabetes, school-age Children from kindergarten age to about age 11 or 12 who have diabetes (pre-adolescents). Children may have either Type 1 or Type 2 diabetes. Type 1 diabetes, formerly called JUVENILE ONSET DIABETES is more common among children but researchers are finding an increasing incidence of Type 2 diabetes among children and adolescents. According to the American Diabetes Association, about one in 600 children develops Type 1 diabetes.

Children with Type 1 Diabetes

White children have a greater risk of developing Type 1 diabetes than children of other races, although the incidence of the disease varies greatly from country to country. (See chart in this entry.) Children diagnosed with Type 1 diabetes must receive daily doses of insulin, either through injections or via an insulin pump. Most children who take injections can manage on two to three insulin shots per day, although some children need even more daily injections.

Because of the need for not only monitoring blood but also administering injections (or having someone else test the child's blood and give the shots), school can become a much bigger problem for children with Type 1 diabetes than for those with Type 2 diabetes.

The primary risks for school-age children with Type 1 diabetes are DIABETIC KETOACIDOSIS (DKA), among newly diagnosed children and HYPOGLYCEMIA, among children whose glucose levels are out of control because they are ill or for another reason.

Children with Type 2 Diabetes

Children who are African American have a higher risk of having or developing Type 2 diabetes. Children in some Native American tribes, particularly PIMA INDIANS, are at very high risk of developing Type 2 diabetes.

In general, children 10–19 years old who are diagnosed with Type 2 diabetes are obese and lead sedentary lives. They also often have a parent or parents with diabetes. Many children with Type 2 diabetes have ACANTHOSIS NIGRICANS.

Girls appear to have a higher risk of developing Type 2 diabetes as children than do boys, according to Centers for Disease Control and Prevention researcher Anne Fagot-Campagna, M.D., Ph.D. and her colleagues in their 2000 article for the *Journal of Pediatrics.*

Complications of Diabetes for Children

Children with diabetes have a five times greater risk of developing periodontitis than do non-diabetic children. As a result, parents should ensure that their children have regular visits with their dentist, who should also be told about the diabetes.

Preventing hypoglycemia Parents can be proactive in helping their children avoid hypoglycemia. According to Francine Kaufman, M.D., in her 1999 article in *Diabetes Forecast,* parents should take the following precautions:

- Ensure that the child does not miss meals or snacks. If the child must miss a meal or snack, then blood glucose checks need to be done more frequently. Also, another glucose level should be taken on the child in the middle of the night. If it is under 70 mg/dL, that level is low and should be treated.

- Parents should monitor children's exercise. If a child has more exercise than usual, then extra snacks such as peanut butter and crackers should be given.

- The child's glucose levels should be checked at bedtime. If they are below 100 mg/dL, they should be rechecked in the middle of the night.

- In the event of severely low blood glucose, and if the child is unable to eat or drink, GLUCAGON should be administered.

Children around the Globe

The rates of diabetes vary greatly depending on the country a child lives in. Type 1 diabetes is far more common among children than is Type 2 diabetes and experts have analyzed the incidence of Type 1 diabetes in countries worldwide. (See Table 1.) As you can see from the table, the incidence of Type 1 diabetes in children ranges from a low of 0.1 per 100,000 children in some parts of China to a high of 36.8 per 100,000 children in Sardinia, Italy, and 36.5 in Finland.

Incidence also varies by gender. In some countries, the incidence among boys is higher and in other countries, the incidence among females predominates.

The age of the incidence of Type 1 diabetes in children also varies by country. (See Table 2.) In some countries, there are few or no cases reported for ages 0–4, while in other countries, there are many cases. For example, in Finland, the rate of incidence for both boys and girls is 29.6 per 100,000 for ages 0–4, followed by Sardinia, with 29.2 per 100,000 cases in this age group. The incidence of diabetes rises for Finnish children ages 5–9 to 40.5 per 100,000. It also rises for children in Sardinia to 41.4 per 100,000 for children ages 5–9.

In some countries, the incidence is higher for younger children than older children; for example, in some parts of Portugal. As a rule, however, the incidence is greater among children ages five and older. This is the pattern followed by children in the US; for example, in Allegheny, Pennsylvania, the incidence is 8.7 per 100,000 for children ages 0–4, more than doubling to 19.3 for children ages 5–9. The rate continues to increase, although much less sharply, to 25.3 for children ages 10–14. (See also ADOLESCENTS, INFANTS, JUVENILE DIABETES RESEARCH FOUNDATION.)

TABLE 1	WORLDWIDE AGE-STANDARDIZED INCIDENCE OF TYPE 1 DIABETES IN CHILDREN ≤ 14 YEARS OF AGE (PER 100,000 PER YEAR)						
Region (country and area)	Incidence			Ratio of Boys:Girls	Cases		
	Boys	Girls	Total		Boys	Girls	Total
Africa							
Algeria							
Oran*	4.4	7.0	5.7	0.6	9	14	23
Tunisia							
Beja*	9.0	6.5	7.8	1.2	22	16	38
Gafsa*	10.0	7.5	8.8	1.3	31	22	53
Kairoan*	5.5	5.9	5.7	0.9	23	23	46
Monastir*	4.7	5.2	4.9	0.8	15	16	31
Sudan							
Gezira	5.6	4.4	5.0	1.3	17	12	29
Mauritius	1.3	1.5	1.4	0.9	10	11	21
Asia							
China							
Wuhan	5.2	3.8	4.6	1.4	13	9	22
Sichuan	1.8	2.7	2.3	0.7	9	13	22
Huhehot	1.1	0.7	0.9	1.6	10	6	16
Dalian	1.1	1.2	1.2	0.9	10	11	21
Guilin	0.6	1.0	0.8	0.6	2	3	5
Beijing*	0.7	1.1	0.9	0.6	38	52	90
Shanghai	0.7	0.7	0.7	1.0	24	23	47
Chang Chun	0.6	1.1	0.8	0.5	7	11	18

TABLE 1   WORLDWIDE AGE-STANDARDIZED INCIDENCE OF TYPE 1 DIABETES
IN CHILDREN ≤ 14 YEARS OF AGE (PER 100,000 PER YEAR) *(continued)*

Region (country and area)	Incidence			Ratio of Boys:Girls	Cases		
	Boys	Girls	Total		Boys	Girls	Total
Nanjing	0.6	1.1	0.8	0.5	7	13	20
Jinan	0.4	0.4	0.4	1.0	12	11	23
Jilin	0.4	0.8	0.6	0.5	8	14	22
Shenyang	0.4	0.5	0.5	0.8	12	13	25
Lanzhou	0.5	0.3	0.4	1.7	5	3	8
Harbin	0.3	0.3	0.3	1.0	18	17	35
Nanning	0.3	0.7	0.5	0.4	4	10	14
Changsha	0.3	0.2	0.3	1.5	10	7	17
Zhengzhou	0.2	1.0	0.6	0.2	2	8	10
Hainan	0.1	0.2	0.2	0.5	6	11	17
Tie Ling	0.2	0.2	0.2	1.0	5	3	8
Zunyi	0.1	0.1	0.1	1.0	1	2	3
Wulumuqi	0.9	0.8	0.8	1.1	5	4	9
Hong Kong*	0.6	2.1	1.3	0.3	4	13	17
Kuwait	19.2	17.3	18.3	1.1	82	71	153
Israel[†]	5.5	6.6	6.0	0.8	167	194	361
Japan							
Chiba*	1.2	1.6	1.4	0.8	27	34	61
Hokkaido	2.2	2.1	2.2	1.0	45	44	89
Okinawa	1.0	1.8	1.4	0.6	6	11	17
Pakistan							
Karachi	0.5	0.9	0.7	0.6	9	16	25
Russia							
Novosibirsk	5.7	6.4	6.0	0.9	90	101	191
Europe							
Austria[†]	9.8	9.3	9.6	1.1	348	312	660
Belgium[†]							
Antwerpen	10.5	12.8	11.6	0.9	44	51	95
Bulgaria							
Varna	5.9	7.6	6.8	0.8	82	100	182
West Bulgaria	9.9	10.0	9.9	1.0	131	125	256
Denmark[†]							
4 counties	16.4	14.5	15.5	1.1	96	81	177
Estonia*	9.9	11.2	0.5	0.9	85	93	178
Finland*	37.0	36.0	36.5	1.0	915	853	1,768
France[†]							
4 regions	8.7	8.3	8.5	1.0	372	337	709
Germany[†]							
Baden-Württemberg	11.0	10.9	11.0	1.0	463	440	903
Greece[†]							
Attica	10.2	9.1	9.7	1.1	149	124	273
Hungary[†]							
18 counties	8.7	9.6	9.	0.9	337	360	697
Italy							
Sardinia[†]	43.6	29.5	36.8	1.5[‡]	337	211	548
Eastern Sicily[†]	13.4	9.9	11.7	1.4	75	53	128
Pavia	11.6	11.9	11.7	1.0	17	17	34
Marche	10.5	8.9	9.7	1.2	55	44	99
Turin	11.9	10.1	11.0	1.2	86	69	155

Region (country and area)	Incidence			Ratio of Boys:Girls	Cases		
	Boys	Girls	Total		Boys	Girls	Total
Lazio*[†]	8.0	8.3	8.1	1.0	164	162	326
Lombardia[†]	7.6	6.8	7.2	1.1	239	204	443
Latvia	7.0	5.7	5.9	1.2	59	47	106
Lithuania	7.7	7.1	7.4	1.1	162	145	307
Luxemburg[†]	12.6	10.2	11.4	1.2	22	17	39
The Netherlands[†]							
5 regions	12.9	13.2	13.0	1.0	178	175	353
8 counties	22.4	19.9	21.2	1.1	222	187	409
Poland							
Krakow*	6.1	6.1	6.1	1.0	134	126	260
Wielkopolska	4.1	6.0	5.0	0.7	28	40	68
Portugal							
Algarve[†]	16.3	12.9	14.6	1.3	26	19	45
Coimbra	9.4	9.9	9.7	0.9	19	19	38
Madeira Island[†]	6.9	7.5	7.2	0.9	10	11	21
Portalegre[†]	15.9	26.7	21.1	0.6	9	14	23
Romania[†]							
Bucharest	4.2	5.9	5.0	0.7	52	65	117
Slovenia[†]	6.8	9.0	7.9	0.8	70	88	158
Slovakia	7.9	9.1	8.5	0.9	261	289	550
Spain							
Catalonia	12.5	12.6	12.5	1.0	358	338	696
Sweden*	28.1	26.9	27.5	1.0	1,135	1,031	2,166
U.K.							
Aberdeen	32.5	15.0	24.0	2.2	16	7	23
Leicestershire[†]	15.4	15.3	15.3	1.0	70	66	136
Northern Ireland[†]	20.1	19.3	19.7	1.0	202	185	387
Oxford*[†]	20.1	15.3	17.8	1.3[‡]	266	191	457
Plymouth	16.5	18.1	17.3	0.9	63	65	128
North America							
Canada							
Alberta	23.4	24.7	24.0	0.9	87	88	175
Prince Edward Island*	28.0	20.8	24.5	1.3	17	12	29
U.S.							
Allegheny, PA	19.1	16.4	17.8	1.2	112	94	206
Jefferson, AL*	14.6	15.4	15.0	0.9	50	51	101
Chicago, IL[§]	10.2	13.3	11.7	0.8	131	169	300
South America							
Argentina							
Avellaneda	5.6	7.5	6.5	0.7	11	15	26
Córdoba	6.2	7.9	7.0	0.8	21	26	47
Corrientes	2.9	5.7	4.3	0.5	4	8	12
Tierra del Fuego	20.2	0	8.0	4		0	4
Brazil							
São Paulo	6.9	9.1	8.0	0.8	15	19	34
Chile							
Santiago	1.7	1.5	1.6	1.1	66	56	122
Colombia							
Santa Fe de Bogotá	4.7	2.9	3.8	1.6[‡]	35	21	56
Paraguay*	1.0	0.8	0.9	1.3	45	34	79

TABLE 1   WORLDWIDE AGE-STANDARDIZED INCIDENCE OF TYPE 1 DIABETES
IN CHILDREN ≤ 14 YEARS OF AGE (PER 100,000 PER YEAR) *(continued)*

Region (country and area)	Incidence			Ratio of Boys:Girls	Cases		
	Boys	Girls	Total		Boys	Girls	Total
Peru							
Lima	0.2	0.6	0.4	0.3	4	12	16
Uruguay							
Montevideo	8.3	8.3	8.3	1.0	13	13	26
Venezuela							
Caracas							
(second center)*	0.1	0.2	0.1	0.5	18	25	43
Central America and West Indies							
Barbados*	2.4	1.6	2.0	1.5	3	2	5
Cuba	2.5	3.4	2.9	0.7	152	197	349
Dominica	6.6	4.9	5.7	1.5	3	2	5
Mexico							
Veracruz				1.5	3	6	9
Puerto Rico (U.S.)	16.2	18.7	17.4	0.9	398	445	844
Virgin Islands (U.S.)*	14.7	11.5	13.1	1.4	9	7	16
Oceania							
Australia							
New South Wales	13.1	15.9	14.5	0.8	335	387	722
New Zealand							
Auckland	12.3	13.6	12.9	0.9	65	70	135
Canterbury	23.9	19.8	21.9	1.2	43	35	78

*Primary source only; [†]EURODIAB ACE Study; [§]African-American and Hispanic

TABLE 2   WORLDWIDE AGE-SPECIFIC INCIDENCE OF TYPE 1 DIABETES
IN CHILDREN ≤ 14 YEARS OF AGE (PER 100,000 PER YEAR)

Region (country and area)	Boys			Girls			Total		
	0–4 Years	5–9 Years	10–14 Years	0–4 Years	5–9 Years	10–14 Years	0–4 Years	5–9 Years	10–1 Years
Africa									
Algeria									
Oran*	2.8	4.3	6.1	5.8	5.8	9.4	4.3	5.0	7.8
Tunisia									
Beja*	11.0	6.1	10.0	1.4	6.4	11.6	6.3	6.2	10.8
Gafsa*	3.1	9.6	17.3	2.2	6.0	14.3	2.7	7.8	15.8
Kairoan*	6.4	4.7	10.9	1.0	9.1	13.5	3.8	6.8	12.1
Monastir*	1.9	3.6	8.5	2.9	1.8	11.0	2.3	2.7	9.7
Sudan									
Gezira	1.2	3.7	11.9	0.6	2.1	10.4	0.9	2.9	11.2
Mauritius	0.8	0.4	2.5	0.8	1.3	2.2	0.8	0.9	2.4
Asia									
China									
Wuhan	3.6	6.8	5.3	2.0	3.6	5.8	2.8	5.2	5.6
Sichuan	0.5	0.5	4.5	0.5	2.3	5.3	0.5	1.4	4.9

Region (country and area)	Boys			Girls			Total		
	0–4 Years	5–9 Years	10–14 Years	0–4 Years	5–9 Years	10–14 Years	0–4 Years	5–9 Years	10–1 Years
Huhehot	0.0	1.9	1.5	0.4	1.1	0.8	0.2	1.5	1.2
Dalian	0.5	0.9	2.1	1.0	0.9	1.8	0.7	0.9	1.9
Guilin	0.0	0.0	1.9	0.0	1.0	2.0	0.0	0.5	1.9
Beijing*	0.4	0.7	1.0	0.3	1.0	2.1	0.4	0.8	1.5
Shanghai	0.7	0.7	0.6	0.4	0.8	0.9	0.5	0.8	0.8
Chang Chun	1.1	0.3	0.6	0.3	1.1	1.8	0.7	0.7	1.1
Nanjing	0.2	0.5	1.0	1.3	1.0	1.1	0.7	0.7	1.0
Jinan	0.1	0.2	0.9	0.2	0.6	0.4	0.1	0.4	0.7
Jilin	0.5	0.5	0.3	0.2	0.5	1.7	0.3	0.5	1.0
Shenyang	0.2	0.4	0.7	0.2	0.6	0.6	0.2	0.5	0.6
Lanzhou	0.0	0.5	0.8	0.4	0.3	0.0	0.2	0.4	0.4
Harbin	0.2	0.3	0.3	0.0	0.3	0.5	0.1	0.3	0.4
Nanning	0.0	0.2	0.6	0.2	1.2	0.6	0.1	0.7	0.6
Changsha	0.2	0.2	0.5	0.1	0.0	0.6	0.2	0.1	0.6
Zhengzhou	0.3	0.4	0.0	0.3	0.8	2.0	0.3	0.6	1.0
Hainan	0.00	0.05	0.28	0.06	0.21	0.38	0.03	0.13	0.33
Tie Ling	0.13	0.30	0.25	0.00	0.32	0.13	0.07	0.31	0.19
Zunyi	0.00	0.17	0.00	0.00	0.00	0.28	0.00	0.09	0.13
Wulumuqi	0.0	0.6	2.1	0.5	0.6	1.1	0.3	0.6	1.6
Hong Kong*	0.5	0.5	0.9	0.0	3.0	3.4	0.3	1.7	2.1
Kuwait	16.2	17.0	24.4	10.0	18.6	23.3	13.2	17.8	23.8
Israel[†]	2.4	5.6	8.4	2.5	7.8	9.5	2.5	6.7	8.9
Japan									
Chiba*	0.8	0.7	2.0	1.2	1.6	2.0	1.0	1.2	2.0
Hokkaido	1.9	1.5	3.1	0.6	2.3	3.5	1.3	1.9	3.3
Okinawa	1.6	0.0	1.4	0.6	1.0	3.9	1.1	0.5	2.6
Pakistan									
Karachi	0.2	0.9	0.3	0.5	0.3	2.0	0.3	0.6	1.1
Russia									
Novosibirsk	5.8	5.5	5.8	2.8	8.0	8.3	4.3	6.7	7.0
Europe									
Austria[†]	5.9	11.4	12.1	4.7	9.8	13.3	5.3	10.6	12.7
Belgium[†]									
Antwerpen	6.3	10.2	15.3	6.6	12.9	19.1	6.4	11.5	17.2
Bulgaria									
Varna	3.3	5.5	9.0	4.4	7.7	10.8	3.8	6.6	9.9
West Bulgaria	5.9	10.6	13.0	7.3	9.0	13.5	6.6	9.8	13.3
Denmark[†]									
4 counties	8.6	16.5	24.2	6.4	14.9	22.2	7.5	15.7	23.3
Estonia*	8.1	8.1	13.5	7.4	9.7	16.4	7.8	8.9	14.9
Finland*	28.5	40.6	41.8	30.7	40.3	37.1	29.6	40.5	39.6
France[†]									
4 regions	4.6	9.9	11.6	4.8	8.7	11.4	4.7	9.3	11.5
Germany[†]									
Baden-Württemberg	6.7	10.5	15.8	7.6	11.6	13.5	7.1	11.1	14.7
Greece[†]									
Attica	6.6	8.3	15.7	7.0	9.6	10.8	6.8	8.9	13.3
Hungary[†]									
18 counties	5.7	9.2	11.1	5.8	10.1	12.8	5.8	9.6	11.9
Italy									
Sardinia[†]	32.6	48.3	49.9	25.7	34.1	28.6	29.2	41.4	39.6

TABLE 2   WORLDWIDE AGE-SPECIFIC INCIDENCE OF TYPE 1 DIABETES IN CHILDREN ≤ 14 YEARS OF AGE (PER 100,000 PER YEAR) *(continued)*

Region (country and area)	Boys 0–4 Years	Boys 5–9 Years	Boys 10–14 Years	Girls 0–4 Years	Girls 5–9 Years	Girls 10–14 Years	Total 0–4 Years	Total 5–9 Years	Total 10–1 Years
Eastern Sicily[†]	10.5	18.1	11.6	7.7	11.1	11.1	9.1	14.7	11.3
Pavia	8.8	13.1	12.8	2.3	13.9	19.4	5.7	13.5	16.0
Marche	7.7	13.2	10.6	4.8	13.3	8.6	6.3	13.3	9.6
Turin	9.3	12.2	14.0	9.8	8.8	11.7	9.5	10.5	12.9
Lazio*[†]	6.5	9.0	8.4	6.7	9.8	8.4	6.6	9.4	8.4
Lombardia[†]	6.6	7.9	8.4	5.1	7.0	8.3	5.9	7.5	8.3
Latvia	3.3	5.6	12.0	3.1	4.8	9.3	3.2	5.2	10.7
Lithuania	4.7	8.0	10.3	3.1	8.7	9.4	3.9	8.3	9.9
Luxemburg[†]	9.5	10.4	18.0	8.3	11.0	11.3	8.9	10.7	14.7
The Netherlands[†] 5 regions	9.3	12.3	17.1	9.7	15.0	14.8	9.5	13.6	15.9
Norway[†] 8 counties	14.3	23.0	29.8	10.1	20.9	28.6	12.3	22.0	29.2
Poland Krakow*	3.0	5.7	9.6	3.5	7.3	7.5	3.2	6.5	8.6
Wielkopolska	2.9	4.2	5.2	2.0	6.9	9.0	2.5	5.5	7.1
Portugal Algarve[†]	12.8	8.1	28.0	11.1	15.0	12.6	12.0	11.4	20.5
Coimbra	3.8	11.4	13.1	2.0	15.5	12.2	2.9	13.4	12.7
Madeira Island[†]	9.1	6.1	5.5	7.1	2.2	13.2	8.1	4.2	9.3
Portalegre[†]	5.1	27.7	19.3	11.2	44.8	30.4	8.0	35.9	24.8
Romania[†] Bucharest	0.9	4.3	7.5	3.6	9.7	4.4	2.2	6.9	6.0
Slovakia	6.3	7.3	10.1	6.5	9.7	11.2	6.4	8.5	10.6
Spain Catalonia	5.6	12.8	18.9	5.0	13.5	19.2	5.3	13.1	19.0
Sweden*	19.6	28.9	35.7	17.4	31.8	31.5	18.5	30.3	33.7
U.K. Aberdeen	24.1	30.4	43.0	12.6	25.8	6.5	18.5	28.2	25.3
Leicestershire[†]	6.2	16.8	23.1	10.6	15.0	20.1	8.4	15. 9	21.7
Northern Ireland[†]	11.4	22.4	26.6	10.4	22.4	25.1	10.9	22.4	25.9
Oxford*[†]	15.6	19.0	25.6	12.4	12.5	21.1	14.0	15.8	23.5
Plymouth	15.5	16.5	17.6	12.2	19.3	22.7	13.9	17.9	20.1
North America Canada Alberta	9.0	26.0	35.2	19.1	24.4	30.7	13.9	25.2	33.0
Prince Edward Island*	15.0	34.6	34.4	10.5	25.8	26.1	12.8	30.3	30.3
U.S. Allegheny, PA	7.4	19.4	30.4	10.1	19.2	20.0	8.7	19.3	25.3
Jefferson, AL*	9.7	13.8	20.3	6.5	15.1	24.6	8.1	14.4	22.4
Chicago, IL[‡]	4.4	9.1	16.9	5.0	12.4	22.6	4.7	10.7	19.8
South America Argentina Avellaneda	2.1	2.4	8.3	0.0	24.7	2.8	1.1	13.4	5.6
Córdoba	3.6	6.0	9.0	2.2	11.4	10.0	2.9	.8.7	9.5

Region (country and area)	Boys			Girls			Total		
	0–4 Years	5–9 Years	10–14 Years	0–4 Years	5–9 Years	10–14 Years	0–4 Years	5–9 Years	10–1 Years
Corrientes	3.9	0.0	4.7	6.0	6.7	4.6	5.0	3.3	4.6
Tierra del Fuego	0	0	60.6	0	0	0	0	0	30.3
Brazil									
São Paulo	4.1	6.9	9.8	5.6	8.5	13.0	4.8	7.7	11.4
Chile									
Santiago	1.5	3.1	4.1	1.4	1.3	5.0	1.5	2.2	4.6
Colombia									
Santa Fe de Bogotá	3.0	3.9	7.3	2.0	2.8	3.9	2.5	3.3	5.6
Paraguay*	0.7	0.6	1.8	0.5	1.0	0.8	0.6	0.8	1.3
Peru									
Lima	0.1	0.0	0.4	0.4	0.7	0.6	0.3	0.4	0.5
Uruguay									
Montevideo	0.0	3.6	21.2	2.0	14.8	7.9	1.0	9.1	14.7
Venezuela									
Caracas (second center)*	0.1	0.2	0.0	0.1	0.2	0.2	0.1	0.2	0.1
Central America and West Indies									
Barbados*	2.5	4.7	0.0	0.0	2.3	2.3	1.3	3.5	1.2
Cuba	1.1	2.9	3.5	1.9	3.8	4.5	1.5	3.3	4.0
Dominica	0.0	8.2	13.5	0.0	0.0	14.6	0.0	4.0	14.1
Mexico									
Veracruz							0.5	2.0	2.1
Puerto Rico (U.S.)	12.1	16.6	19.8	9.8	21.9	24.2	11.0	19.2	22.0
Virgin Islands (U.S.)*	15.9	14.3	13.9	10.8	9.7	14.1	13.4	12.0	14.0
Oceania									
Australia									
New South Wales	8.1	12.3	18.9	10.1	16.8	20.8	9.1	14.5	19.8
New Zealand									
Auckland	4.5	18.7	13.8	8.8	14.0	17.9	6.6	16.4	15.8
Canterbury	12.6	31.2	28.0	19.6	15.9	24.0	16.0	23.7	26.1

‡ Statistically significant.

Permission granted to reprint tables by Marjatta Karvonen, Ph.D., senior researcher, Department of Epidemiology and Health Promotion, National Public Institute, Helsinki, Finland.

American Diabetes Association, "Type 2 Diabetes in Children and Adolescents," *Pediatrics* 105, no. 3 (March 2000): 671–680.

William L. Clarke, M.D., "Advocating for the Child with Diabetes," *Diabetes Spectrum* 12, no. 4 (1999): 230.

Anne Fagot-Campagna, M.D., Ph.D., et al., "Type 2 Diabetes Among North American Children and Adolescents: An Epidemiological Review and a Public Health Perspective," *Journal of Pediatrics* 136, no. 5 (May 2000): 664–672.

Marjatta Karvonen, Ph.D., et al., "Incidence of Childhood Type 1 Diabetes Worldwide," *Diabetes Care* 23, no. 10 (October 2000): 1516–1526.

Francie Ratner Kaufman, M.D., et al., "Association Between Diabetes Control and Visits to a Multidisciplinary Pediatric Diabetes Clinic," *Pediatrics* 103, no. 5 (May 1999): 948–951.

Francine Kaufman, M.D., "Preventing Hypoglycemia (Low Blood Glucose) in Children," *Diabetes Forecast* (June 1999): 77–79.

Myriam Rosilio, M.D., et al., "Factors Associated with Glycemic Control: A Cross-Sectional Nationwide Study in 2,579 French Children with Type 1 Diabetes," *Diabetes Care* 21, no. 7 (July 1998): 1146–1153.

Carla R. Scott, et al., "Characteristics of Youth-Onset Noninsulin-Dependent Diabetes Mellitus and Insulin-Dependent Diabetes Mellitus at Diagnosis," *Pediatrics* 100, no. 1 (July 1997): 84–91.

cholesterol (good cholesterol/bad cholesterol)

One of several fats (lipids) that circulate in the body as lipoproteins, including low density lipoproteins (LDL) and high density lipoproteins (HDL). Although most people think of all cholesterol as "bad," it is LDL that is considered a "bad" form of cholesterol, while HDL is "good." Very simply put, HDL removes cholesterol from the blood vessels, while LDL clogs the vessels.

People with diabetes, even when they are adolescents or young adults (and the risk increases for middle-aged individuals and those who are older), are at risk for having abnormal LDL and low HDL. According to the National Cholesterol Education Program, people with diabetes have "diabetic dyslipidemia" when they have high triglycerides, low HDL, and small dense LDL.

Excessive levels of LDL can cause fatty deposits to collect within the arteries and can then result in medical problems such as strokes or heart attacks. People with diabetes are already at higher risk for cardiac ailments and strokes, even if their cholesterol levels are at optimal levels. In one study done in Finland, patients with diabetes who had never had a heart attack had a higher risk of having a heart attack than did nondiabetic patients who had already had one or more previous heart attacks. Thus, patients with diabetes must keep their LDL levels as low as possible and their HDL levels as high as possible.

Testing Cholesterol Levels and Cholesterol Guidelines Created in 2001

To test for lipoproteins, physicians order a lipoprotein profile, which will provide data on levels of LDL, total cholesterol, HDL, and triglyc-erides (another fatty substance found in the blood).

In 2001, new guidelines were released by the National Cholesterol Education Program, coordinated by the National Heart, Lung, and Blood Institute (NHLBI). Earlier guidelines had been issued in 1993. These guidelines reinforced the concept that diabetes is a major risk factor for developing dyslipidemia as well as clinical heart disease. Other risk factors for the development of coronary heart disease are:

- Cigarette smoking
- High blood pressure
- Low HDL cholesterol (under 40 mg/dL)
- Family history of early heart disease
- Age: men 45 or older and women 55 or older

According to the National Cholesterol Education Program guidelines, LDL should be less than 100 mg/dL in patients with diabetes (either type). Some research suggests that all patients with diabetes might benefit from an even lower level of less than 100, although this is a very controversial area. Conversely, high density lipoprotein levels (HDL) should be greater than 40 mg/dL.

In the Scandinavian Simvastatin Survival Study (the 4-S Study), patients with diabetes who reduced their cholesterol levels had a 54 percent risk reduction in major coronary events (fatal and near fatal myocardial infarctions) while the patients without diabetes had only a 32 percent risk reduction. This study yet again proved the importance of cholesterol levels to the person with diabetes.

Treatment of High Cholesterol Levels

Dietary adjustments can lower LDL levels; for example, foods that are high in starch and fiber can help to lower the LDL level, as well as foods that are low in fat and cholesterol. It's also important to supplement changes in diet with an increase in exercise and weight loss for those who are overweight. Generally diet and exercise will lower total cholesterol levels by 5 to 20 percent, with 10 percent being a typical response. Given this fairly small effect, most patients with diabetes and dyslipidemia will require the use of cholesterol-lowering medications. For most patients with diabetes, the first class of medication that is usually considered is an HMG CoA reductase inhibitor drug, (or "statin"), such as pravastatin (Pravachol) or simvastatin (Zocor). These medications can lower LDL cholesterol levels by about 15–40 percent.

In 2001, the FDA removed Baycol (cerivastatin), a cholesterol-lowering drug, from the market after it was linked to deaths in 40 people worldwide. The drug resulted in rhabdomyolysis in a small number of people, which is muscle damage leading to pain and possible kidney failure. This problem has not been as severe in the five other HMG CoA reductase inhibitor medications that remain on the market. Mild myalgias (muscle aches) are not uncommon with this class of drugs, but usually are not severe enough to change muscle enzyme levels or to affect kidney function. Often a physician will change a patient from one drug to another if this occurs, as the effect is unpredictable; i.e., it may occur with one of the five and none of the other four medications.

Another treatment for high cholesterol levels is intermediate-release niacin, which can often be used, albeit with caution. Physicians and patients need to be aware that niacin can affect glucose levels and it can also increase uric acid levels, leading to the development of gout (a very painful acute inflammation of a joint, often in the foot). Prescribed niacin may also cause upset to the stomach, and it can affect liver function tests. In addition, it may cause an intense flushing syndrome; however, this reaction can be avoided with the use of aspirin 30 minutes prior to taking the niacin.

One study, reported in the *Journal of the American Medical Association* in 2000, found a positive effect with high doses of niacin on patients who had been diagnosed with peripheral arterial disease. Of the 468 patients who were studied, 125

of them had Type 2 diabetes and the other patients were nondiabetic. The study lasted for 60 weeks.

The researchers found that after 30 weeks, the niacin significantly increased the HDL levels of the patients with diabetes by 29 percent and decreased their triglycerides by 23 percent, both positive findings. They concluded,

Our study suggests that lipid-modifying dosages of niacin can be safely used in patients with diabetes and that niacin therapy may be considered as an alternative to statin drugs or fibrates for patients with diabetes in whom these agents are not tolerated or fail to sufficiently correct hypertriglyceridemia or low HDL-C [cholesterol] levels.

CLASSIFICATION OF LDL, TOTAL CHOLESTEROL, AND HDL CHOLESTEROL (MG/DL)

LDL Cholesterol	
100	Optimal
100–129*	Near optimal/above optimal
130–159	Borderline high
160–189	High
190 and higher	Very high

* Among people with diabetes, the recommended LDL is under 100.

Total Cholesterol	
200	Desirable
200–239	Borderline high
240 or higher	High

HDL Cholesterol	
40	Low
60 or higher	High

Source: National Cholesterol Education Program, 2001.

(See also DYSLIPIDEMIA, HDL, LDL, TRIGLYCERIDES.)

William P. Castelli, M.D., and Glen C. Griffin, M.D., *Good Fat, Bad Fat: Reduce Your Heart-Attack Odds* (Tucson, Ariz.: Fisher Books, 1997).

Marshall B. Elam, Ph.D., M.D., et al., "Effect of Niacin on Lipid and Lipoprotein Levels and Glycemic Control in Patients with Diabetes and Peripheral

Arterial Disease: The ADMIT Study: A Randomized Trial," *Journal of the American Medical Association* 284, no. 13 (2000): 1263–1270.

National Cholesterol Education Program, National Heart, Lung, and Blood Institute, "Detection, Evaluation, and Treatment of High Blood Cholesterol in Adults (Adult Treatment Panel III): Executive Summary," NIH Publication No. 01-3670, May 2001.

chromium supplements Additional portions of chromium that are taken as dietary supplements. Some preliminary research has indicated that it is possible that diabetes may deplete the body or at least be associated with lower levels of important trace elements such as chromium and ZINC. As a result, supplements may be needed. However, individuals with diabetes should not take any dietary supplements without first consulting with their physicians.

In recent years, there has been a tremendous amount of interest in the trace mineral chromium. Much of this stems from basic research into the mechanism by which insulin is released from the beta cells in islets (ISLETS OF LANGERHANS) of the PANCREAS. When islet cells are cultured in a laboratory, if the media in which they are maintained is depleted of chromium, then the cells do not secrete insulin very well. If chromium is added back, the cells begin to secrete insulin robustly. Obviously, however, it is a large leap from animal islet cells grown in a laboratory to making assumptions about a human being.

There has also been interesting data from rural China, where subjects with diabetes received chromium supplements and their glucose levels subsequently improved. However, people in China eat a diet that is far different from what most people in America, Canada, and Europe consume, thus, these results are not easily generalized to Western cultures.

At the present time, there is no conclusive test for chromium deficiency in humans. In addition, it may be some time before the true impact of chromium on diabetes is answered definitively.

It is also very difficult to measure chromium levels in humans. What we really need to know is the concentration of chromium in the tissues and specifically the concentration at the cellular levels, as opposed to the blood levels. At this time, such techniques are not readily available.

Studies have been done on genetically insulin-resistant rats whose insulin resistance decreased with supplementation with chromium picolinate. But there are no data on safe levels of chromium in the body and what medical problems that long-term exposure or build-up in tissues may lead to.

According to Richard Eastman, M.D., an endocrinologist at the National Institute of Diabetes and Digestive and Kidney Diseases (NIDDK), overweight people who have Type 2 diabetes can gain the same modest benefits as the Chinese subjects did with chromium supplements by losing some weight.

clinical studies/research Controlled experiments or studies that are usually peer-reviewed or evaluated by others who are expert in the field. Clinical studies are the basis for much of modern medical science, as well as the basis for the approval and introduction of new medications and treatments. Clinical studies may last as little as hours or days, or they may last as long as years.

Sometimes scientists return to the people in a previously studied clinical trial, as long as 10 years later, and follow-up on them or perform new studies on this group; however, such long-term followups are not the norm because they are very costly. One example of such a followup/new research study group is the Epidemiology of Diabetes Interventions and Complications (EDIC) Research Group. In 1999, the EDIC Research Group reported that they had received permission from 96 percent of the Diabetes Control and Complications Trial (DCCT) subjects to study them further.

In general and in its simplest form, researchers study medications or treatments in an experimental group (the group that receives the medication or treatment) versus a control group which does not receive it, and the results are then compared to determine any significant differences.

Sometimes more than two groups are involved; for example, some researchers may compare a group of individuals with Type 1 diabetes to a group with Type 2 diabetes and sometimes to a third nondiabetic control group as well.

Some studies compare only people with Type 1 or Type 2 diabetes to a nondiabetic group. Or individuals with Type 1 or Type 2 diabetes may be separated into different groups and the results of the therapy or medication will be compared. Most studies are limited to using adult subjects, however, increasingly more studies are performed on children and adolescents who have diabetes. There are many possible combinations of groups that may be used to study a broad array of treatments and medications for diabetes.

Prior to publication in a professional medical journal, most clinical studies are "peer-reviewed," which means that individuals who are knowledgeable in the same field read the study to see if it seems feasible and logical and if enough information is provided so that others could duplicate the study. Scientists know they will be reviewed and this helps to ensure their carefulness (although not all clinical studies are rigorously performed).

For a new medication to obtain the approval of the FDA, in most cases, 2,000–10,000 patients must be studied to verify that the medication is not only safe but also efficacious. Researchers also look for possible side effects that the new medication may have.

Researchers seek to find statistical "significance." This means that statistical techniques are used to determine if the findings are more than what would occur with just random chance.

Individuals who do clinical studies also review what studies have gone on before them, not only so that they can learn from previous experience, but also because they may attempt to design their study in such a way as to avoid errors or problems that may have occurred in the past.

Clinical studies are vitally important to those interested in diabetes because researchers are constantly seeking to learn more about treatments and medications that directly impact people with diabetes. Researchers also study issues such as risk of developing diabetes or complications of diabetes, so that physicians can identify people who are most likely to develop specific medical problems. If they can act ahead of time, doctors may be able to advise their patients how to act to avoid the problem or at least limit its severity if it cannot be avoided.

There have been hundreds and probably thousands of studies on diabetes in recent years. Several prominent and often cited diabetes studies involved large numbers of individuals who were studied over extended periods of time; for example, the DIABETES CONTROL AND COMPLICATIONS TRIAL (DCCT) was a 10-year federally funded study of individuals with Type 1 diabetes in North America which ran from 1983 to 1993. The National Institute of Diabetes and Digestive and Kidney Diseases (NIDDK) conducted the study.

The DCCT was profoundly important because it conclusively proved that tight glucose control in patients with Type 1 diabetes could greatly reduce the risk of the development or slow progression of microvascular complications from diabetes, such as DIABETIC RETINOPATHY, kidney disease, and DIABETIC NEUROPATHY. As a direct result of this study, physicians now urge their patients to control their glucose levels as tightly as possible. If patients need proof for why they should take this action, doctors can justify their advice with the findings of this study.

The UNITED KINGDOM PROSPECTIVE DIABETES STUDY (UKPDS) was another major clinical study of diabetes. It was performed in the United Kingdom and concentrated on the impact of tight glucose control on individuals who had Type 2 diabetes. The study also conclusively proved that tight glucose control greatly decreased the likelihood of later microvascular complications from diabetes.

coma An extended loss of consciousness that may last for days, weeks, or much longer. A coma may stem from glucose levels that are either too low (HYPOGLYCEMIA) or too high (HYPERGLYCEMIA). (See also HYPEROSMOLAR COMA.) Some individuals do not recover from a diabetic coma, and they die.

Coma may occur because the person did not adequately pay attention to diet or it could be due to other controllable or noncontrollable circumstances such as medication, illness, and excessive exercise.

The comatose individual needs emergency treatment and usually requires hospitalization. (See also COMPLICATIONS, DIABETIC KETOACIDOSIS [DKA].)

complications of diabetes Diseases or conditions that are caused or exacerbated by the underlying diabetes. Some severe examples are AMPUTATION, DIABETIC RETINOPATHY or BLINDNESS, CARDIOVASCULAR DISEASE, CORONARY HEART DISEASE, END-STAGE RENAL DISEASE, ERECTILE DYSFUNCTION, DIABETIC NEPHROPATHY, STROKE and other medical problems.

Large-scale studies, such as the DIABETES CONTROL AND COMPLICATIONS TRIAL (DCCT) and the UNITED KINGDOM PROSPECTIVE DIABETES STUDY (UKPDS), have definitively proven that for both patients with TYPE 1 DIABETES and the far more common TYPE 2 DIABETES, tight glucose control can greatly decrease the risk for microvascular complications of diabetes. In addition, if complications have already occurred, glycemic control can often delay a worsening of the problem.

The Diabetes Control and Complications Trial Research Group, "Effect of Intensive Diabetes Treatment on the Development and Progression of Long-Term Complications in Adolescents with Insulin-Dependent Diabetes Mellitus: Diabetes Control and Complications Trial," *The Journal of Pediatrics* 125, no. 2 (August 1994): 177–188.
Marvin E. Levin, M.D., and Michael A. Pfeiffer, M.D., *The Uncomplicated Guide to Diabetes Complications*

(Alexandria, Va.: American Diabetes Association, 1998).

Congressional Diabetes Caucus A bipartisan group of congresspersons that was formed in 1995 with the commitment to improving the lives of Americans who have diabetes. Approximately 275 Congressional members serve on the caucus. As of this writing, the group is chaired by Rep. George Nethercutt (R-WA) and Rep. Diana DeGette (D-CO), along with co-vice chairs Curt Weldon (R-PA) and John LaFalce (D-NY).

The mission of the group is to increase awareness of diabetes in Congress and promote greater research on diabetes and its complications.

One result of their efforts was the creation by Congress of the Diabetes Research Working Group, a group of scientific and lay experts, and leaders of major diabetes organizations. In 1999, this group released "Summary of the Report and Recommendations of the Congressionally-Established Diabetes Research Working Group: A Strategic Plan for the 21st Century." The Caucus also was successful in its effort to expand Medicare coverage to include diabetes self-management education, glucose testing strips, and glucose monitors. More information is available at www.house.gov/nethercutt/diabetes.html.

continuous glucose monitoring system A glucose sensor, created by MiniMed, Inc., that will measure glucose levels every five minutes for 72 hours. It consists of a small catheter that is inserted into subcutaneous tissue and then taped down. The catheter continuously measures subcutaneous fluid glucose levels, which are registered in a small device about the size of a pager. It can be attached to a belt or bra or kept in the pocket.

After three days, the patient returns to the physicians' office and hands in the device. Results from the device are downloaded and then printed out. The continuous glucose monitoring system can often discover times of asymptomatic hypoglycemia and hyperglycemia that can help guide changes in patient management. For example, based on the results, the physician may change the dosages of insulin or oral medications, or may make recommendations on nutrition or exercise.

For patients with wide swings in glucose levels or unexplained hypoglycemia or HYPO-GLYCEMIC UNAWARENESS, the information provided by a continuous glucose monitoring system can be very helpful.

coronary heart disease (CHD)   Diseases of the heart, such as MYOCARDIAL INFARCTION (heart attack) and/or ANGINA PECTORIS (chest pains from heart disease) that are due to blockages in the coronary arteries. Also known as coronary artery disease. People with diabetes have a much higher risk for CHD than nondiabetics, and thus, a diagnosis of diabetes is considered a major risk factor for developing CHD. Other risk factors for heart disease are high levels of LDL cholesterol, HYPERTENSION, SMOKING, and OBESITY.

The CENTERS FOR DISEASE CONTROL AND PREVENTION (CDC) reports that about 12 million Americans have CHD, and in 1998, about 460,000 died of coronary heart disease. There were dramatic differences of death rates among states; for example, the age-adjusted death rate ranged from a low of 208.1 per 100,000 people in New Mexico to a high of 440.6 in New York.

Diabetes and Heart Disease

Based on an analysis of ten studies by Warren Lee and his colleagues and also reported in *Diabetes Care* in 2000, women who have diabetes experience more than a two and a half times greater risk of coronary death than nondiabetic women. Men with diabetes have about twice the risk of death as nondiabetic men.

Coronary artery disease (CAD) may result in a sudden heart attack (MYOCARDIAL INFARCTION) or a sudden cardiac death. According to experts, CAD is the cause of death in more than half of all patients who have diabetes. CAD also causes disability in many others.

In the UNITED KINGDOM PROSPECTIVE DIABETES STUDY (UKPDS), researchers studied the effect of the drug METFORMIN on patients with diabetes and made the dramatic finding that the drug resulted in significantly lower death rates from heart disease among all treatment groups.

This was very valuable data because, according to the report "Conquering Diabetes: A Strategic Plan for the 21st Century," released in 1999 by the Diabetes Research Working Group, a Congressionally established group, individuals with diabetes are two to four times more likely to suffer from a variety of cardiac problems than are those who are nondiabetic. In addition, people with diabetes have a higher DEATH rate from heart problems than do their nondiabetic peers.

Studies have also shown that African American WOMEN WITH DIABETES are at particular risk for suffering from coronary disease and death. Clearly, cardiac conditions are an area of concern for the person with diabetes as well as his or her family members.

For further information, contact:

The American Heart Association
7272 Greenville Avenue
Dallas, TX 75231-4596.
(800) AHA-USA1 (242-8721; toll-free)
www.americanheart.org

(See also CARDIOVASCULAR DISEASE, DIURETICS, DIGAMI STUDY.)

American Heart Association, *2001 Heart and Stroke Statistical Update*, American Heart Association, 2000.

David Bell, S.H., M.B., and Ovalle, Fernando, M.D., "Diabetes as a Risk Factor for Ischemic Heart Disease," *Clinical Reviews* (Spring 2000): 88–92.

Zachary Bloomgarden, M.D., "Cardiovascular Disease in Type 2 Diabetes," *Diabetes Care* 22, no. 10 (1999): 1739–1744.

Centers for Disease Control and Prevention, "American Heart Month—February 2001," *Morbidity and Mortality Weekly Report* 50, no. 6 (February 16, 2001): 89–93.

Stephanie Cooper, M.D., and James H. Caldwell, M.D., "Coronary Artery Disease in People with Diabetes: Diagnostic and Risk Factor Evaluation," *Clinical Diabetes* 17, no. 2 (1999).

Warren L. Lee, M.D., et al., "Impact of Diabetes on Coronary Artery Disease in Women and Men," *Diabetes Care* 23, no. 7 (July 2000): 962–968.

counterregulatory hormones Reactive hormones such as cortisol (the body's natural cortisone), GLUCAGON, EPINEPHRINE, and GROWTH HORMONE. HYPOGLYCEMIA leads to a release of these hormones. For example, if a person develops hypoglycemia, then glucagon should be released to counteract the low blood sugar by helping stimulate the breakdown of glycogen from the liver. Unfortunately, within five years of the diagnosis of diabetes, most patients lose the ability to secrete glucagon in response to hypoglycemia.

If the body no longer releases glucagon in response to hypoglycemia, then epinephrine may be released to protect the body. If the hypoglycemia continues, then cortisol and growth hormone may be released, although they take a much longer time to become effective.

Some people with diabetes have reduced rates of responses from their counter-regulatory hormones. This can be due to tight glycemic control or autonomic neuropathy. This will cause HYPOGLYCEMIC UNAWARENESS, a state when the person does not have identifiable symptoms of hypoglycemia. Most of the typical symptoms of hypoglycemia, such as shakiness, sweating, nausea, and nervousness, are caused by epinephrine.

C-peptide The "connecting peptide" that is derived from pro-insulin after it is cleaved to form insulin. A peptide is a protein or part of a protein that is made from amino acids. The body releases C-peptide in equal proportions to the amount of insulin that is also released.

A laboratory test for C-peptides can determine how much insulin the body is releasing; however, it is only rarely used by physicians to make clinical decisions. C-peptide may be measured to determine if a patient still makes insulin. It is also measured in cases of severe HYPOGLYCEMIA, to determine if patients are making too much insulin (high C-peptide) or if they have been surreptitiously taking insulin by injection (causing low C-peptide levels). Some individuals who are weight lifters, but who do not have diabetes, use insulin illegally, as do others for a variety of reasons.

As of this writing, MEDICARE requires a C-peptide test with a specific result before it will approve the payment for an insulin pump.

creatinine A body chemical that is found in the blood and that is excreted through the urine. It is a measure of kidney function and the higher the creatinine level, the worse the kidney function. Creatinine as measured in the blood stream is also proportional to muscle mass, and more muscle mass means a higher creatinine level. As a result, because men generally have larger muscle masses than women, they also have higher creatinine levels, although men do not necessarily have lesser kidney function than women do.

Typically, creatinine levels in a healthy person range from approximately 0.5 to 1.5 mg/dL. Physicians caring for patients with diabetes should measure this blood level at least one time per year to monitor their patients' renal (kidney) function. When the creatinine measure is greater than or equal to 1.8 to 2.0 mg/dL, then it is appropriate to refer the patient to a NEPHROLOGIST (another member of the diabetes care team), because of his or her expertise in kidney diseases.

It is important to understand that because a referral to a nephrologist (physician expert in kidney disease) is made does not automatically mean that the patient is in dire straits. Instead, the specialist's insights into kidney function are sought, to ensure that both the referring M.D. and the patient are doing all they can to stabilize and protect the remaining kidney function. Some examples of actions that may be taken are to adjust medications (especially antihypertensive drugs), suggest dietary changes, and look for other possible risk factors that can be adjusted/corrected, such as avoidance of non-steroidal antiinflammatory medications.

A 24-hour urine collection may also be ordered. This test will provide a better estimate of kidney function (creatinine clearance) as well as measure if excess amounts of protein are being lost in the urine. Test results will show exactly at what level the kidneys are functioning. Since many people with diabetes also suffer from kidney disease, but often they have no symptoms, this is an important test.

critically ill non-diabetic patients who become hyperglycemic Severe life-threatening illness may induce diabetes in some patients and can contribute to their deaths, if not treated. According to a study reported in the *New England Journal of Medicine* in 2001 by physicians in a Belgium hospital, this HYPERGLYCEMIA may lead to complications and even death. Patients were assigned to either the intensive therapy group or the conventional therapy group.

Researchers instituted intensive insulin therapy in 765 critically ill patients, and found that deaths (mortality) were reduced to 4.6 percent from 8.0 percent for patients with conventional care. In terms of numbers, 35 patients died in the intensive treatment group, versus 63 patients in the conventional treatment group. The patients suffered from a variety of medical problems including cardiac surgery, neurologic disease, cancer and other illnesses.

The authors concluded,

The use of intensive insulin therapy to maintain blood glucose at a level that did not exceed 110 mg per deciliter substantially reduced mortality in the intensive care unit, in-hospital mortality, and morbidity [sickness] among critically ill patients admitted to our intensive care unit.

Greet Van Der Berge, M.D., Ph.D., et al., "Intensive Insulin Therapy in Critically Ill Patients," *New England Journal of Medicine* 335, no. 19 (November 8, 2001): 1359–1367.

Cushing's syndrome/Cushing's disease Any syndrome, regardless of the source, that leads to excess cortisol levels. Cushing's disease results from the pituitary gland making excessive levels of ACTH. It is also known as hypercortisolism. Hyperglycemia (a high glucose level) is one sign that is found in adults with Cushing's syndrome, along with other symptoms that may accompany the illness.

Cushing's syndrome is a rare endocrine disease caused by the excessive secretion of cortisol, a hormone that is released by the adrenal glands. It has a prevalence of about 10–15 cases per million people each year. In 90 percent of the cases, the patient is an adult and in 10 percent of the cases, the patient is a child or an adolescent.

Symptoms of Cushing's Syndrome in a Child or Adolescent Include:

- Delayed growth
- Excessive weight gain, particularly in the face, neck, and abdomen (also called central obesity)
- Hypertension
- Either delayed or very early onset of puberty in a child or adolescent
- Amenorrhea (missed periods in females)
- Extreme fatigue

Symptoms of Cushing's Syndrome in an Adult Include:

- Sleep disorders
- Hyperglycemia
- Menstrual disturbances
- Osteoporosis
- Muscle weakness (more prominent in the shoulder and hip girdle muscles)
- Depression
- Thin skin that is easily bruised
- Hirsutism (excess hair growth and in atypical areas) in women, especially on the face, neck, chest, and abdominal area
- Decreased fertility among men and/or lack of interest in sex and diminished libido

Causes of Cushing's Syndrome

The disease may result from a variety of causes, including:

- Long-term use of steroids such as prednisone
- Cancerous tumors in other parts of the body which cause the adrenal glands to overproduce cortisol
- Benign or cancerous tumors of the adrenal glands

Diagnosis

The illness is diagnosed through laboratory tests such as measurement of urinary free cortisol and the dexamethasone suppression test. Other radiologic tests may be ordered, such as computerized tomography (CT) scans of the adrenal glands and magnetic resonance imaging (MRI) scans of the pituitary.

Treatment

Once diagnosed, the treatment depends on the underlying cause. Cushing's can be treated with medication, chemotherapy, radiation treatments, surgery, or a variety of other treatments. Sometimes surgery is indicated, especially when the patient has a cancerous tumor. If the primary cause is steroid use, often the medication level is steadily reduced to the lowest dose the physician considers efficacious for the other illness the patient may have (rheumatoid arthritis, lupus, etc.).

cystitis   An inflammation of the bladder and a medical problem that is commonly caused by a urinary tract infection (UTI). Cystitis is a frequent complication of individuals with diabetes, particularly females. (Women in general are more likely to suffer from cystitis than men.)

The key symptoms of cystitis are: frequency of urination, urgency, burning (dysuria), and incontinence. Afflicted individuals also often strain when they are urinating. However, there may be no symptoms and asymptomatic bacteriuria (bacteria found in the urine) is actually more common among people with diabetes than in non-diabetics.

The physician may choose to culture the urine or may decide to treat the patient immediately, based on the cloudy appearance of the urine, microscopically visible bacteria, and the patient's symptoms. There may also be visible or microscopic blood found in the urine.

Treatment of a urinary tract infection is best done with an antibiotic with a narrow spectrum of efficiency or one that is picked based on urine culture results. Treatment of UTIs in patients with diabetes is not only done to alleviate infection but also to protect the kidneys from damage.

Once diagnosed, treatment usually involves prescribing an antibiotic that may be taken for as few as one to three days. Longer courses of treatment may be used for patients who have frequent infections or who have structural abnormalities or resistant bacteria.

Some individuals with undiagnosed diabetes, as well as patients with poorly controlled diabetes, may suffer from recurrent bouts of cystitis. (See also BLADDER PROBLEMS, INFECTIONS, NEUROGENIC BLADDER, URINARY TRACT INFECTION (UTI).)

Endre Ludwig, M.D., Ph.D., "Bacteriuria in Women with Diabetes Mellitus," *Infections in Urology* 13, Supp. 5A (2000): S3–S6.

dawn phenomenon   A sudden rise in the blood glucose level of patients with diabetes, usually between 2 A.M. and 8 A.M., and prior to eating. Individuals with Type 1 diabetes may experience this early morning hyperglycemia, but it is less common in those who have Type 2 diabetes. Individuals with BRITTLE DIABETES are prone to suffering from this condition, although all patients experience the dawn phenomenon to some extent.

The dawn phenomenon is caused by the effects of counterregulatory hormone levels, such as adrenaline/epinephrine, noradrenaline/norepinephrine, and so forth. These hormone levels rise in the early morning and enable the individual to awake and "face the day." However, at the same time, they also lead to increased levels of glucose and blood pressure. These hormones do this by counteracting the effects of insulin and causing a rise in glucose as the person sleeps. Many people mistakenly believe that early morning hyperglycemia is mainly caused by what the individual ate the night before. Much of the excess morning hyperglycemia is due to the overproduction of glucose from the liver partly due to this dawn phenomenon.

The increases in counterregulatory hormones, which lead to increased glucose levels, increased blood pressure, elevated heart rate, and changes in lipids and in blood clotting, are why more heart attacks and strokes occur in the early morning than at other times.

For people with Type 1 diabetes who experience a problem with dawn phenomenon, physicians may suggest taking a long-lasting insulin before bedtime. They may also be good candidates for an INSULIN PUMP.

death   Cessation of life. People with diabetes have a higher death rate (mortality rate) than those who don't have diabetes. Of course, all people must eventually die. A higher mortality rate in this case means that people with diabetes are statistically more likely to die at a younger age from a variety of different ailments than are those who don't have diabetes.

Individuals with diabetes are also particularly at risk of death from CARDIOVASCULAR DISEASE, as revealed in study after study, especially among WOMEN WITH DIABETES. In addition, African-American women are at particularly high risk, in part because of the high incidence of diabetes among black women.

Among children and adolescents with diabetes, of the few numbers of deaths that occur, most are caused by either DIABETIC KETOACIDOSIS or HYPOGLYCEMIA, both conditions in which blood glucose levels are out of control.

Statistics on Death and Diabetes
According to data released by the Centers for Disease Control and Prevention (CDC) in their 1999 report, "Chronic Diseases and Their Risk Factors: The Nation's Leading Causes of Death," 2.7 percent of all deaths in 1996, or 61,768, were attributed to diabetes. Diabetes is believed to be underreported as the cause of death on death certificates, thus the numbers of deaths associated with diabetes are likely to be much higher. Diabetes was one of four chronic diseases that together comprised nearly 72 percent of the

causes of all deaths in the United States. (The other diseases were cardiovascular diseases, cancers, and chronic obstructive pulmonary diseases.) Also in this report, the CDC said that diabetes was a contributing cause to an additional 131,300 deaths.

Death rates from diabetes, state by state   In considering a state by state rate of deaths from diabetes per 1,000 deaths in the United States in 1996, the CDC found the highest rates were as follows: Louisiana (32.5), District of Columbia (28.7), West Virginia (25.1), Ohio (24.5), and Maryland (24.2). The CDC did not speculate on why rates of death from diabetes were high in some states and low in others.

In contrast, the lowest death rates were found in Hawaii (14.6), Nevada (14.5), Nebraska (13.7), Iowa (13.6), and Colorado (13.2).

Male/female death rates, state by state   In comparing male to female death rates from diabetes, the overall rate for the United States was 20.1 for men and 17.2 for women.

In looking at men only, men had the highest death rates from diabetes in the following states: Louisiana (31.5), District of Columbia (27.3), New Hampshire (26.6), West Virginia (26.6), and Ohio (26.5). Men had the lowest rates in the following states: Wyoming (12.6), Colorado (14.1), Iowa (15.7), New York (15.7), and Hawaii (15.9).

In looking at women only, women had the highest death rates from diabetes in the following states: Louisiana (32.8), District of Columbia (29.5), West Virginia (23.6), Ohio (22.9), and Maryland (22.1). Women had the lowest death rates from diabetes in the following states: North Dakota (12.0), Iowa (12.0), Nebraska (12.2), Colorado (12.3), and Massachusetts (12.9).

Death rates among people with diabetes   Some individuals with diabetes have a greater mortality risk than others. For example, according to 1997 statistics reported in *Healthy People 2010,* the total death rate for people with diabetes is 8.8 per 1,000 people. However, the rate is 9.0 for non-Hispanic whites and 8.9 per 1,000 for whites. The rate for African Americans is 8.1. (See Table 1.)

TABLE 1

Persons with Diabetes, 1997	Diabetes-Related Deaths
	Rate per 1,000
TOTAL	8.8
Race and ethnicity	
American Indian or Alaska Native	3.3
Asian or Pacific Islander	5.4
Asian	6.3
Native Hawaiian and other Pacific Islander	2.5
Black or African American	8.1
White	8.9
Hispanic or Latino	7.4
Gender	
Female	8.6
Male	9.5
Select populations	
Age groups (not age adjusted)	
Under 45 years	2.0
45 to 64 years	7.7
65 to 74 years	20.1
75 years and older	73.4

DNA = Data have not been analyzed. DNC = Data are not collected. DSU = Data are statistically unreliable.
Note: Age adjusted to the year 2000 standard population.

Death rates for Asian/Pacific Islanders with diabetes were lower, at 5.4 per 1,000 and death rates were lower still for American Indians/Alaska Natives with diabetes, at 3.3 per 1,000. Males with diabetes had a higher death risk than females, at 9.5 per 1,000 compared to 8.6 per 1,000 for women. Age is clearly linked to death rate, as can be seen from Table 1.

Women and diabetes deaths   An article in a 2000 issue of the *Journal of Clinical Epidemiology* reported on a study that looked at 1,035 African-American women and 5,732 white women ages 25–74, including women with and without diabetes. The women were followed for about 20 years. The researchers found that black women with diabetes had a significantly higher risk of coronary heart disease, cardiovascular disease, and death. In fact, diabetes was a predictor of disease and death. It was also a predictor of death for white women but the relationship was weaker for the African-American women. Among African-American women, the risk for coronary heart disease was 8.7 percent versus the risk of 6.1 percent for white women.

State by state numerical data The CDC also provided narrative data on the number of adults diagnosed with diabetes in each state as well as the number who died from diabetes and in whom the underlying cause of death was diabetes. In looking at the five states with the highest rates of death from diabetes, based on CDC data, the following chart provides a numerical breakdown on adult deaths of people with diabetes in these states.

TABLE 2

ADULTS WITH DIABETES AS THE CAUSE OR CONTRIBUTING CAUSE OF DEATH

	Adults with Diabetes in 1996	Underlying Cause of Death	Contributing Cause of Death
LA	187,297	1,624	1,282
DC	21,892	202	340
WV	77,972	669	1,462
OH	383,551	3,611	7,568
MD	191,827	1,413	3,026

Source: "Chronic Diseases and Their Risk Factors: The Nation's Leading Causes of Death," U.S. Center of Health and Human Services, Centers for Disease Control and Prevention, December 1999.

Death from Cardiovascular Causes

In study results of 1,694 deaths of people who were diagnosed with diabetes, reported in a 2000 issue of *Diabetes Care*, researchers found that nearly half (49 percent) of the deaths were caused by cardiovascular disease. Cardiovascular disease is also a major killer among nondiabetic males, where it represents the cause in 36 percent of all deaths.

A U.S.-based study of 2,468 elderly women and men were studied for mortality risks by the American Diabetes Association and the World Health Organization (WHO). Researchers reported that individuals with diagnosed diabetes had a four to five times greater risk of death from all causes, including cardiovascular diseases.

Researchers reported that many individuals with diabetes also have other risk factors for cardiovascular diseases. These include:

• Elevated fasting plasma glucose levels (in patients with diabetes, the higher the fasting plasma glucose level, the higher the risk of coronary heart disease)

• Hypertension

• High cholesterol and triglycerides

• Obesity

One study revealed a link between death from cardiovascular problems and DIABETIC RETINOPATHY. Rajala et al. identified and studied men and women in Finland with visual impairment in 1993, including diabetic and nondiabetic subjects. The researchers followed up the subjects until the end of 1997. Their findings were reported in a 2000 issue of *Diabetes Care*.

There were two separate groups of people with diabetes and retinopathy, including one group with diabetic retinopathy treated with lasers and another group whose members had been diagnosed using fundus photography. The third group did not have diabetes.

Researchers found that 10 of the nondiabetic subjects had died by the end of the study and 91 of those with diabetes had died. According to the researchers the mortality rate for the group whose members had had their retinopathy treated with lasers was 224 per 1,000. The rate was 150 per 1,000 for the fundus photography group. The rate was 94 per 1,000 for the nondiabetic group with visual impairment.

The researchers said, "The survival of diabetic subjects with visual impairment caused by DR [diabetic retinopathy] was poor. The high mortality rate was attributed mainly to cardiovascular diseases. Therefore, severe retinopathy proves to be a risk marker of cardiovascular death in diabetic patients."

Annika M. Adlerberth, M.D., et al., "Diabetes and Long-Term Risk of Mortality from Coronary and Other Causes in Middle-Aged Swedish Men," *Diabetes Care* 21, no. 4 (1998): 539–545.

Femmie de Vegt, M.Sc., et al., "Similar 9-Year Mortality Risks and Reproducibility for the World Health Organization and American Diabetes Association Glucose Tolerance Categories: The Hoorn Study," *Diabetes Care* 23, no. 1 (January 2000): 40–44.

Richard F. Gillum, M.D., et al., "Diabetes Mellitus, Coronary Heart Disease Incidence, and Death from All Causes in African American and European American Women: The NHANES I Epidemiologic Follow-up Study," *Journal of Clinical Epidemiology* 53, no. 5 (May 2000): 511–518.

Ken Gu, Ph.D., et al., "Mortality in Adults with and Without Diabetes in a National Cohort of the U.S. Population, 1971–1993," *Diabetes Care* 21, no. 7 (July 1998): 1138–1145.

Rebecca Lipton, B.S.N., M.P.H., Ph.D., "Ethnic Differences in Mortality from Insulin-Dependent Diabetes Mellitus among People Less Than 25 Years of Age," *Pediatrics* 103, no. 5 (May 1999): 952–956.

Christopher Morgan, et al., "Relationship between Diabetes and Mortality," *Diabetes Care* 23, no. 8 (August 2000): 1103–1107.

Ulla Rajala, Ph.D., et al., "High Cardiovascular Disease Mortality in Subjects with Visual Impairment Caused by Diabetic Retinopathy," *Diabetes Care* 23, no. 7 (July 2000): 957–961.

Lise Tarnow, M.D., et al., "Cardiovascular Morbidity and Early Mortality Cluster in Parents of Type 1 Diabetic Patients with Diabetic Nephropathy," *Diabetes Care* 23, no. 1 (January 2000): 30–33.

dehydration   Severe and harmful lack of fluid, with the primary symptoms of thirst, dry skin and mucous membranes, lightheadedness, and nausea. HYPERGLYCEMIA is one cause of dehydration because excessive levels of glucose filtered through the kidneys pulls water out in a process that is called an "osmotic diuresis."

The primary causes of dehydration are as follows:

- Inadequate fluid intake
- Vomiting
- Diarrhea
- Diuretic medications
- High glucose levels (hyperglycemia)
- Bleeding

Dehydration is treated by determining the cause of the problem and by replacing fluids to an adequate level. The dehydrated person may need to be hospitalized, depending on the severity of the dehydration.

Dehydration can become a serious problem if untreated, and dehydration may lead to or definitely contribute to and exacerbate DIABETIC KETOACIDOSIS (DKA) or HYPEROSMOLAR COMA. (See also HYPOGLYCEMIA.)

dementia   A process that leads to very diminished cognitive ability, behavioral changes, and the inability to perform activities of daily living. The person may have ALZHEIMER'S DISEASE or he or she may have another form of dementia. Often the person may have emotional outbursts or rages. Some studies indicate that people with diabetes are at greater risk for developing dementia than are nondiabetics. In a study reported by Ott et al., in a 1999 issue of *Neurology*, the researchers described their findings on dementia drawn from the Rotterdam study, a study of 6,370 older people and chronic disorders. Of the total, there were 692 patients who had diabetes.

The subjects were followed for about two years and 126 of the patients with diabetes developed dementia. Of these, 89 developed Alzheimer's disease. Researchers found that subjects with diabetes had nearly double the risk of developing dementia over those who did not have diabetes, although they could not identify the underlying cause for this occurrence. Patients with newly diagnosed diabetes had a lower probability of developing dementia, while those who were receiving insulin were most likely to be diagnosed with dementia. This does not indicate that insulin was the cause of dementia. Instead, it was likely that these patients had diabetes for a longer period and required more therapy.

Signs of Dementia

The person with dementia and diabetes often cannot recognize the signs and symptoms of low and high glucose levels and often cannot respond appropriately because the person's brain is not functioning well. Wide swings in glucose levels may also exacerbate acute changes in cognitive skills and behavior.

The ill person with severe dementia may not recognize her own children, may not know the purpose of a wristwatch, and may experience paranoia, hallucinations, and other psychotic behaviors. These individuals are extremely difficult to care for in a home environment and may require care in an ASSISTED LIVING FACILITY or a SKILLED NURSING FACILITY.

Often medical doctors allow patients with dementia to have slightly higher levels of glucose (in the 120 to 250 range) to try to avoid HYPOGLYCEMIA, a problem that is more frequent with tight control. (See also ALZHEIMER'S DISEASE, ELDERLY.)

A. Ott et al., "Diabetes Mellitus and the Risk of Dementia: The Rotterdam Study," *Neurology* 53 (1999): 1937–1942.

denial (of diabetes)

denial (of diabetes)   Refusal to accept that one has diabetes and/or refusal to accept that actions must be taken as a result of the disease. When a child, adolescent, or adult is first diagnosed with diabetes, it may be very difficult for the individual and other family members to accept the illness and the steps that must be taken to control it. The person and his or her loved ones may also fear immediate death, although such a consequence is rare. They may also worry about or resent the idea of taking lifelong medications, having to periodically check their BLOOD GLUCOSE levels and, in some cases, needing to self-inject with INSULIN.

It's important for newly diagnosed individuals with diabetes to receive a complete EDU-CATION about their illness, including a general overview of either Type 1 or Type 2 diabetes (whichever they are diagnosed with), as well as an explanation of what medications will be needed and what lifestyle changes are recommended.

The individual needs to be shown how to test his or her own blood and to understand what the meanings are of the findings. If the person must self-inject insulin, then he or she must be taught how to prepare the tools they need and where they can be obtained, and how to self-inject and they also must be taught how to identify and react to immediate symptoms or problems that may sometimes occur subsequent to injections.

If the denial persists, the physician may refer the patient to a social worker, psychologist, psychiatrist, or other mental health professional.

depression   A continued feeling of severe and profound sadness and hopelessness, which, in its most extreme state, can lead an individual to contemplate or even to carry out a plan for suicide. Also known as depressive disorder or major depressive disorder. People with diabetes are about three times more likely to suffer from depression than nondiabetics. WOMEN WITH DIABETES are more likely to be diagnosed with depression than men with diabetes. (Women in general are more frequently diagnosed with depression than men.)

According to the *Diagnostic and Statistical Manual of Mental Disorders, DSM-IV-TR* (American Psychiatric Association, 2000), a reference source used by many psychiatrists, "Up to 20–25 percent of individuals with certain general medical conditions (e.g., diabetes, myocardial infarction, carcinomas, stroke) will develop Major Depressive Disorder during the course of their general medical conditions."

In looking specifically at people diagnosed with diabetes, including both Type 1 and Type 2, studies have revealed that such patients are more prone to depression than are nondiabetics, particularly if their life activities are severely limited. According to a 2000 report on depression published by the National Academy on an Aging Society, in looking at individuals aged 51–61, 13 percent report experiencing four or more symptoms of depression, versus 6 percent of nondiabetics who report such symptoms. Others say the rate is much higher.

Risk Factors for Depression among People with Diabetes

Research has indicated that people with diabetes are more prone to depression if they are not high school graduates and/or they suffer from two or more medical complications associated with diabetes. Type 2 patients who also suffer from depression are more likely to have a weight problem and to be using insulin rather than oral medications.

The divorce or death of a spouse are other factors that have been found to be associated with depression among those with diabetes. (This is a problem for people who don't have diabetes as well.) Some studies have found retirement from work to be significantly related to the presence of depression among individuals with diabetes.

One very important factor linked to depression is poor GLYCEMIC CONTROL. Experts are not sure whether poor glucose control might be a result of depression or whether poor glycemic control could actually precipitate a depression.

According to Patrick Lustman, professor of medical psychology in the department of psychiatry at Washington University School of Medicine, St. Louis, in a 1999 lecture at the American Diabetes Association meeting,

> Those who are depressed are more likely to have poor blood glucose control even after you factor out that depressed people are less likely to take good care of themselves. It is possible that the hormonal impact of depression, which affects cortisol levels, may worsen insulin resistance and potentiate the atherogenic effects of diabetes.

Racial and Ethnic Groups and Depression

Some racial and ethnic groups are more likely to suffer from depression than others; for example, African Americans are highly prone to problems with depression. In one study of 183 African Americans with diabetes, reported in a 2000 issue of *Diabetes Care*, researchers found that 30 percent of the subjects had symptoms of depression. Because African Americans are also more likely than other ethnic groups to experience complications from diabetes and to suffer from amputations, this may account for at least part of the high rate of depression.

Mexican Americans with diabetes also have a high rate of depression. In one study of 636 older Mexican Americans with diabetes, compared to a control group of 2,196 nondiabetics and reported in a 1999 issue of *Diabetes Care*, Mexican Americans with diabetes had a significantly higher rate of depression than the nondiabetics.

Thirty-one percent of diabetic Mexican Americans had depressive symptoms compared to 24 percent in the control group. Among diabetics, women were more likely to be depressed, as were non–high school graduates. Unmarried people with diabetes were also more likely to experience depressive symptoms.

A Treatable Illness

Depression is highly treatable in most cases, according to most psychiatrists. Studies on depressed individuals who have diabetes have revealed that a class of antidepressant medications called "serotonin selective reuptake inhibitors" (SSRIs) are highly effective in treating depression. This class includes medications such as Prozac (fluoxetine) and Zoloft (sertraline).

Psychiatrists are medical doctors who treat emotional disorders such as depression. Although any physician may treat depression, psychiatrists are generally the most knowledgeable about medications and treatments. Of course, it's very important for the psychiatrist to coordinate any prescribed medication with the diabetic person's primary care physician and ensure that any problem with medication interactions are prevented or minimized.

Many people have an unfairly negative and fearful view of psychiatrists, assuming, for example, that psychiatrists only treat individuals who are severely mentally ill. The reality is that most patients of psychiatrists experience common and treatable ailments such as depression and anxiety and few patients are psychotic.

Some people with diabetes may benefit from seeing a psychologist or social worker in order to gain insight to their feelings and learn better coping skills. Some individuals also benefit from joining support groups where they can not only empathize with other people in a similar situation but also learn practical and useful information from other members.

For further information, contact the following organizations:

American Psychological Association
750 Frost Street, NE
Washington, DC 20002
(202) 336-5500
www.apa.org

American Psychiatric Association
1400 K Street, NW
Washington, DC 20005
(202) 682-6000
www.psycho.org

(See also EMOTIONAL PROBLEMS.)

Tiffany L. Gary, M.H.S., et al., "Depressive Symptoms and Metabolic Control in African-Americans with Type 2 Diabetes," *Diabetes Care* 23, no. 1 (January 2000): 23–29.
Patrick J. Lustman, Ph.D., "Fluoxetine for Depression in Diabetes," *Diabetes Care* 23, no. 5 (May 2000): 618–623.

diabetes A condition in which insufficient or no insulin is available to the body. In the case of TYPE 1 DIABETES, the individual's body produces no insulin and insulin must be taken to survive. In the case of TYPE 2 DIABETES, the body is unable to use the insulin that is produced. The individual needs to take medications to boost the body's use of insulin.

Diabetes Control and Complications Trial (DCCT) An extremely important federally funded study of individuals with Type 1 diabetes which studied 1,441 subjects and followed them from 1983 to 1993, amassing enormous amounts of data and analyzing the many ramifications and effects of the illness among adults. The Diabetes Control and Complications Trial Research Group in Bethesda, Maryland conducted the study, under the auspices of the National Institute of Diabetes and Digestive and Kidney Diseases (NIDDK).

The study information has been used by many different medical experts and some subgroups have also been contacted for further studies. In addition, an outgrowth of this study, the Epidemiology of Diabetes Interventions and Complications (EDIC) Research Group, continues to study the DCCT group. In 1999, the EDIC Research Group reported that they had received permission from 96 percent of the DCCT subjects to study them further.

This clinical study was the largest diabetes study that has ever been performed. It was carried out in 29 medical centers in the United States and Canada. Although the design changed somewhat from the onset, it ultimately involved patients who were divided into two groups.

One group was given traditional diabetes therapy, which generally involved one insulin injection per day. The glucose was initially monitored with urine glucose testing and later, with once per day blood glucose monitoring. The other group received intensive control, involving multiple daily blood glucose measurements (four or more times per day) and insulin that was delivered either four times daily through injections or administered continuously through an insulin pump.

The intensively managed group also received a diet and exercise plan. In addition, members of this group received weekly phone calls from educators, monthly visits with a team comprised of a doctor, a nurse, a dietitian and also a therapist, all assets that were not provided to the group receiving the standard therapy. The intensively treated group had an average HgbA1c that was 2 percent lower than the other group. (Seven percent versus nine percent.)

The Results

The DCCT study clearly established that tight control of blood glucose decreased the probability of complications related to diabetes. For example, the risk of eye disease was reduced by 76 percent with tight control. In addition, the group that successfully tightly controlled their diabetes had a 50 percent reduced risk for kidney disease and a 60 percent reduced risk for nerve disease. These are very dramatic results and people in the medical community took notice.

Problem with Tight Control

One problem with very tight control is that it is very difficult for most patients to achieve. Most people with diabetes find it hard to test their blood four times a day and self-inject four times. Also, few patients have monthly access not only to a doctor but also to a team of interested and highly motivated specialists.

Another problem with attempting very tight control is that it also involves a greater risk of the development of severe HYPOGLYCEMIA. The intensively treated group had three times the rate of severe hypoglycemia as that experienced by the standard-treatment group. As a result of this risk, physicians as of this writing do not recommend such tight control for the following groups of people:

- Those with severe diabetic complications
- Those with hypoglycemic unawareness
- Those with an inability to monitor glucose levels
- Those with autonomic neuropathy

A related study, the UNITED KINGDOM PROSPECTIVE DIABETES STUDY (UKPDS), studied tight glucose control in individuals with Type 2 diabetes.

Importance of Team Approach to Treatment

The DCCT illustrated to physicians the important role of the diabetes team approach in assisting people with diabetes to maintain good glycemic control. It also became clear that dietitians should be a part of the team.

Relatives of DCCT Subjects

In a subsequent study based on the relatives of DCCT subjects, published in a 1997 issue of *Diabetes,* the researchers located biological relatives of the subjects and found a high degree of illness among them. Of 448 relatives with diabetes who were identified, about half (45 percent) had Type 1 diabetes and about half (45 percent) had Type 2 diabetes. (It was unknown what type of diabetes the remaining 10 percent had.)

The researchers contacted 241 relatives who provided further information. They learned that when the DCCT subjects had DIABETIC RETINOPATHY, about 40 percent of their relatives with diabetes also had retinopathy.

When the DCCT subjects had MICROALBUMINURIA, about 62 percent of the relatives with diabetes also had microalbuminuria. It seems clear that there are familial risks, not only to diabetes but also to the complications of diabetes. It is also likely that there may be other commonalities that will be discovered in the future.

The DCCT also showed that there did not appear to be a numerical threshold for glycemic complications below which level one is "safe" and above which one is at risk. Instead, there appears to be a continuous and graded relationship between the A1c level and the risk of development or progression of a complication.

The economic analysis of the DCCT showed that although the initial cost of therapy is higher than standard therapy costs, the benefits that accrue with tight glycemic control mean that the individual is less likely to require kidney dialysis because he is less likely to experience END-STAGE RENAL DISEASE (ESRD). The person is also less likely to face an amputation of a limb due to neuropathy. Thus, the long-term savings in both dollars, human lives, and suffering make tight control worth the expenses involved.

American Diabetes Association, "Implications of the Diabetes Control and Complications Trial," *Diabetes Care* 24, Supp. 1 (2001): S25–27.

Diabetes Control and Complications Research Group, "Baseline Analysis of Renal Function in the Diabetes Control and Complications Research Trial," *Kidney International* 43 (1993): 668–674.

Diabetes Control and Complications Research Group, "Clustering of Long-Term Complications in Families with Diabetes in the Diabetes Control and Complications Trial," *Diabetes* 46 (November 1997): 1829–1839.

Diabetes Control and Complications Research Group, "Effect of Intensive Diabetes Management on Macrovascular Events and Risk Factors in the Diabetes Control and Complications Trial," *The American Journal of Cardiology* 75 (May 1, 1995): 894–903.

Diabetes Control and Complications Research Group, "Effect of Intensive Diabetes Therapy on the Development and Progression of Neuropathy," *Annals of Internal Medicine* 122, no. 8 (April 15, 1995): 561–568.

Diabetes Control and Complications Research Group, "Effect of Intensive Diabetes Treatment on the Development and Progression of Long-Term Complications in Adolescents with Insulin-Dependent Diabetes Mellitus: Diabetes Control and Complications Trial," *The Journal of Pediatrics* 125, no. 2 (August 1994): 177–188.

Diabetes Control and Complications Research Group, "Effect of Intensive Therapy on the Development and Progression of Diabetic Nephropathy in the Diabetes Control and Complications Trial," *Kidney International* 47 (1995): 1703–1720.

Diabetes Control and Complications Research Group, "Effect of Intensive Treatment of Diabetes on the Development and Progression of Long-Term Complications in Insulin-Dependent Diabetes Mellitus," *The New England Journal of Medicine* 329 (September 30, 1993): 977–986.

Diabetes Control and Complications Research Group, "Epidemiology of Severe Hypoglycemia in the Diabetes Control and Complications Research Trial," *The American Journal of Medicine* 90 (April 1991): 450–459.

Diabetes Control and Complications Research Group, "Expanded Role of the Dietitian in the Diabetes Control and Complications Trial: Implications for Clinical Practice," *Journal of the American Dietetic Association* 93 (July 1993): 758–764.

Diabetes Control and Complications Research Group, "Factors in Development of Diabetic Neuropathy: Baseline Analysis of Neuropathy in Feasibility Phase of Diabetes Control and Complications Trial (DCCT)," *Diabetes* 37 (April 1998): 476–481.

Diabetes Control and Complications Research Group, "Hypoglycemia in the Diabetes Control and Complications Trial," *Diabetes* 46 (February 1997): 271–286.

Diabetes Control and Complications Research Group, "Progression of Retinopathy with Intensive versus Conventional Treatment in the Diabetes Control and Complications Trial," *Ophthalmology* 102, no. 4 (April 1995): 647–661.

Epidemiology of Diabetes Control and Complications (ERIC) Research Group, "Epidemiology of Diabetes Interventions and Complications," *Diabetes Care* 22 (January 1999): 99–111.

Epidemiology of Diabetes Control and Complications (ERIC) Research Group, "Progression of Retinopathy in the DCCT Cohorts After 4 Years. Followup in the Epidemiology of Diabetes Interventions and Complications (ERIC) Study," *Diabetologia* 41, Supp. 1 (1998): A281.

diabetes insipidus A rare metabolic disease stemming from the kidneys or pituitary gland rather than the pancreas, and completely unique from Type 1 or Type 2 diabetes mellitus. Some forms of this disease are hereditary while other forms occur subsequent to brain surgery or an injury. The symptoms of the person with diabetes insipidus may be similar to those of the person with Type 1 or Type 2 diabetes, such as frequent urination, fatigue, and excessive thirst. However, the person with diabetes insipidus does not have HYPERGLYCEMIA, the hallmark feature of diabetes mellitus. Unless the person drinks copious quantities of fluid, he or she will become severely dehydrated and constipated.

The disease may occur abruptly in individuals of any age. If infants with the disease are not treated quickly, they may suffer from brain damage or developmental delays such as mental retardation. Symptoms of diabetes insipidus in a baby are fever, vomiting, and convulsions with high levels of sodium found in the blood upon laboratory examination.

Diabetes insipidus is usually treated with desmopressin acetate (DDAVP), a hormone that is available as a nasal spray, liquid, or tablets. Drugs are also prescribed to limit excessive urination. Paradoxically, diuretic drugs, usually effective in increasing urination, will reduce urine volume in the person with diabetes insipidus, in whom the cause is a kidney problem.

diabetes mellitus A general name that encompasses both Type 1 and Type 2 diabetes, although the causes of the two illnesses are very different. Their common denominator is that the body is unable to function properly because of inadequate use or supply of insulin. In the case of individuals with Type 1 diabetes, their pancreas no longer produces insulin and it must be supplemented in order for them to survive. Conversely, people with Type 2 diabetes may produce enough insulin but they have an INSULIN RESISTANCE and are unable to use the insulin properly.

Diabetes Prevention Trials Refers to two large clinical trials launched by the National Institutes of Health in the 1990s including the Diabetes Prevention Trial for Type 1 Diabetes (DPT-1) and the Diabetes Prevention Program (DPP) for people with Type 2 diabetes. The DPT-1 is an ongoing study and the DPP ended in 2001. The purpose of these studies was to screen people who are at high risk for developing either Type 1 or Type 2 diabetes, to provide treatments, and to determine which approach is most effective at preventing the development of diabetes.

The DPT-1 Study

The purpose of this study is to screen for autoimmune abnormalities that predispose people to developing Type 1 diabetes. In the North American and Puerto Rican sites of the DPT-1 study, nondiabetic relatives of patients with Type 1 diabetes were recruited from nine centers. Eligible subjects were required to have impaired first phase insulin response (which means that they did not secrete insulin appropriately), a pre-diabetic condition, and also to have islet cell antibodies with a normal or impaired glucose tolerance test. These individuals are anticipated to have a 50 percent chance of developing Type 1 diabetes within five years.

In this phase, 89,827 relatives were screened. About 4 percent tested positive for islet cell antibodies. Of these, 338 were enrolled in the study, including 169 to the therapy group and 169 to the control group, which will be observed only.

Subjects in the treatment group receive insulin intravenously for four days each year and also receive ultralente insulin twice each day. They receive oral glucose tolerance tests every six months.

Preliminary results for this study have shown that there are risk factors for the rapid development of Type 1 diabetes including:

• Younger age
• Positive blood tests for more than one islet cell antibody
• A history of impaired glucose tolerance (IGT)

The subjects are closely followed. Individuals whose laboratory tests show that they have antibodies to insulin but their insulin levels are still in the normal range are treated with oral medications. Preliminary results have shown that small doses of insulin do not appear to prevent the development of Type 1 diabetes in susceptible individuals.

The DPP

Individuals who were at risk for developing Type 2 diabetes were the volunteers for the DPP, including women who have had GESTATIONAL DIABETES, members of ethnic groups with high rates of diabetes, people with a family member who has Type 2 diabetes, and others. Individuals are tested to determine if they have abnormal glucose levels but have not yet developed diabetes. Those who don't have diabetes are placed into one of three groups and followed up.

One group provided members with lifestyle recommendations and a placebo (sugar pill). The second group was given an even more intensive lifestyle management program that emphasized exercise and a personal trainer. The third group received an oral antidiabetic medication, either a sulfonylurea drug or metformin. The goal was to determine which of these three approaches is most effective at prevention.

The DPP ended in 2001 and Allan Spiegel, director of the National Institute of Diabetes and Digestive and Kidney Diseases (NIDDK) said that its results offered hope to an estimated 10 million Americans who were not diabetic but were "perilously close to the brink."

The study found that a relatively small weight loss of 10 to 15 pounds, accompanied by exercise for 30 minutes each day, enabled the subjects to reduce their risk for developing diabetes by a dramatic 58 percent. The study also found that metformin taken twice a day reduced the risk of developing diabetes by nearly one-third (31 percent). The drug worked best in obese and younger individuals ages 25–44.

diabetic cheirarthropathy Limited joint mobility causing an inability to fully extend the fingers. A classic sign of this disorder is the inability to flatten out or to touch the palms together with fingers spread, the diagnostic "prayer sign." This disorder is found primarily among children and adults with Type 1 diabetes but it is also seen in those with Type 2 diabetes. From 10 to 50 percent of patients with diabetes experience diabetic cheirarthropathy.

It is characterized by a limited mobility of extension of the small joints of the hands and also by thickening and stiffness of the overlying skin. Diabetic cheirarthropathy may be related to changes in collagen that are induced by higher glucose levels. The condition may improve with better GLYCEMIC CONTROL. No treatment is known or required.

A. Rosenbloom et al., "Diabetes, Short Stature and Joint Stiffness: A New Syndrome," *Clinical Research* 22 (1974): 92A.
J. H. Silverstein et al., "Long-term Glycemic Control Influences the Onset of Limited Joint Mobility in Type 2 Diabetes," *Journal of Pediatrics* 132, no. 6 (1998): 944–947.

diabetic glomerulosclerosis Scarring and hardening of the tiny blood vessels inside the kidneys of a person with diabetes. (A similar condition can also be caused by a disease such as lupus.) This can harm the kidneys to the extent that they stop functioning and the patient has END-STAGE RENAL DISEASE (ESRD). At that point, in order to live, the person will need to have either kidney dialysis or a kidney transplant.

Glomerular disease is diagnosed with laboratory tests that measure protein in the urine, or PROTEINURIA, as well as blood in the urine (hematuria). The doctor will also check for fluid retention (edema). The patient should report to the doctor such symptoms as foamy urine (which may indicate proteinuria), blood that is pink or dark-colored, or signs of edema such as swelling around the hands or ankles.

diabetic ketoacidosis (DKA) An acute metabolic complication of diabetes that involves a combination of HYPOGLYCEMIA and DEHYDRATION. Often caused by an illness such as the flu, DKA can be very severe and may lead to COMA and DEATH. In 1996, DKA was the first listed diagnosis for 100,000 hospital discharges. It was also a secondary diagnosis in 122,000 hospital discharges. DKA is seen primarily in people with Type 1 diabetes rather than Type 2 diabetes.

DKA is one of the two leading causes of death among children and adolescents with Type 1 diabetes. (Hypoglycemia is the other leading cause.)

Patients with Type 2 diabetes who experience DKA will need insulin. If they had previously been maintained on oral medication, they may be able to return to oral medications at a later date if their glycemic control improves and stabilizes.

DKA is very serious and experts report a mortality rate of 5–10 percent. The blood glucose level of the afflicted person is very high and chemicals known as KETONES can be found in the urine. In most cases, the patient will need to be hospitalized, usually in the intensive care unit, in order to stabilize and carefully monitor the person.

Patients who have been hospitalized for DKA should be very carefully followed by their doctors and should also be extremely vigilant with regard to monitoring their blood glucose levels. Fluid and electrolyte levels should be closely monitored as well.

Major Risk Factors for DKA

Ethnicity is a factor in DKA: Blacks were more than twice as likely to be admitted to the hospital for DKA as whites. DKA is also a more common problem among older people of all races and people over age 75 had the highest death rates. However, Centers for Disease Control and Prevention researchers also found that death rates for people with diabetes who were age 45 were higher in 1996 than in 1980 for all groups except white females.

Symptoms of DKA

Some common symptoms of DKA are BLURRED VISION, nausea, abdominal pains, and a lack of appetite. The individual may also experience increased urination and great thirst.

Treatment of DKA

In the 1970s and earlier, physicians favored very high doses of insulin (20–100 U/h) to treat this condition; however, the current medical thinking is to provide lower doses of insulin, such as 5–10 U/h, in order to alleviate the risk of an immediate fall in blood glucose levels, which may also be dangerous to the patient. In addition to the administration of insulin, an aggressive program of "rehydration" or providing adequate fluids and replenishing potassium levels of the patient, is also instituted as a standard part of the treatment.

Poor Glycemic Control Can Lead to DKA

A study in Germany of 114 patients with Type 1 diabetes and who experienced occurrences of severe DKA over the period 1986–1997 was reported in a 1999 issue of *Diabetes Care* and provided important data.

The researchers found that in 26 percent of the cases, the DKA stemmed from the patients' failure to adjust their insulin dosages when they were ill with an infection. Apparently these subjects had not prepared or complied with the SICK DAY RULES recommended by physicians for patients with diabetes.

Also, in 17 percent of the cases, the patients were not adequately monitoring their glucose levels. The largest cause of DKA (61 percent) was found in patients who were receiving incorrect dosages of insulin because of a pump or catheter defect or an incorrect insulin dose.

Studies indicate that patients with DKA and who are seen by ENDOCRINOLOGISTS have a briefer and less costly stay than do patients who are treated by general practitioners. Endocrinologists order fewer tests and are apparently more confident about their treatment plan than general practitioners.

Terri D'Arrigo, "Ketoacidosis: The Snake in the Grass," *Diabetes Forecast* 54, no. 7 (July 2001): 71–72, 74.

Susan Grinslade, and Elizabeth A. Buck, "Clinical Care: Diabetic Ketoacidosis: Implications for the Medical-Surgical Nurse," *Med Surg Nursing* 8, no. 1 (1999): 37–45.

Arnd Wagner, M.D., et al., "Therapy of Severe Diabetic Ketoacidosis: Zero-Mortality Under Very-Low-Dose Insulin Application," *Diabetes Care* 22, no. 5 (May 1999): 674–677.

diabetic nephropathy Kidney damage that may lead to kidney failure. Patients with diabetic nephropathy account for about 42 percent of all cases of END-STAGE RENAL DISEASE (ESRD) in the United States and diabetic nephropathy is the underlying cause for an estimated 100,000 people each year who need either kidney dialysis or a kidney transplant. Unfortunately, kidney disease usually has no symptoms until less than 25 percent of kidney function remains.

Causes of Nephropathy

The combination of diabetes and HYPERTENSION is a very dangerous one and a key cause of rapid renal damage and destruction. When patients have hypertension and diabetes, and they develop nephropathy, their mortality risk increases by 37 times. For this reason, it is critically important for hypertensive diabetes patients to comply with medical regimens for decreasing high blood pressure, including taking medication, losing weight, and following other medical advice.

Other Symptoms

Most patients with diabetic nephropathy also have RETINOPATHY as well. If a patient is diagnosed with DIABETIC RETINOPATHY, he or she should be evaluated for kidney disease.

Genetic Risks

Researchers have found that the siblings of patients with both diabetes and kidney disease have five times the risk of also developing nephropathy themselves.

(See also END-STAGE RENAL DISEASE, HYPERTENSION, SYNDROME X.)

Joan H. Aiello, "Preventing Diabetic Nephropathy: The Role of Primary Care," *The Nurse Practitioner* 23, no. 2 (1998): 11–13, 17–18, 23–24.

Timothy C. Evans, M.D., et al., "Diabetic Nephropathy," *Clinical Diabetes* 18, no. 1 (Winter 2000): 278–285.

Irl B. Hirsch, M.D., Editor, "Diabetic Nephropathy: Why Are We Seeing More," *Clinical Diabetes* 18, no. 1 (Winter 2000): 97–98.

diabetic neuropathy Refers to nerve damage directly caused by diabetes. Almost any part of the nervous system can be affected, although it is rare for the brain and spinal cord to be involved. Neuropathy is usually classified by the type of nerve that is affected, whether it is a PERIPHERAL NEUROPATHY, AUTONOMIC NEUROPATHY, cranial mononeuropathies, radiculopathies, or other focal neuropathies.

Diabetic neuropathy may result in a variety of ailments, including a loss of feeling in the feet or hands, the delayed digestion of food (GASTROPARESIS DIABETICORUM), ERECTILE DYSFUNCTION, and other medical problems. An estimated 60–70 percent of those with diabetes suffer from mild to severe neuropathy.

Diabetic neuropathy may also cause chronic and sometimes severe pain, and people with diabetes may need medications or creams. Many clinicians prescribe antiseizure medication such as NEURONTIN (gabapentin) as well as antidepressants to help treat chronic pain.

In one study, reported in the *British Journal of Clinical Pharmacology* in 2000, the researchers reported that patients' pain was reduced with a cream made from a combination of capsaicin and doxepin. Either of these two substances alone also provided pain relief, but the relief was greater and occurred faster when they were combined into one component.

Cranial Mononeuropathies

When the nerves of the face are affected, it can mimic symptoms of a stroke and may also cause a facial droop similar to that found in Bell's palsy. It may also cause an eyelid droop. These type of neuropathies are caused by "nerve attacks," or a sudden blockage of blood flow to the nerve that is similar to what happens in the heart and brain during a heart attack or a stroke. Cranial mononeuropathies often resolve on their own within weeks to months and rarely persist longer than six months.

Radiculopathies

A painful neuropathy in which a nerve root is affected. If the nerve root that is supplying the area is located just below the right lower ribs, it can mimic a gallbladder attack. If it is a lower back nerve root supplying the legs, it can cause sciatica.

Other Focal Neuropathies

Patients with diabetes are more commonly affected than nondiabetics by compression neuropathies, such as carpal tunnel syndrome and tarsal tunnel syndrome. This may be due to the deposit of carbohydrates and protein-like material in the canals where the nerves run. It may also be due to AGE deposition in the tissues as well as abnormal blood flow problems.

Damage to the peroneal nerve in the foot can lead to "foot drop," which is the inability to dorsiflex the foot (point the toes up), causing it to drag when walking.

The Diabetes Control and Complications Trial Research Group, "The Effect of Intensive Diabetes Therapy on the Development and Progression of Neuropathy," *Annals of Internal Medicine* 122 (April 15, 1995): 561–568.

G. McCleane, "Topical Application of Doxepin Hydrochloride, Capsaicin and a Combination of Both Produces Analgesia in Chronic Human Neuropathic Pain: A Randomized, Double-Blind, Placebo-Controlled Study," *British Journal of Clinical Pharmacology* 49, no. 6 (June 2000): 574–579.

diabetic retinopathy   Disease of the retina, stemming from diabetes. Diabetic retinopathy is the most common eye disease complication experienced by people with diabetes. According to the National Institutes of Health (NIH), diabetic retinopathy is also responsible for 12 percent of all new cases of BLINDNESS each year and is the leading cause of adult onset blindness. Diabetic retinopathy is at least partially caused by high levels of glucose that result in varying levels of harm to the blood vessels in the retina. Other factors such as genetic predisposition, HYPERTENSION, SMOKING, HYPERLIPIDEMIA, and renal insufficiency may exacerbate the retinopathy.

Early diagnosis with a dilated eye examination and treatment can prevent the loss of sight for over 90 percent of patients with diabetes. However, according to the National Institutes of Health, less than half (47 percent) of patients with diabetes have annual eye examinations. Only an early eye examination will detect possible problems because the early stages of the disease produce no symptoms. In its Healthy People 2010 plan, the federal government has set a goal to have 75 percent of all adults with diabetes obtain a dilated eye examination per year.

One hopeful note is the NATIONAL DIABETES EYE EXAMINATION PROGRAM. If the patient with diabetes is over age 65 and on MEDICARE, this program between national eye professionals organizations and the Centers for Medicare and Medicaid Services (CMS), formerly the Health Care Financing Administration (HCFA) will help patients find an OPHTHALMOLOGIST in their area who will provide a dilated eye examination at no cost.

Risk Factors for Diabetic Retinopathy

People with Type 1 diabetes are at greater risk for developing retinopathy than are those with Type 2 diabetes. Experts report that nearly everyone who has had Type 1 diabetes for 15 or more years has some degree of retinopathy. Patients with Type 2 diabetes who require insulin are also likely to develop retinopathy. (Ninety-seven percent of patients on insulin have some retinopathy after 15 years, and 80 percent of those not requiring insulin have some retinal changes.)

AFRICAN AMERICANS with Type 1 diabetes are particularly at risk for developing diabetic retinopathy. HISPANICS with diabetes, especially Mexican Americans, are also at high risk for developing retinopathy. In addition, it is also possible for children who have diabetes to suffer from diabetic retinopathy, although the risk appears to be low, especially prior to puberty.

The people with diabetes who are the most likely to suffer from diabetic retinopathy include those who fit the following profile:

- Did not control their diabetes in the first years after diagnosis
- Have had diabetes for 17 or more years
- Experience high blood pressure
- Are African American, Native Indian, or Hispanic
- Have high cholesterol levels
- Have had GESTATIONAL DIABETES
- Are smokers
- Abuse alcohol
- Have other illnesses, such as kidney disease
- Have a genetic risk for eye disease

Symptoms of Diabetic Retinopathy

There are few symptoms of early diabetic retinopathy that are detectable to the patient. This is why screening examinations are critical. Some early symptoms may be worsening of peripheral (side) vision, or worsening color vision. A dilated eye examination performed by an ophthalmologist should reveal the problem. When there are symptoms, often they may be mistakenly ignored as minor or a sign of aging.

Diagnosis of Diabetic Retinopathy

Diabetic retinopathy is identified with a dilated eye examination. The eye care expert puts special drops in the eyes so that the pupils will enlarge. This enables the examiner to see the back of the eye easier and to notice any signs of disease. Experts say that the dilated eye examination gives the examiner a clear view of the retina, much like looking through an open door. Without the dilated eye examination, it is like trying to see by peering through the shuttered windows of a house.

If a physician other than an ophthalmologist/optometrist performs the examination, a device called an ophthalmoscope is usually used. Endocrinologists and other physicians will screen their patients in the office with these hand-held devices. However, several studies have shown that even experienced examiners generally only detect approximately 30–50 per-

cent of the pathology that is present. This is why dilated exams by the ophthalmologists and optometrists are critical.

Eye professionals can use the ophthalmoscope as well but usually they will use a device called a slit lamp. This device will allow the expert to look at the retina with both eyes simultaneously, i.e., with depth perception. In contrast, the lack of depth perception that is missing when a physician uses a hand-held ophthalmoscope makes the early diagnosis of MACULAR EDEMA very difficult. The device used by the ophthalmologist provides binocular views of the eye.

In 1999, eye doctors began using laser technology to enable them to diagnose retinopathy at the earliest stages. The equipment is very costly and was used infrequently; however, eye experts said the cost would come down and they anticipate laser screening should become common by 2010.

Stages of Diabetic Retinopathy

Retinopathy is broken down into two major classes, including background diabetic retinopathy (BDR) and proliferative retinopathy.

In the early stages of the disease, some vessels inside the retina of the eye narrow while others become enlarged. The doctor may refer to microaneurysms, blot and dot hemorrhages, and hard exudates (leakage of protein and fat into the retina). At this point, the disease is called "nonproliferative retinopathy." Background retinopathy may wax and wane from week to week and month to month.

A scary and perplexing observation made in the past 20 years is that tightening of GLYCEMIC CONTROL actually may lead to a transient worsening of background diabetic retinopathy. It is important for the patient to know that good glycemic control can cause *temporary* problems and for the ENDOCRINOLOGIST or primary care provider to be in contact with the ophthalmologist so that this information can be passed along.

Some patients with BDR will develop leakage or EDEMA. This occurs when the lining of the capillaries in the retina are damaged. As a result, these vessels leak and fluid accumulates in the retina. This leakage is called "clinically significant edema," when it threatens the macula or the center of the retina.

Longer-term follow-up on patients with good glycemic control has revealed that their retinopathy improved. Consequently, in the long term, it is always better to have tighter glycemic control.

At this stage, the individual's eyesight may not be in serious danger, and there may be no noticeable changes in vision; however, it's best that diagnosis and treatment begin at this point. When the eye doctor first notices changes in the retina, he or she may ask the patient to have a follow-up appointment sooner, for example, in three to six months versus the usual 12 months, to see if the problem is progressing.

Once the part of the eye known as the "macula," which controls our sharpest and central vision, becomes involved, vision loss is a threat to the patient. Thus, even small amounts of leakage and/or hemorrhage around this area may lead the eye doctor to recommend therapy.

A more severe state of retinopathy is "proliferative diabetic retinopathy," which involves the growth of abnormal vessels that can rupture and cause retinal detachments, significant transient visual loss, and finally blindness. The doctor may refer to new vessel growth or neoproliferative disease. "Cotton wool spots" can be seen, which are white spots seen on the retina that represent areas of severely decreased blood flow. The patient in this stage of the disease is now usually aware that he or she has a problem.

Patients with this type of retinopathy need to discuss the type of physical exercise they intend to do with their eye doctor because isometric type exercises such as weight lifting can cause a severe increase in the pressure in the tiny vessels of the eye and may actually precipitate a hemorrhage.

Treatment of Diabetic Retinopathy

If the retinopathy is in the early stages, the patient may be able to improve his or her condi-

tion with tight glycemic control. According to ophthalmologists Fong and Ross in their book, *The Diabetes Eye Care Sourcebook,* there are no medications that can effectively treat diabetic retinopathy. Aspirin was tested as a possible remedy but was not found effective at preventing retinopathy (however it also did not worsen retinopathy). Instead, the best "medicine" is to maintain good glucose control. The key reason for this is that often it was HYPERGLYCEMIA that caused and also escalated the retinopathy.

If the retinopathy is advanced, then laser surgery, also known as photocoagulation, may be recommended. The physician will use a laser to make tiny burns over the surface of the retina in order to destroy blood vessels growing over the surface of the eye or stop leakage from retinal vessels.

Lasers have been the mainstay treatment of diabetic retinopathy since the 1970s. Laser photocoagulation reduces the risk of blindness in people with diabetes by approximately 50 percent. The laser makes burns in the eye area where the doctor directs it. The advantages of laser therapy are that no incision is required and that it is a procedure that can be performed on an outpatient basis. It's best done when eyesight is still normal or near normal.

There are a variety of forms of laser treatments. Focal laser, for example, is used to seal off leaky blood vessels. Another form of treatment is scatter photocoagulation or panretinal photocoagulation. In this laser procedure, the ophthalmologist uses hundreds of applications. The procedure may need to be repeated more than once.

Sometimes surgery requiring an incision must be performed. The vitrectomy is a surgical procedure that removes old blood and scar tissue from within the eye, all of which resulted from the disease. The doctor may also seek to reattach the retina with a gas bubble. As of 2001, this procedure is successful in 90 percent of the cases where it is attempted.

Research on alternative remedies Some preliminary research performed at the JOSLIN DIA-

BETES CENTER in Boston and released in 1999 indicated that very high doses of vitamin E might help reduce already-existing eye damage. This issue needs further study before physicians can recommend this treatment. It's also unwise for people with diabetes to self-medicate with vitamin E without first discussing this plan with their physician.

Leptin and eye disease Preliminary studies performed at Yale University and reported in 2000 have indicated that high levels of LEPTIN, a substance known to exist in fatty tissue, was also present in patients with diabetic retinopathy. Apparently, excessive leptin may cause blood vessels to grow. This finding is still being evaluated for its ramifications, and further study is anticipated.

Screening Children with Diabetes for Diabetic Retinopathy

The sections of endocrinology and ophthalmology of the American Academy of Pediatrics discussed screening in a 1998 issue of *Pediatrics*. It was recommended that children with Type 1 diabetes and no symptoms of eye disease should receive an examination within the first year of diagnosis of diabetes and then at three- to five-year intervals for children who are over the age of nine years.

Prevention of Retinopathy

The American Academy of Ophthalmology regularly releases their assertion that it is necessary for individuals with diabetes to receive annual eye screenings by an ophthalmologist. (This is a disputed contention and some experts do not agree that screenings must be annual or that they must be performed by an ophthalmologist.)

Patients with diabetes are well advised to take the following actions:

- Strictly control glucose levels. The DIABETES CONTROL AND COMPLICATIONS TRIAL (DCCT) revealed that those patients who kept their hemoglobin A1c at 7 percent had $^1/_4$ the rate of retinopathy experienced by those whose

A1c was at 9 percent. (i.e., a 76 percent reduction). Similar results were seen in the UNITED KINGDOM PROSPECTIVE DIABETES STUDY (UKPDS) in which patients with Type 2 diabetes were studied.

- Control hypertension. High blood pressure contributes to eye problems. The goal is less than 135/85

- Stop smoking

- See an ophthalmologist if pregnant or hoping to become pregnant, to detect any early indications of eye problems

- Go to the ophthalmologist if vision is blurred, you have double vision, or you feel pressure in the eye. Other indicators of possible problems are diminished peripheral (side) vision or lines that appear wavy to the patient when they are actually straight.

Blurred Vision and Diabetic Retinopathy

Dramatic swings in glucose levels from low to high and vice versa can lead to very blurry vision and this is yet another reason to maintain good glycemic control. The lens of the eye does not need insulin to take up glucose. Glucose enters the lens and is converted to SORBITOL, an osmotically active particle. It then draws water into the lens and causes blurred vision.

Patients are advised to avoid getting new glasses or contact lenses until they have stabilized their glycemic control for at least four to six weeks.

Exercise Precautions for People with Diabetic Retinopathy

According to the American Diabetes Association, there are some physical activities that should be discouraged among patients with moderate-to-severe diabetic retinopathy. Some examples are power lifting, boxing, weight lifting, jogging, high-impact aerobics, and racquet sports (tennis/badminton/squash/racquetball). Trumpet playing (or playing of similar instruments) should also be avoided.

Some activities that are recommended even with severe diabetic retinopathy, are swimming, walking, stationary cycling, and low-impact aerobics. Activities that have less pressure and less up and down motion are recommended.

For further information, contact:

American Academy of Ophthalmology
655 Beach Street
San Francisco, CA 94109-7424
(415) 561-8500
www.eyenet.org

National Eye Health Education Program
2020 Vision Place
Bethesda, MD 20892-3655

(See also BLINDNESS, BLURRED VISION, CATARACTS, EYE PROBLEMS, GLAUCOMA, and MACULAR EDEMA.)

American Academy of Pediatrics, "Screening for Retinopathy in the Pediatric Patient with Type 1 Diabetes Mellitus," *Pediatrics* 101, no. 2 (February 1998): 313–314.
American Diabetes Association, "Diabetes Mellitus and Exercise," *Diabetes Care* 24, Supp. 1 (2001): 551–555.
Centers for Disease Control and Prevention and the National Institutes of Health, "Diabetes," in *Healthy People 2010,* 2000.
The Diabetes Control and Complications Trial Research Group, "Early Worsening of Diabetic Retinopathy in the Diabetes Control and Complications Trial," *The Archives of Ophthalmology* 116 (1998): 874–886.
Donald S. Fong, M.D., M.P.H., and Robin Demi Ross, M.D., *The Diabetes Eye Care Sourcebook.* (Los Angeles, Calif.: Lowell House, 1999).
Maureen I. Harris, Ph.D., M.P.H., "Is the Risk of Diabetic Retinopathy Greater in Non-Hispanic Blacks and Mexican Americans Than in Non-Hispanic Whites with Type 2 Diabetes?" *Diabetes Care* 21, no. 8 (August 1998): 1230–1235.
Gareth Williams and John C. Pickup, *Handbook of Diabetes* (Oxford, England: Blackwell Science, 1999).

diabetologist A physician who specializes in the diagnosis and treatment of people who have diabetes. This is a descriptive title but it is not an officially recognized specialty by the American Board of Internal Medicine. Most ENDOCRINOLOGISTS are also diabetologists.

Some internists take an extra year of training to learn more about diabetes. Most endocrinologists take a two- to three-year fellowship to master diabetes and endocrinology.

diagnosis (of diabetes) A medical doctor's determination that a person has diabetes and/or another illness. The decision to test for diabetes may be made as a result of SYMPTOMS a person is experiencing that indicate the possibility of diabetes (such as extreme thirst and/or hunger, repeated minor infections, frequent urination, etc.) A preliminary diagnosis of diabetes is also considered based on underlying risk factors that the patient has (OBESITY, sedentary lifestyle, ethnicity, steroid use, family history of diabetes, etc.).

These risk factors may be discovered as a part of a planned office visit, or during a routine annual checkup, or during an employment physical examination. These risk factors are particularly significant if the patient is older than about age 45.

Important Elements of a Diagnosis

This diagnosis should result from the following elements:

- A careful medical history, including questions about the patient's biological relatives (particularly parents and siblings), the presence of gestational diabetes, the past delivery of large babies or information on whether the patient was a large or small baby

- A physical examination

- A review of any symptoms the patient may exhibit, such as extreme thirst, frequent urination, slow healing cuts/wounds, blurred vision, unexplained weight loss, and other symptoms that are typically found among people who have diabetes

- Blood glucose testing. The doctor may also choose to order other tests.

CHARACTERISTICS OF INDIVIDUALS WITH DIAGNOSED DIABETES IN THE UNITED STATES, 1997

Total Population, 1997	Overall Cases of Diagnosed Diabetes
	Rate per 1,000
TOTAL	40
Race and ethnicity	
Black or African American	74
White	36
Hispanic or Latino	61
Gender	
Female	40
Male	39
Education level (aged 25 years and older)	
Less than high school	95
High school graduate	58
At least some college	44
Geographic location	
Urban	40
Rural	38
Disability status	
Persons with disabilities	87
Persons without disabilities	28
Select populations	
Age groups (not age adjusted)	
18 to 44 years	15
45 to 64 years	76
65 to 74 years	143
75 years and older	117

Diagnosing Type 1 diabetes   Individuals who have Type 1 diabetes are usually easier to diagnose because their bodies produce *no* insulin and thus they are typically in a more acute state with more symptoms and are often sicker. Their symptoms of thirst, extreme urination, and other typical symptoms cannot be ignored by any competent physician.

Diagnosing Type 2 diabetes   Making the diagnosis of Type 2 diabetes can be a much more difficult task because the person with Type 2 diabetes may be exhibiting no symptoms or, if symptoms are present, they may be mild. Many people with Type 2 diabetes are not diagnosed for years after the onset of the illness. Unfortunately, if the disease progresses for years without diagnosis or treatment, serious complications can occur as well.

Knowing the risk factors for diabetes helps doctors determine if a person is a likely candidate to develop the illness. Obesity and a family history for the disease are the two major risk factors and if a patient is obese and has parents or siblings with diabetes, physicians should check for the illness. In addition, as people age, they are more at risk for developing the disease.

People from certain ethnic groups are at particular risk for developing Type 2 diabetes, such as African Americans, Hispanics, and some Native American tribes. However, a person who is white, of medium or even small build, and who is not obese can still have Type 2 diabetes—it is less likely to be seen, however, than in a person who fits the various risk categories.

ADA criteria for diagnosing diabetes   As of this writing (2001), the American Diabetes Association criteria for the diagnosis of diabetes is as follows:

A blood test that is done without regard to the time of the last meal (fasting is not required), with a resulting plasma glucose level that is equal to or greater than 200 mg/dL. With this criteria, the doctor will be looking for symptoms such as frequent urination (polyuria), frequent drinking of fluids or intense thirst (polydipsia) or an unexplained weight loss. Another sign of diabetes is a fasting plasma glucose level that is equal to or greater than 126 mg/dL OR a plasma glucose level that is measured after the patient takes 75 g oral glucose. The level for diabetes must be equal to or greater than 200 mg/dL 2 hours after taking the oral glucose.

Confirmation on a later day with one of these tests is also required before diabetes can be diagnosed with certainty.

A fasting plasma glucose of 110–125 mg/dL is now classified as impaired fasting glucose and glucose levels between 140–199 mg/dL on a 2-hour OGTT are classified as having impaired glucose tolerance (IGT).

Physicians and patients need to be attuned to the risk factors that would place a patient at a much higher risk and to screen these patients. It is also clear that the scientific community should continue to work on diagnostic tests and schemes that will allow physicians to identify people with diabetes at a much earlier stage.

When screening can occur   Diabetes can be screened for at any time of the day. The first abnormality seen prior to the development of overt diabetes is an abnormal increase in the glucose levels after a meal. Thus, many physicians favor an oral glucose tolerance test in an attempt to diagnose and ascertain the risk early: Does the person have euglycemia (normal glucose levels), impaired glucose tolerance (IGT), impaired fasting glucose (IFG), or overt diabetes mellitus? As a practical matter, many patients are screened at the time of an office visit via fingerstick glucose and thus many are being checked after a meal.

Many experts suggest that if the fasting glucose level is 100–110, then the person should be tested with an oral glucose tolerance test (OGTT). The reason for this is that there is a progressive risk for people with impaired glucose tolerance to progress to overt diabetes. The OGTT can better screen for those people who fall into this category. Also, more people have impaired glucose tolerance than have impaired fasting glucose.

The Diabetes Prevention Program of over 3,000 patients with impaired glucose tolerance (68 percent female) showed that 150 minutes of exercise per week and 5–7 percent weight loss led to a 58 percent decrease in the numbers of subjects who progressed to overt Type 2 diabetes. The group treated with METFORMIN (glucophage) had a 33 percent decrease in the risk of progression.

The DECODE trial from Europe showed that patients with impaired glucose tolerance appear to have a higher risk of developing cardiovascular disease. This may confirm earlier observations that seem to suggest that elevated postprandial glucose levels (levels taken after a meal) are a better predictor of the development of coronary heart disease than the level of the fasting glucose.

Traits of individuals diagnosed with diabetes
Most people with diabetes have Type 2 diabetes. Researchers have also looked at overall characteristics of individuals diagnosed with diabetes. (See table.) As seen from the chart, blacks and Hispanics have a much higher rate of Type 2 diabetes than whites, or 74 cases per 1,000 for blacks, 61 for Hispanics or Latinos, and 36 for whites.

People with less than a high school education have the highest rate of diabetes, or 95 cases per 1,000. The rate drops to 58 cases per 1,000 for high school graduates and still further to 44 per 1,000 for individuals with some college education. It is unclear why this discrepancy exists, although perhaps more educated people have more healthful habits and are less prone to developing Type 2 diabetes.

When it comes to age, the rate is only 15 cases per 1,000 for people ages 18 to 44 years, rising dramatically to 76 cases per 1,000 for those who are 45 to 64, and rising yet again to 143 for those ages 65 to 74 years. The rate then drops to 117 per 1,000 for those ages 75 and older. It is unclear why the rate drops, although perhaps many individuals with diabetes have died by that time from the COMPLICATIONS of the illness, such as CARDIOVASCULAR DISEASE, END-STAGE or RENAL DISEASE.

(See also EARLY DETECTION, IMPAIRED GLUCOSE TOLERANCE, SYMPTOMS.)

A. J. G. Hanley, S. B. Harris, and B. Zinman, "Application of the Revised American Diabetes Association Criteria for the Diagnosis of Diabetes in a Canadian Native Population," [letter] *Diabetes Care* 21 (1998): 870–871.

G. Ko, J. C. N. Chan, and V .T. F. Yeung, et al. "Combined Use of a Fasting Plasma Glucose Concentration and HgbA1c or Fructosamine Predicts the Likelihood of Having Diabetes in High-risk Subjects," *Diabetes Care* 21, no. 8 (1998): 1221–1225.

Expert Committee on the Diagnosis and Classification of Diabetes Mellitus. Report of the Expert Committee on the Diagnosis and Classification of Diabetes Mellitus, *Diabetes Care* 20 (1997): 1183–1197.

dialysis   See END-STAGE RENAL DISEASE (ESRD).

diastolic blood pressure   Blood pressure maintained by the heart between heart contractions and the lower number or denominator when blood pressure results are reported. In contrast, systolic pressure is the peak pressure generated by the left ventricle as the heart contracts and is the numerator or top number that is reported. The heart spends about $2/3$ of its time in diastole and $1/3$ in systole.

Individuals with both Type 1 and Type 2 diabetes are at high risk for developing high levels of both diastolic and systolic blood pressure, or HYPERTENSION. When combined with diabetes, hypertension can often lead to severe COMPLICATIONS, such as BLINDNESS, NEPHROPATHY (kidney disease), STROKE, and even DEATH. (See also SYSTOLIC PRESSURE.)

diet   Planned intake of food. May also refer to patterns of foods eaten by an individual, such as a low-fat diet, a high carbohydrate diet, and so forth. There is no one diet for people with diabetes because people vary greatly in their nutritional needs, depending on size, age, and many other factors. As a result, people with diabetes need to work with a registered dietitian to plan a diet that would work best for them to keep their glucose levels as close to normal as possible.

The daily diet is an extremely important aspect of the lives of most people with diabetes because their diet is a key factor in helping to improve (or worsen) their GLYCEMIC CONTROL. In the early stages of Type 2 diabetes, careful attention to diet alone may often be sufficient to keep the illness in check. People with Type 1 diabetes, however, require insulin to remain alive, and they also need to carefully monitor their diets.

Although it is no longer considered necessary for a person with diabetes to give up all sweets forever, it's a good idea to restrict their consumption, not only to keep glucose levels as close to normal as possible, but also to limit the risk of OBESITY, which in itself creates more problems. However, many patients with diabetes report that they resent it when others snatch high-calorie or sugary food away from them because such foods are considered "bad." It's important for the person with diabetes to control his or her own diet to the greatest extent possible.

As a result, dietitians and diabetes experts have created listings or exchanges for the grams of carbohydrates and fats in a wide variety of foods, so that a person with diabetes can make personal choices. This means that if the individual wishes to have a small piece of cake, then he or she would avoid another carbohydrate, such as rice or potato.

Typical meal plans or diets for patients with diabetes contain less than 30 percent of their calories from fat, 50–60 percent from carbohydrates, and 10–20 percent of calories from protein.

For further information, contact:

American Dietetic Association
216 West Jackson Boulevard
Suite 800
Chicago, IL 60606
(312) 899-0040 or (800) 366-1655
(Consumer Nutrition Hotline from 9 A.M.–4 P.M. Central Time, Monday–Friday only)

(See also CARBOHYDRATE COUNTING, DIETITIAN, HYPOGLYCEMIA, MEAL PLANNING, NUTRITION.)

dietitian   Person who is registered in and an expert on nutrition and can advise on healthy eating habits. Upon diagnosis, people with diabetes should receive their health care from a team of experts, including a dietitian. Dietitians can help the patients with meal planning and weight control, and may also assist with any problematic eating patterns. They help patients develop a meal/nutrition plan that they can live with and one that is adapted to an individual's needs and special circumstances. Annual referrals to a dietitian may be advisable, depending on the individual and his or her ability to adapt to the illness.

People with diabetes should look for RDs, or registered dietitians, and, if possible, for one who is also a certified diabetes educator or C.D.E.

Many insurance plans will now cover some consultation on a yearly basis with a registered dietitian. Patients are advised to resubmit claims if they are denied or to appeal the denial, backed up with an accompanying letter from their medical doctor that this education will improve control, prevent complications, and will also save money.

DIGAMI Study   Refers to the Diabetes Mellitus Insulin Glucose Infusion in Acute Myocardial Infarction (DIGAMI) study. Diabetes patients have a two to four times greater risk for death from a myocardial infarction than nondiabetics. The DIGAMI study group looked at the impact of very tight glucose control on the patients' subsequent cardiac history and the researchers found that a significant impact resulted from intensive control.

In this study, 620 Swedish patients with diabetes and an acute myocardial mellitus syndrome were divided into two groups. The first group, 306 patients, received standard intravenous glucose and insulin infusions followed by insulin injection therapy, and the remaining 314 patients received standard diabetes care, mainly the use of oral diabetes medications. These patients were followed by an average of 3.4 years, The insulin-treated group had a 33 percent mortality, and the control group had a 44 percent mortality—an absolute decrease of 11 percent and a relative decrease of 25 percent. Despite this impressive result, experts in the United States disagree about whether it was the early and intensive sulfonylureas medications in the treatment group or another factor that resulted in the difference.

Jennifer Cummings, M.D., et al. "A Review of the DIGAMI Study: Intensive Insulin Therapy During and After Myocardial Infarctions in Diabetic Patients," from *Diabetes Spectrum* 12, no. 2 (1999), in *Annual Review of Diabetes 2000* (Alexandria, Va: American Diabetes Association, 2000).

digestive disorders   Dysfunctions of the various parts of the digestive system, primarily including the esophagus, stomach, and small and large intestine. Individuals with diabetes, particularly those who have had long-term diabetes, are at risk for a variety of digestive disorders. Although many people believe that it is only people with Type 1 diabetes who have digestive disorders, studies have revealed that many people with Type 2 diabetes also experience gastrointestinal problems, ranging from mild to very severe ailments.

In an article for a 1999 issue of *Diabetes Reviews,* author Dr. Aaron Vinik and his colleagues say that as many as 75 percent of all patients with diabetes eventually develop some form of esophageal (food tube) motor disorders.

Other digestive disorders that people with diabetes often experience are GASTROESOPHAGEAL REFLUX DISEASE (GERD), also commonly called "heartburn," and ulcer disease.

According to Doctors Wolosin and Edelman, in their article on digestive disorders in a 2000 issue of *Clinical Diabetes,* up to 75 percent of patients receiving treatment at diabetes clinics will suffer from significant gastrointestinal symptoms at some point.

The authors say,

The entire GI tract can be affected by diabetes from the oral cavity and esophagus to the large bowel and anorectal region. Thus, the symptom complex that may be experienced can vary widely. Common complaints may include dysphagia [difficulty swallowing, possibly due to a narrowed esophagus], early satiety [fullness], reflux [GERD], constipation, abdominal pain, nausea, vomiting, and diarrhea. Many patients go undiagnosed and undertreated because the GI tract has not been traditionally associated with diabetes and its complications.

The most commonly seen digestive disorders among people with diabetes are:

- slow stomach emptying (GASTROPARESIS)
- constipation (colonic dysmotility)
- diabetic diarrhea (often nocturnal and uncontrolled)
- candida esophagitis (yeast infection of the esophagus)

Some other digestive problems that patients with diabetes may experience are:

- Yeast infections in the GI tract and mouth
- abdominal pain and bloating
- pancreatic dysfunction (primarily found in patients with Type 1 diabetes)
- fatty liver

Gastroparesis and Diabetes

About 25 percent of those with diabetes have gastroparesis (slow stomach emptying), which itself may lead to or be associated with other medical problems such as severe chronic heartburn/GERD and may make glycemic control difficult. For example, insulin is injected and food is eaten, but when the person has gastroparesis, the food is moved forward and digested at a slower or more sporadic rate. This may lead to hypoglycemia.

Problems with Constipation

Constipation is another very common digestive problem, found in about 25 percent of patients with diabetes. When it becomes severe, fecal matter may become impacted and medical attention is required at that point. Diarrhea is also a problem that is experienced by about 20 percent of people with diabetes. It may result from bacterial overgrowth, malabsorption, and other problems stemming from diabetic neuropathy. Many people with diabetes suffer from intermittent bouts of both constipation and diarrhea. They may have typical irritable bowel syndrome (IBS), although IBS does not appear to be more common among patients with diabetes than among those in the general population.

Poor Glycemic Control Is a Risk Factor

Individuals with poor GLYCEMIC CONTROL and/or DIABETIC NEUROPATHY are more likely to experience digestive disorders. Chronic hyperglycemia leads to AUTONOMIC NEUROPATHY which causes the stomach to empty at a slower than normal rate (GASTROPARESIS DIABETICORUM). This delayed emptying is initially a problem in just the digestion of solid foods but it can later deteriorate to include a slowed digestion of liquids as well.

Acute Digestive Problems

Sometimes diabetes can lead to acute digestive problems. Doctors Mesiya and Minocha say, in their 1998/1999 article for *Clinical Reviews*, "Acute problems include acute stress gastritis during ketoacidosis, acute pancreatitis and acute cholecystitis [gallbladder inflammation]. Most problems, are however chronic, and may manifest with remissions and relapses." In addition patients with DIABETIC KETOACIDOSIS (DKA) often have upper abdominal (epigastric) pain of unclear etiology that clears up when the DKA improves. It is often mistaken for an ulcer or pancreatitis. The illness may stem from abnormal movements in the gut with subsequent stretching of the bowel and stimulation of nerve fibers that transmit pain. It may also stem from the direct effects of the elevated glucose or the ketoacids.

To treat the digestive disorder, prescribed or over-the-counter medications may also be used, depending on the specific digestive problem, its severity, and the health of the patient. In rare cases, surgery may be required.

Lifestyle Changes May Help

To help resolve or improve their digestive problems, many doctors recommend that patients with diabetes institute a diet that is high in FIBER and that they also eat small and frequent meals rather than "three square meals" per day. However, some experts caution that high amounts of fiber may create more problems in some individuals with diabetes, particularly those who have gastroparesis. Each person with diabetes should consult with their physician to determine whether extra fiber is best in their case. It's also better for everyone to eat the larger meal at lunch rather than in the evening, so that most of the meal is digested before the person goes to bed.

Doctors strongly advise their patients who smoke to stop as soon as possible, especially when they have both diabetes and digestive problems. Smoking further aggravates many digestive disorders.

Jeffrey L. Barnett, "Gut Reactions (How Diabetes Can Affect the Gastrointestinal Tract)," *Diabetes Forecast* 50, no. 8 (August 1997): 26–30.

Gerald Bernstein, M.D., "The Diabetic Stomach: Management Strategies for Clinicians and Patients," *Diabetes Spectrum*, 12 (2000): 11–20.

Sikander A. Mesiya, M.D., and Anil Minocha, M.D., F.A.C.P., F.A.C.G., "Gastrointestinal Disease in Diabetes Mellitus," *Clinical Reviews* (Winter 1998/1999): 33–38.

Aaron Vinik, M.D., Ph.D., F.C.P., F.A.C.P., et al., "Gastrointestinal, Genitourinary, and Neurovascular Disturbances in Diabetes," *Diabetes Reviews* 7, no. 4 (1999): 346–366.

James D. Wolosin, M.D., F.A.C.P., and Steven V. Edelman, M.D., "Diabetes and the Gastrointestinal Tract," *Clinical Diabetes* 18, no. 4 (Fall 2000): 148–151.

disability/disability benefits A disability is a medical problem that makes it difficult or impossible for a person to perform tasks that others of about the same age and abilities could perform without difficulty. Disability benefits are the financial or medical benefits received by such a person from the federal or state government or from a private employer.

According to the CENTERS FOR DISEASE CONTROL AND PREVENTION (CDC), people with diabetes have a higher rate of disability than nondiabetics. About half of those diagnosed with diabetes (4.1 million) reported a disability that limited their activities in 1996. Of these 4.1 million people, 65 percent said they were limited because of their diabetes.

In 1996, people with diabetes averaged about 36 days per year when they had to restrict their activities. Of these 36 days, 17 days were spent in bed. On average, black patients had a greater number of restricted activity and bed days than whites. When considering gender, females had a greater number of restricted activity and bed days than males.

Disability Benefits

The illness may have been caused by the job or it may be completely independent of work, such as with the development of diabetes or other ailments. The individual who is disabled may be able to collect short-term or long-term disability from an employer, depending on many different factors.

The federal government also has several disability programs. Social Security Administration Disability is one major program and was created for people who have worked for a sufficient time in the past. Another program is the Supplemental Security Insurance (SSI) program for disabled children and adults who have either never worked or who have not worked for enough time.

The person alleging disability must obtain medical documentation on the existence of the disability, how long it is expected to last or if it is considered indefinite, and other related issues. It may take months or even years before the federal government adjudicates the disability.

In the case of a disability approved and acknowledged as valid by the Social Security Administration, the amount paid will date back to the date of application. However, in many cases of SSA disability, the claimant will have contracted with an attorney to document and prove his or her case. At the time of adjudication, the attorney is then entitled to some percentage of the lump sum payment that dates back to the point of application.

For further information, contact:

Disability Rights Education and Defense
  Fund, Inc.
2212 6th Street
Berkeley, CA 94710
(510) 644-2555 or (800) 466-4232 (Toll-free)

(See also AMERICANS WITH DISABILITIES ACT, FAMILY AND MEDICAL LEAVE ACT, EMPLOYMENT, SSI.)

Edward W. Gregg, Ph.D., et al., "Diabetes and Physical Disability Among Older U.S. Adults," *Diabetes Care* 23, no. 10 (October 2000): 1272–1277.

diuretics Also known as "water pills," these are medications that are taken to rid the body of excess fluids and sodium by increasing the amount of urine excreted by the kidneys. Diuretics may be extremely helpful for those who have CORONARY HEART DISEASE (CHD), HYPERTENSION, or congestive heart failure.

Such medications generally cause a loss of salt and water and may be helpful in low doses to treat patients with edema. However, they can also cause decreased levels of insulin secretion and worsen hyperglycemia. Most people with diabetes can take diuretic medications if they are used judiciously and under the watchful care of a physician who is knowledgeable about diabetes.

Studies such as the Systolic Hypertension in the Elderly Program (SHEP) have proven that diuretic medications can reduce the risk of STROKE among patients with diabetes. Because people with Type 2 diabetes have from two to three times the risk of death from CARDIOVASCULAR DISEASE compared to the general population, a diuretic may be a lifesaving drug for such patients.

Timothy C. Fagan, M.D., and James Sowers, M.D., "Type 2 Diabetes Mellitus. Greater Cardiovascular Risks and Greater Benefits of Therapy," *Archives of Internal Medicine* 159, no. 10 (May 24, 1999): 1033–1034.

driving   Legally operating a motor vehicle.

Most adults with diabetes drive without incident; however, if the individual becomes dehydrated or overly tired, he or she is more likely to be impaired. It's very important for the person in such a case to pull over and treat himself or herself and also to assess possible indications of HYPOGLYCEMIA.

Some people with diabetes are denied a commercial driver's license because of the stated or unstated fear that the person might have a severe attack of hypoglycemia and, consequently, could become disoriented or even unconscious. This apparently rarely happens and most people with diabetes recognize hypoglycemic symptoms that indicate that their glucose levels are out of control, and they are able to act immediately.

There are, however, a small number of people who have HYPOGLYCEMIC UNAWARENESS, which means that they have no prior symptoms before severe hypoglycemia suddenly occurs. Such people often have repeated bouts of severe hypoglycemia.

According to an article in a 1999 issue of the *Journal of the American Medical Association (JAMA)*, in their report on driving by people with Type 1 diabetes, researchers stated that these individuals "may not judge correctly when their blood sugar levels are too low and may consider driving with a low BG [blood glucose level]." The researchers considered less than 70 mg/dL to be low.

Confusing Hypoglycemia with Alcohol Intoxication

In some cases, a person with diabetes and who is suffering from hypoglycemia may be mistaken for a drunk driver by a police officer. There have been reported cases in which people with diabetes were placed in jail and not given the medical treatment they needed because of the appearance of drunkenness. For this reason, a medical identification bracelet is very important for all individuals who have diabetes. Of course, everyone with diabetes should have a plan for what to do should their blood glucose levels swing dangerously out of control.

An Action Plan for Drivers with Diabetes

Experts such as Santa Monica, California, attorney Kriss Halpern, himself an individual with Type 1 diabetes and who assists people with diabetes with alleged discrimination claims, has recommended that individuals with Type 1 diabetes take the following actions to deal with possible hypoglycemia:

- If you prefer to treat hypoglycemia with liquids, keep a fluid with sugar that doesn't spoil quickly such as apple juice in the car. Some individuals prefer to use candy or gel packs of glucose.
- If the individual with Type 1 diabetes begins to feel that his or her blood sugar is low, then he or she should pull over immediately.
- Have testing equipment readily accessible (not in the trunk of the car).
- The individual with a low blood glucose problem should not immediately return to the road after treatment. Instead, he or she should wait until blood glucose levels are normal, and they also feel completely recovered. This may take 20–45 minutes.

After treatment with juice, candy, or glucose gels, it is important to follow up with more food containing protein and/or fat, in addition to carbohydrates, such as crackers, milk, or sandwiches. This is done to prevent the recurrence of low blood sugar, particularly if the individual is on a long drive.

Claire Laberge-Nadeau M.D., M.Sc., et al., "Impact of Diabetes on Crash Risks of Truck-Permit Holders and Commercial Drivers," *Diabetes Care* 23, no. 5 (May 2000): 612–617.

Gerald McGwin, Jr., Ph.D., et al., "Diabetes and Automobile Crashes in the Elderly," *Diabetes Care* 22, no. 2 (1999): 220–227.

drug interactions   See MEDICATION INTERACTIONS.

dry skin (xerosis)   An extremely common problem experienced by people with diabetes. Dry skin may be treated with a variety of creams and lotions. These are available either over the counter or by prescription. Dry skin may also become itchy and inflamed and could also become infected. Sometimes as a result of DIABETIC NEUROPATHY, the patient may experience no sweating (anhidrosis), which further increases the problem of dry skin.

Many individuals with diabetes have a problem with dry skin on their feet which leads to cracks in the skin, especially in the heels, predisposing the patients to pain and infection.

As a result, it is very important, especially for those with Type 1 diabetes, to keep the feet clean and moisturized, except between the toes, which should be kept dry to avoid maceration of skin tissue leading to fungal infections and skin breakdown. Thus, daily vigilance to foot care cannot be overemphasized. Patients should also use super-fatted soaps. (See also SKIN PROBLEMS.)

dyslipidemia   An imbalance of serum lipoproteins, such as high density lipoprotein cholesterol (HDL) and low density lipoprotein cholesterol (LDL). Dyslipidemia can lead to ATHEROSCLEROSIS, STROKE, and other serious ailments. People with Type 2 diabetes are more prone to suffering from dyslipidemia than nondiabetics. They are especially prone to high triglyceride levels and lower HDL cholesterol levels.

When dyslipidemia is combined with other risk factors (such as OBESITY or SMOKING), the risk for severe disease is further accelerated.

American Diabetes Association, "Position Statement: Management of Dyslipidemia in Adults with Diabetes," *Diabetes Care* 24, Supp. 1 (2001): S58–S61.

Paul S. Jellinger, M.D., F.A.C.E., Chairman, "The American Association of Clinical Endocrinologists Medical Guidelines for Clinical Practice for the Diagnosis and Treatment of Dyslipidemia and Prevention of Atherogenesis," *Endocrine Practice* 6, no. 2 (March/April 2000): 162–213.

early detection   The diagnosis of diabetes in an early stage of the disease before the onset of complications caused by the disease. This is very important because when detected in the early stages, diabetes is far more manageable and far less likely to cause the severe damage that late-diagnosed diabetes may have already and irreversibly caused, such as diseases of the kidney or other organs.

The UNITED KINGDOM PROSPECTIVE DIABETES STUDY definitively showed that at the point of diagnosis with Type 2 diabetes, most patients had already lost half their ability to secrete insulin, and they were likely to have metabolic abnormalities that had been present for five to seven years prior to diagnosis. Thus, looking at risk factors and screening appropriate populations of individuals at risk for diabetes is critically important. The American Diabetes Association has a diabetes Alert Day every year in March to continue to try and teach the public about risk factors and to push those with significant risk to have screening tests.

It seems clear that the Oral Glucose Tolerance Test (OGTT) and also screening for postprandial (after a meal) hyperglycemia may allow physicians to diagnose diabetes sooner than if they relied upon measuring fasting plasma glucose levels. The older that patients are, the more true that this becomes, that is, they are more likely to have isolated postprandial hyperglycemia.

Some physicians believe that an early detection of TYPE 1 DIABETES may enable physicians to extend the HONEYMOON PHASE, or that time during which there is still some insulin produced by the pancreas.

The DIABETES PREVENTION TRIALS, studies being performed by the National Institutes of Health (NIH), seek to determine what actions may delay the onset of diabetes in individuals who show indications of developing Type 1 diabetes.

Damage That May Occur without Early Detection

Sometimes, by the time a person is diagnosed, very serious damage has occurred, such as the onset of DIABETIC RETINOPATHY. In addition, the female patient may have had frequent vaginal infections and the male patient may have had many urological infections (especially Candida BALANITIS).

eating disorders   Abnormal eating patterns, usually either eating too little or nothing at all (anorexia) or overeating and then inducing vomiting (bulimia). Many studies indicate that people with diabetes, particularly adolescent girls who have Type 1 diabetes, may be at an increased risk for developing eating disorders, including anorexia and bulimia. Eating disorders are associated with poor GLYCEMIC CONTROL. Some adolescent girls purposely withhold their insulin to try to manipulate their weight.

Adolescents with diabetes who seek tight glycemic control are at risk for gaining weight, which is one reason why some may develop eating disorders. Of the adolescents who were part of the DIABETES CONTROL AND COMPLICATIONS TRIAL (DCCT), nearly half (48 percent) gained enough weight to be considered overweight or obese, compared to only 28 percent of adolescents who became overweight while on conventional therapy.

According to Patricia Colton and her colleagues, authors of an article that appeared in a 1999 issue of *Psychiatric Annals,* eating disorder problems among adolescents with diabetes were first reported in the 1970s. Some researchers reporting on adolescents with Type 1 diabetes in 2001 challenge whether adolescent girls with diabetes are at greater risk for having eating disorders, finding few cases of such problems in their study. They did recommend, however, that adolescent females and young adults be screened for eating disorders.

Manipulation of Body Weight through Manipulation of Insulin

One eating disorder-related problem that is unique to girls who have diabetes, and which distresses the medical community, is either purposefully withholding their insulin or decreasing their prescribed insulin dose. This is done in order to lose weight. Adolescents often control their own insulin intake, with variable levels of supervision. As a result, it is possible for them to limit or altogether fail to take their medication, unbeknownst to adults in the adolescent's family or to their physicians—until they come in the doctor's office with significant weight loss or a very high hemoglobin A1c (indicating hyperglycemia).

Of course, sometimes adolescents fail to take their insulin for reasons other than a desire for weight loss. For example, they may be in DENIAL about their illness or may have a fear of low blood sugars (HYPOGLYCEMIA). They may also dislike or fear glucose testing or self-injections. Teenagers may also check their blood glucose levels less frequently than suggested by their physician or fail to check them at all. They may also simply forget or delay taking their insulin. Adolescents have a characteristically poor record with regard to testing their blood as often as they should and recording and acting upon the information.

A study reported in a 2000 issue of the *British Medical Journal* compared 356 adolescent girls in Canada between the ages of 12–19 years who had Type 1 diabetes to 1,098 nondiabetic girls in the same age group to determine the level of eating disorders in each group.

The researchers found that about 10 percent of the diabetic adolescents had an eating disorder problem versus only about 4 percent of the nondiabetic girls. They also found that about 11 percent of the girls with diabetes reported taking a below-normal dose of insulin as a weight loss remedy. (Some girls used this method intermittently in order to lose weight.) As might be expected, the mean blood A1c level was higher in the girls with diabetes who had an eating disorder than it was in the diabetic girls who did not have an eating disorder.

The researchers also found a higher percentage (14 percent) of the girls with diabetes who had a "subthreshhold" eating disorder. This is an abnormal eating pattern that meets some, but not all, of the criteria for a diagnosable disorder. About 8 percent of the nondiabetic girls had a subthreshhold eating disorder.

The worsening in glycemic control during adolescence may be attributed to hormonal changes. However, as mentioned earlier in this essay, it is also purposeful for some girls. The authors said in the *Psychiatric Annals* article,

> A subset of adolescent girls tend to be less compliant with a strict diabetic treatment regimen because of their body dissatisfaction, drive for thinness, and associated dietary dysregulation. Indeed 45–80 percent of adolescent girls with DM [diabetes mellitus] admit to binge eating, and 13 percent to 36 percent regularly omit or decrease their prescribed insulin dose in an attempt to control their weight and to compensate for binge eating. By decreasing or omitting their insulin dosage, individuals with DM cause their circulating blood sugar levels to rise, and a large number of calories, in the form of sugar [glucose], are lost in the urine. The frequency of this behavior is surprising and disturbing in view of the extensive education these individuals receive about the serious adverse health consequences of poor blood sugar control.

The authors pointed out circumstances in which purposeful insulin dosage manipulation should be suspected in an adolescent who may have an undiagnosed eating disorder that needs treatment. Some possible indicators they listed are:

- an unexplained high blood glucose level
- recurrent incidents of diabetic ketoacidosis (DKA) or hospitalizations
- frequent cases of hypoglycemia
- delayed growth and/or delayed puberty

Another study of adolescents with eating disorders concentrated on adolescents with diabetes and sought to determine whether eating disorders were linked to poor glycemic control (reported in a 2001 issue of *Diabetes Care*). The researchers studied 152 adolescents ages 11–19 years old. In general, the researchers did not find a pattern of eating disorders among adolescents with diabetes and found that some adolescents had more body satisfaction than a control group of nondiabetic adolescents. When they did find eating disorders, however, they also found poor glycemic control.

The researchers found a subset of teenagers who were at risk for eating disorders especially bulimia: females ages 13–14. There were also several other predictors for an eating disorder, such as a higher BODY MASS INDEX (BMI). Length of disease was also a predictor, with overweight adolescents who had had the illness for years at greater risk than newly diagnosed adolescents.

The researchers said,

It is interesting to note that male subjects did not report clinically significant symptoms of bulimia in any of the age-groups studied. Clearly, females seem to have more difficulty adapting to hormonal and physical changes associated with puberty and the onset of adolescence.

A Chronology of the Problem

When a young woman who is very slender due to undiagnosed diabetes is then placed on insulin therapy, she may begin to regain the lost weight because she has better blood glucose levels. There is no longer a loss of a considerable amount of calories in her urine and the patient goes from a breakdown type metabolism (catabolic) to a build up state (anabolic). This means her body is now able to store amino acids in protein, fatty acids into triglycerides, and glucose into glycogen.

In addition, the patient's appetite may improve when she is less ill, leading to a larger caloric intake. The increased weight may cause great consternation to a female adolescent, who may now find herself heavier than her friends (in contrast to prediagnosis, when she was probably thinner than average).

To attempt to regain her former weight, an adolescent may radically reduce the amount of food she eats, or she may manipulate her insulin dosages to cause a weight loss. Some adolescents with diabetes binge on food and then purge, although such behavior does not appear to be characteristic for the adolescent with diabetes, perhaps because, as experts speculate, she can manipulate her weight through withholding her insulin.

As a result, it is up to parents or guardians to challenge a sudden weight loss, or the presence of one or more of the previously mentioned indicators of a possible eating disorder. The short- and long-term consequences of eating disorders can be very serious for the adolescent, up to and including death.

Treatment of Eating Disorders

Individuals with eating disorders need help from experienced clinicians, usually a team that includes a mental health professional, registered dietitian, certified diabetes educator, and medical doctor. People with eating disorders may also need day treatment in a hospital or even need to be admitted to a hospital. The individual may also benefit from receiving cognitive-behavioral psychotherapy from a trained psychologist or therapist, who teaches the patient how to challenge unreasonable and unrealistic ideas, such as the importance of attaining a perfect body, and the idea that someone who is not slender is therefore a worthless person.

Can Diabetes Itself Trigger an Eating Disorder?

Some psychiatrists have speculated that the dietary and glycemic management that individuals with Type 1 diabetes need to practice may trigger an eating disorder. They further report that an intense emphasis on tight glycemic control might exacerbate the problem even further because such people may become extremely preoccupied with food and their body. Such individuals need to learn to manage their diabetes without becoming obsessed with the illness or with food, and that is why a trained and experienced diabetes care team is the best choice for an adolescent who has an eating disorder. (See also ADOLESCENTS, OBESITY.)

Patricia A. Colton, M.D., et al., "Eating Disturbances in Young Women with Type 1 Diabetes Mellitus: Mechanisms and Consequences," *Psychiatric Annals* 29, no. 4 (April 1, 1999): 213–218.

Lois Javonovic, M.D., "Diabetes in Women Introduction," *Diabetes Spectrum* 10, no. 2 (1997): 178–180.

Jennifer M. Jones et al., "Eating Disorders in Adolescent Females with and without Type 1 Diabetes: Cross Sectional Study," *British Medical Journal* 320, no. 7249 (June 2000): 1563–1566.

Lisa J. Meltzer M.S., et al., "Disordered Eating, Body Mass, and Glycemic Control in Adolescents with Type 1 Diabetes," *Diabetes Care* 24, no. 4 (2001): 678–682.

economic cost of diabetes   The expenses to society for the cost of health care for people with diabetes as well as the cost incurred because people with diabetes are unable to work.

The nationwide cost of diabetes in the United States was estimated at over $105 billion in 2000 and it continues to grow. More than one of every 10 healthcare dollars was spent on diabetes. About 25 percent of Medicare dollars and about 15 percent of all health care dollars are spent on individuals who have diabetes.

When complications from diabetes can be minimized, the economic cost to both the individual and to society is also decreased. This is yet another reason why it is important for the individual to maintain GLYCEMIC CONTROL as close to normal as possible. Studies have clearly proven that tight glycemic control decreases the incidences of complications from diabetes.

A complex cost analysis performed by Dr. Richard Eastman and his colleagues for Type 2 diabetes revealed that "recommended" care (more treatment and evaluation than is currently standard but less than intensive management) reduced the total costs to $29,851 per person per lifetime. This represented $1,000 in savings per person per lifetime compared to the total cost of standard care. Most of the savings were due to fewer problems with kidney and nerve disease.

Richard C. Eastman et al., "Prevention Strategies for Type 2 Diabetes Mellitus: A Health and Economic Perspective," in *Diabetes Mellitus: A Fundamental and Clinical Text* (Philadelphia, Pa.: Lippincott, Williams and Wilkins, 2000).

Gregory Nichols, Ph.D., "Type 2 Diabetes: Incremental Medical Care Costs During the 8 Years Preceding Diagnosis," *Diabetes Care* 23, no. 11 (November 2000): 1654–1659.

edema   An excess of fluid in the body that causes swelling and bloating, often found in areas such as the ankles. Edema may be a sign of kidney disease (NEPHROPATHY) or it may be a side effect of some medications, such as CALCIUM CHANNEL BLOCKERS or THIAZOLIDINEDIONES. Any patient with diabetes should report edema to the doctor. The physician may prescribe a DIURETIC to decrease the fluid.

Patients with chronic edema are usually instructed to weigh themselves daily and to report any changes of three or more pounds (up or down) in any one 24-hour period to their physician.

education about diabetes   Teaching individuals with diabetes and their families about the disease and what is needed to cope with it. Ideally, the person with diabetes would receive education from the team managing his or her case, including such team members as a physician, nurse, and dietitian.

Most diabetes experts believe that education is extremely important for individuals with diabetes and their families as well as for the general public. A key reason for educating the public is that many people (at least half of all those with Type 2 diabetes in the United States) have not yet been diagnosed with the illness. Education and awareness of the symptoms of diabetes can

lead people with the illness to their doctors and result in an earlier diagnosis and treatment. Early diagnosis and treatment is best because individuals may avoid developing complications of diabetes that are caused by nontreatment in the early stages of the disease.

Education of the general public is also important even for those who do not have or do not develop diabetes. For example, many people have a distorted view of the severity of diabetes and may regard a person with diabetes as an invalid. Yet, few people with diabetes require constant bed rest or frequent hospitalization (although people with diabetes are hospitalized more frequently—for brief periods—than nondiabetics). Instead, most people with diabetes are active individuals who are employed, have spouses and children, and lead full lives. Members of the general public should also be aware of HYPOGLYCEMIA and its treatment, so that they do not mistake the symptoms of hypoglycemia for intoxication or drug use.

Despite the importance of education about diabetes, researchers have found that less than half (45 percent) of the people who are actually diagnosed with diabetes have received education about their disease. As a result, these individuals are less likely to take actions necessary to control their disease effectively and to minimize the risk for COMPLICATIONS. They may not realize that taking such actions as performing regular foot examinations, having dilated eye examinations, and undergoing annual dental examinations can all screen for early signs of complications.

One of the "Healthy People 2010" federal government goals is that 60 percent of people with diabetes will receive education about their illness. Of course, 100 percent would be better, but that is not a feasible goal at this time.

According to the information provided in the table, both blacks and whites are about equally ill-informed about diabetes, although Hispanics with diabetes have an even lower percentage (34 percent). Females (49 percent) are more likely to be educated than males (42 percent), but the majority of women do not receive diabetes edu-

PERSONS WITH DIABETES AND PERCENTAGE RECEIVING EDUCATION ON DIABETES IN 1998	
Persons With Diabetes, 1998	**Diabetes Education**
TOTAL	45
Race and ethnicity	
Black or African American	45
White	46
Hispanic or Latino	34
Gender	
Female	49
Male	42
Education level (aged 25 years and older)	
Less than high school	26
High school graduate	43
At least some college	56
Geographic location	
Urban	49
Rural	37
Disability status	
Persons with disabilities	87
Persons without disabilities	28
Select populations	
18 to 44 years	48
45 to 64 years	47
65 to 74 years	40
75 years and older	27

Note: Age adjusted to the year 2000 standard population.

cation. Formal education is clearly related to diabetes education, and people with diabetes who have had at least some college education are the most likely (56 percent) to have received diabetes education. People in urban settings (49 percent) are more likely to receive diabetes education than people in rural settings (37 percent).

Sadly, as people age, they are less likely to receive diabetes education. Those who are ages 18–44 have the highest rate (48 percent) and the rate declined to 40 percent of those who are ages 65–74 and only 27 percent of those who are 75 years or older. Yet, it is older people who are most at risk for the complications of diabetes.

Most states now require insurance companies to pay for both initial and ongoing education for people with diabetes.

Maria L. De Alva, "Education: A Liberating Tool," *Diabetes Spectrum* 12, no. 3 (1999): 132.

elderly   People who are over age 65. Older individuals may have Type 1 diabetes, although they are a small subset of the group and instead, older people stand a much greater risk for developing or already having Type 2 diabetes than younger individuals. As individuals continue to age, the probability of being diagnosed with Type 2 diabetes increases each year. Graydon S. Meneilly and Daniel Tessier said, in their article on diabetes in elderly adults for a 2001 issue of the *Journal of Gerontology,*

> Because elderly patients with diabetes are living longer and are likely to use increasing amounts of scarce health care resources in the next several decades, diabetes in aged adults may ultimately prove to be the most important epidemic of the 21st century.

Who among the Elderly Has Diabetes

Overall, about 11 percent of all Americans ages 65–74 years have diabetes. About 20 percent of those who live to age 75 have diabetes, although about half of them are unaware that they have the disease. The rates of diabetes are significantly higher for African Americans, Hispanics, and Native Americans in the same groups. (See the

separate essays on these groups.) Diabetes is also a risk for older individuals in countries around the world, and will become an increasing burden over the next 20 years.

Diabetes Is Not "Normal" for Older People

Although about 20 percent of those over 75 have diabetes, this also means that about 80 percent do *not* have the illness. Thus, diabetes is not an inevitable consequence of aging. It is also true that among older people who do have diabetes, there are many positive actions that an individual can take to limit the often severe complications stemming from diabetes. Good GLYCEMIC CONTROL and exercise are as important to the person who is 80 years old (or older) as they are for the person who is 40 years old. (Of course, exercise must be tailored to the capabilities of the individual.)

Dr. Petrella said in his 1999 article on the elderly for *Physician & Sportsmedicine,*

> It is commonly believed that the elderly cannot respond to lifestyle interventions and that aging and chronic disease are inevitable, even though both perceptions have been disproved . . . Moreover, patients who adopt interventions can increase active life expectancy, decrease disability, and reduce healthcare costs. Although many questions remain about implementation, strategies for lifestyle change and exercise programs can mitigate the effects of chronic disease in older persons.

Different Symptoms from Younger People with Diabetes

According to authors Meneilly and Tessier, often hyperglycemia is not the key symptom of diabetes among older individuals. Instead, elderly people are more likely to be diagnosed with diabetes after they have been hospitalized for a complication of diabetes such as a STROKE or heart attack. Older individuals with diabetes are more likely to have PERIPHERAL NEUROPATHY. Also, malignant otitis externa, an ear infection caused by *Pseudomonas*, is seen most commonly among elderly people with diabetes.

High Risk of Hypoglycemia

Elderly individuals with diabetes have an elevated risk of HYPOGLYCEMIA, due to three key factors: first, their lack of knowledge of the early stages of hypoglycemia and second, their reduced awareness of these symptoms. Third, experts say that the symptoms of hypoglycemia are often less intense among older individuals.

Elderly Deaths from Diabetes

Diabetes is one of the six leading causes of death among people over age 65 in the United States. In fact, the death rate from diabetes is probably considerably underestimated since death certificates are often incomplete and inaccurate.

Deaths from diabetes were 107 per 100,000 in 1980 and steadily increased to 141 per 100,000 by 1997. The only other illness with deaths that went up more significantly was chronic obstructive pulmonary disease, which increased 57 percent over the same timeframe.

There are still greater numbers of elderly people who are dying from heart attacks and strokes than from diabetes but those numbers have gone down dramatically, according to the Federal Interagency Forum on Aging-Related Statistics in their report *Older Americans 2000: Key Indicators of Well-Being.*

As mentioned earlier, it is also true that some racial groups are more affected by diabetes than others, at all age levels. Among older Americans, diabetes is the third leading cause of death (after heart disease and cancer) for Native Americans and Alaska Natives. It is also the fourth leading cause of death for Hispanics. For whites, blacks, and Asian/Pacific Islanders, diabetes is the sixth leading cause of death.

Complications from Diabetes

Elderly individuals are more likely to suffer from the complications that are related to diabetes, such as BLINDNESS, CARDIOVASCULAR DISEASE, END-STAGE RENAL DISEASE (ESRD), and DIABETIC NEUROPATHY. According to the CENTERS FOR DISEASE CONTROL AND PREVENTION (CDC), lower extremity AMPUTATIONS are more common among people with dia-

betes who are over age 65. In fact, individuals in this group represent 64 percent of all amputations.

According to John R. White Jr. and R. K. Campbell, authors of the chapter on managing Type 2 diabetes in the book *Diabetes Mellitus in the Elderly,*

> The [older] patient with diabetes is 25 times more likely to become blind, 17 times more likely to develop kidney disease, 20 times more likely to develop gangrene, and 2 times more likely to suffer a stroke or a heart attack than aged matched cohorts without diabetes. However, recent studies have demonstrated a tight correlation between development and progression of most of the chronic complications of diabetes and strict glycemic control.

This means that the risks for complications are reduced with good glycemic control. In addition, elderly individuals with diabetes are more likely to suffer from DEPRESSION than are their nondiabetic age counterparts.

Costs of Diabetes

Diabetes is an expensive disease, particularly for those who pay the costs for elderly individuals with diabetes.

According to the Centers for Disease Control and Prevention (CDC), $32 billion represented the total direct medical expenditures that could be attributed to diabetes among people ages 65 and older in 1997. Key reasons for the high cost were hospitalizations, emergency room visits, and frequent outpatient visits.

Dr. Krop and colleagues, in their 1998 article for *Diabetes Care,* reported that the health care costs for the average older adult who has diabetes costs Medicare about 1.5 times more than that expended for other Medicare beneficiaries. (See also ECONOMIC COST.)

Misconceptions About Elderly with Diabetes

Because most discussions and written materials on Type 2 diabetes repeatedly state that obesity can lead to Type 2 diabetes, and also urge obese people to lose weight, many people then mistakenly conclude that thin people cannot develop diabetes. However, experts say that among older individuals, obesity should not be the primary criteria for determining whether diagnostic testing should occur, because slender people who are elderly may, in fact, have Type 2 diabetes. (Some experts believe that when diabetes occurs among thin elderly people, it is a form of the illness that actually falls between Type 1 and Type 2 diabetes, and they say it could be considered more of a "Type 1 1/2 diabetes.")

According to Dr. Mooradian and his colleagues in their 1999 article for *Diabetes Spectrum,* "obesity is not that common among older diabetes patients. In nursing homes [skilled nursing facilities], the problem of being underweight is as common as that of being overweight."

Other atypical symptoms found among older individuals with diabetes are as follows:

- anorexia
- incontinence
- falls
- behavioral or cognitive changes
- pain intolerance

Some individuals have none of the typical or atypical symptoms; however, most people do have some symptoms.

Exercise

It need not be strenuous to be effective. Exercise that is as simple as walking can be very beneficial to older people with diabetes. Most experts recommend low-impact aerobic EXERCISE. All older individuals should check with their doctors before initiating any exercise program. It's also good to test glucose levels before exercising, in case a snack is needed beforehand.

Disability

Some older individuals with diabetes have a high level of disability and may find it very difficult to exercise. They need a limited program tailored to their abilities.

In an article on physical disability and older people with diabetes in the United States, reported in a 2000 issue of *Diabetes Care,* researchers found that 32 percent of females and 15 percent of males with diabetes in their study were unable to walk 1/4 mile, climb stairs, or do house-work. This was in sharp contrast to a similar group of nondiabetic older people, of whom only 14 percent of women and 8 percent of the men were found unable to perform the same tasks.

Diabetes and Cognitive Abilities

Experts have found that diabetes has an effect on the thinking abilities of older people. In a study reported in a 2000 issue of the *Archives of Internal Medicine,* researchers tested the cognitive abilities of nearly 10,000 women who were age 65 and older, including 682 diabetic women. The researchers retested the same women again over the next 3–6 years.

The women with diabetes had a significant decline in their thinking and were more impaired than the nondiabetic women in several of the tests. As a result, researchers determined that older women with diabetes were at greater risk for cognitive difficulties than other aging women who are nondiabetic.

Treatment for Elderly Individuals with Diabetes

Older individuals with diabetes can show considerable improvements with some medications. For example, such studies as the Systolic Hypertension in the Elderly Program (SHEP) study demonstrated that among older individuals with HYPERTENSION and diabetes, those who used DIURETICS dramatically reduced their risk for STROKE. In addition the Heart Outcomes Prevention Evaluation (HOPE) study demonstrated that angiotensin-converting enzyme (ACE) inhibitor medications could reduce the risk of complications and death among elderly individuals with diabetes.

For further information, contact the following organizations:

National Council on Aging
409 3rd Street, SW
2nd Floor
Washington, DC 20024
(202) 479-1200 or (800) 424-9046 (toll-free)
(202) 479-0735 (Fax)

AARP
601 E Street, NW
Washington, DC 20049
(202) 434-2277
(202) 434-2558 (Fax)

(See also AGE, AFRICAN AMERICANS, ASSISTED LIVING FACILITIES, ALZHEIMER'S DISEASE, COMPLICATIONS, DEMENTIA, DEPRESSION, GLYCEMIC CONTROL, SKILLED NURSING FACILITIES.)

Sheri R. Colberg, Ph.D., and David P. Swain, Ph.D., "Exercise and Diabetes Control," *Physician & Sportsmedicine* 28, no. 4 (April 2000): 63.

"Diabetes Among Older Adults: A Heavy Burden and a Great Public Health Opportunity," *Chronic Disease Notes & Reports,* National Center for Chronic Disease Prevention and Health Promotion 12, no. 3 (Fall 1999): 7–9.

"Diabetes Mellitus and Exercise," *Diabetes Care* 24, Supp. 1 (2001): S51–S55.

Edward W. Gregg, Ph.D., et al., "Diabetes and Physical Disability Among Older U.S. Adults," *Diabetes Care* 23, no. 9 (September 2000): 1272–1277.

Liisa Hiltunen, "Self-Perceived Health and Symptoms of Elderly Persons with Diabetes and Impaired Glucose Tolerance," *Age and Ageing* 25, no. 1 (January 1996): 59–67.

Graydon S. Meneilly, and Daniel Tessier, "Diabetes in Elderly Adults," *Journal of Gerontology* 56A, no. 1 (2001): M5–M13.

Robert J. Petrella, M.D., Ph.D., "Exercise for Older Patients with Chronic Disease," *Physician & Sportsmedicine* 27, no. 11 (October 15, 1999): 79.

Matti Vanhanen, M.A., et al., "Cognitive Function in an Elderly Population with Persistent Impaired Glucose Tolerance," *Diabetes Care* 21, no. 3 (March 1998): 398–402.

Jeffrey I. Wallace, M.D., M.P.H., "Management of Diabetes in the Elderly," *Clinical Diabetes* 17, no. 1 (1999): 92–97.

electrolytes Chemicals needed to maintain the normal fluid balance and cellular function of the body. Typically, measured electrolytes are sodium, potassium bicarbonate, chloride, magnesium, and calcium. If a person with diabetes becomes dehydrated, this chemical balance may spin out of control. Electrolytes may be depleted when any individual has severe diarrhea and vomiting leading to dehydration. The problem is further magnified in the person with diabetes.

The individual's condition becomes particularly at risk if insulin levels are deficient and the person suffers from DIABETIC KETOACIDOSIS (DKA). In that case, the person requires hospitalization in order to receive adequate dosages of insulin as well as receive replacement of needed lost fluids and electrolyte levels. Such fluid and insulin replacements are accomplished through intravenous feeding.

In some minor cases of DEHYDRATION, consumption of electrolyte-rich fluids such as Gatorade may help.

emergency medical identification Usually a wearable device that makes it possible to identify a person who cannot provide his name or address or information on a medical condition that he or she has. In general, emergency medical identification refers to an emergency bracelet, necklace, anklet, or other item worn on the body that identifies the individual as a person who has diabetes. An emergency medical ID could also include a tattoo, as long as it is easily visible when the person is fully clothed.

Some people carry emergency medical identification cards in their wallets but these are far less likely to be seen than an emergency bracelet, necklace, or anklet, and as a result, they are far less useful in a medical emergency.

Emergency medical identification is very important because in the event of an emergency and a loss of consciousness, HYPOGLYCEMIA, or a COMA, others who know about the diabetes may not be present or they may be too rattled to report the illness to emergency medical staff.

For further information, contact:

Medic Alert Foundation
P.O. Box 1009
Turlock, CA 95381-1009
(209) 668-3331

(See also HOSPITALIZATION.)

employment   Work for which the individual receives some form of payment.

The ability to work is important to many people in our society; however, sometimes people with diabetes report that they experience difficulties and even discrimination in the workplace. Some studies indicate that people with diabetes may also earn a lower wage than that earned by nondiabetics. According to a 2000 report on diabetes from the National Academy on an Aging Society, the median monthly earnings of people with diabetes for employees ages 18–64 years is $796. In contrast, the median monthly earnings for the same age group for nondiabetics is $1,677, more than double the earnings of the workers with diabetes.

Of course, one major reason for the lower income may be due at least in part to missed workdays. Research indicates that of workers with diabetes who are ages 18–64, 13 percent reported missing work. Nondiabetics in the same age group reported missing work only 6 percent of the time.

Not all studies have found that people with diabetes earn lower wages. In a 1999 study reported in *Diabetes Care* that contrasted 1,502 people with diabetes to 20,405 people without diabetes (all over age 25), the researchers did not find any significant difference in hourly wages. They did find, however, that the people with diabetes had a few more days of lost work per year than the nondiabetics. For example, men with diabetes lost 5.9 days per year versus the 3.9 days lost per year by nondiabetic men. Women with diabetes lost 5.4 days of work per year versus 3.8 days for nondiabetic women.

Fear of Diabetes Status Being Found Out

Sometimes people with diabetes feel that they have to hide their illness from employers. In a study reported in a 1999 issue of *Diabetes Care,* 16 percent of 129 subjects with Type 1 diabetes said that they hid their diabetes from employers because of fear of rejection or discrimination or because of financial concerns. This study also revealed that the support of the supervisor was very important to the worker with diabetes. Since some people take great pains to hide their diabetes from supervisors, it appears that they may be depriving themselves of a happier work relationship.

On the other hand, people with diabetes who wonder about revealing their illness to an employer may be right about the possible negative ramifications of disclosure. Because of some employers' limited experience with people with diabetes—or perhaps because of past experience with a person who had severe complications from diabetes—some supervisors may overreact to the news that a worker has diabetes. They may not realize that today most working age people can readily cope with their blood testing and medication needs, whether they have Type 1 or Type 2 diabetes.

Employers need to stop assuming that all people with diabetes are alike in their problems, any more than all people with arthritis are alike or all people who are African American or Asian are alike. It was hoped that the AMERICANS WITH DISABILITIES ACT would eliminate all or most discrimination against people with diabetes and other medical problems; however, incidents continue to occur and lawsuits are filed and adjudicated.

People with diabetes need to work with their diabetes care team to adjust to night shifts or to erratic work schedules. Workers who travel frequently also need specific help with their meal and medication planning.

Workers should know that sharing information about diabetes with their coworkers and employers can help everyone learn more about diabetes. They can also help others with hypoglycemia symptoms.

The FAMILY AND MEDICAL LEAVE ACT allows workers up to 12 weeks of unpaid leave each year to care for their own serious illness or the illness of a person in their family. Absences may be taken all at once or in smaller increments of time.

For further information, contact:

Equal Employment Opportunity Commission
1801 L Street, NW
Washington, DC 20507
(202) 663-4900 or (800) 669-3362 (for publications.)

(See also AMERICANS WITH DISABILITIES ACT, DISABILITY, DISCRIMINATION, FAMILY AND MEDICAL LEAVE ACT, WORK.)

Jennifer A. Mayfield, M.D., M.P.H., et al., "Work Disability and Diabetes," *Diabetes Care* 22, no. 7 (July 1999): 1105–1109.

Deborah L. Padgett, Ph.D., et al., "Managing Diabetes in the Workplace: Critical Factors," *Diabetes Spectrum* 9, no. 1 (1996): 13–20.

Lee Shirey et al., "Diabetes: A Drain on U.S. Resources," *Challenges for the 21st Century: Chronic and Disabling Conditions* 1, no. 6 (April 2000): 1–6.

Paula M. Trief, Ph.D., et al. "Impact of the Work Environment on Glycemic Control and Adaptation to Diabetes," *Diabetes Care* 22, no. 4 (1999): 569–574.

endocrinologist Physician who is expert in treating endocrine (hormonal) diseases such as diabetes, thyroid ailments, and adrenal difficulties. Most physicians who monitor the healthcare of persons with diabetes are family practitioners or internists who are not endocrinologists; however, it can be difficult for these doctors to stay up to date on the latest treatments and medications for diabetes care or to provide the latest lifestyle advice and recommendations.

Endocrinologists with a major interest in diabetes belong to the AMERICAN DIABETES ASSOCIA-TION as professional members and may also be members of the American Association of Clinical Endocrinology (AACE). Fellowship training for endocrinology takes two to three years, following a three-year residency in internal medicine or pediatrics.

Studies indicate that it is significantly more cost-effective for patients and healthcare companies when endocrinologists are the doctors who see patients with diabetes. One study on the outcomes of hospitalized patients diagnosed with DIABETIC KETOACIDOSIS (DKA), a very dangerous and life-threatening disease, revealed a significant difference in the length of time spent in the hospital and hospital costs, depending on whether the patient was seen by a general practitioner or an endocrinologist.

The study, reported by Dr. Levetan and colleagues in a 1999 issue of *Diabetes Care,* looked at 260 patients hospitalized over a three and a half year period in Washington Hospital, a large hospital in Washington, D.C. The researchers found that although the severity of the illness was about the same for patients, the patients who were seen by general practitioners spent 4.9 days in the hospital versus 3.3 days for the patients of the endocrinologists. The mean general cost for the practitioners' patients was almost double, at about $10,000. The endocrinologists' patients incurred an average hospitalization cost of about $5,500.

Note: these dollar figures may be higher or lower in later years, but what is significant is the ratio of almost two to one in costs, when comparing internists and endocrinologists. The increased number of days in the hospital when under the care of non-endocrinologists also continues to be significant.

One of the reasons for the much higher cost of the practitioners' patients was that they were much more likely to order many tests. For example, only 24 percent of the patients of the endocrinologist had one or more tests during their hospital stay, compared to 49 percent of the general practitioners' patients. The authors said,

Because endocrinologists have additional training in and familiarity with the management of DKA, they may be more confident than generalists in their medical management and may not need to order as many diagnostic procedures. For example, patients with DKA commonly present with symptoms that mimic an acute abdomen. For these patients, physicians who are less familiar with DKA may be more likely to include more comprehensive testing such as abdominal computer tomography or ultrasonography in the initial battery of tests . . . Additionally, endocrinologists may be more comfortable discharging patients earlier and caring for recently hospitalized diabetic patients in an outpatient setting.

It is not clear whether the savings in time and dollars in the hospital can also be extrapolated to general outpatient services, but it would appear to be a logical deduction that it could be. (See also DIABETOLOGIST.)

Claresa S. Levetan, M.D., et al., "Effect of Physician Specialty on Outcomes in Diabetic Ketoacidosis," *Diabetes Care* 22, no. 11 (November 1999): 1790–1795.

end-stage renal disease (ESRD)   Kidney failure. The stage in chronic kidney disease in which either kidney DIALYSIS or the transplantation of a kidney from a recently deceased person or from a live donor is necessary for the person with ESRD to continue to live. People with diabetes have about a 25 times greater risk of developing ESRD than nondiabetics. However, according to the CENTERS FOR DISEASE CONTROL AND PREVENTION (CDC), improvements in blood glucose levels could reduce kidney failures by half, preventing about 16,500 cases per year and avoiding about $2.5 billion in annual MEDICARE costs.

In most cases, patients require dialysis or transplantation when the rate at which the kidneys filter and remove waste products (the GLOMERULAR FILTRATION RATE) falls to less than 10 mL/minute. (Normal values are 100–150 mL/min.)

The U.S. Renal Data System (USRDS), funded by the NATIONAL INSTITUTE OF DIABETES AND DIGESTIVE AND KIDNEY DISEASES (NIDDK) and the Healthcare and Financing Administration, maintains a national database of information on treated chronic kidney failure patients and includes information on an estimated 93 percent of all ESRD patients in the United States.

The USRDS also includes data on the international incidence of ESRD. According to the USRDS, the percentage of patients in whom diabetes was the cause of ESRD was highest in the following countries and in this order: Singapore, New Zealand, and the United States. The lowest incidence of ESRD caused by diabetes was found in Norway, Hungary, Scotland, and the Netherlands.

About 80,000 new cases of ESRD are diagnosed each year in the United States. The most common cause of kidney failure is diabetes, which is responsible for about 43 percent of all cases. ESRD costs about $50,000 per patient per year, and the costs exceed $2 billion dollars for all patients in the United States.

People with HYPERTENSION represent another 26 percent of those with ESRD. Since many people with diabetes also suffer from hypertension, this means that people who have both diabetes and hypertension are at an even higher risk for kidney failure.

Stages of Kidney Failure

Experts say that there are five stages from the beginning of kidney disease to end-stage renal disease. Unfortunately, there are few or no symptoms in the early stage, although diagnostic testing can often determine people who are at risk so that they can be treated early in the disease. Early detection and treatment of kidney disease (DIABETIC NEPHROPATHY) can be lifesaving.

In Stage I, the blood flow through the kidneys is greater than normal and the kidneys become enlarged. Because there is no pain, the patient will not complain to the doctor at this point. If the CREATININE clearance is measured at this time, it is above normal and thus is an early marker of kidney disease.

In Stage II, the blood vessels within the kidney (glomeruli) that filter waste and extra water from the blood and transport them as urine to the kidney start to show wear and tear from the disease. Tiny amounts of albumin can be found in the urine (MICROALBUMINURIA), and this is another early indicator of kidney disease. There is still no pain nor are there any symptoms that are apparent to the patient or physician at this point. As the rate of albuminuria (PROTEINURIA/ALBUMINURIA) increases, however, the albumin may be detected with laboratory tests such as urinalysis or a 24-hour collection of urine to measure creatinine clearance and the loss of protein.

In Stage III of kidney disease, the albumin and other proteins increase even more and they will show up in simple urine tests. At this point, patients who don't already have hypertension may develop it, which harms the kidneys further. Hypertension is both a cause and the result of kidney disease.

In Stage IV, the person is in "advanced clinical nephropathy" and the blood levels of creatinine begin to rise (as kidney function worsens, blood creatinine increases, and creatinine clearance decreases). Large amounts of protein can also be detected in the urine (proteinuria). Patients are not feeling well and they may feel fatigued and have decreased endurance. They may also retain fluid, develop puffy ankles, and have generalized malaise.

The last stage of kidney disease, Stage V, is renal failure or end-stage renal disease. At this point, the patient is experiencing extreme fatigue and malaise, as well as itching and nausea. Increased levels of proteinuria can lead to further swelling (edema), and lack of appetite (anorexia). Patients with ESRD at this stage may lose weight due to malnutrition or they may actually gain weight as a result of fluid retention (EDEMA).

In general, people with Type 1 diabetes may go from Stage I to Stage V in about 23 years, although the disease could progress more rapidly or slower, depending on the individual circumstances.

At Stage V, patients will require either dialysis (the use of a special machine to cleanse toxins from the blood), peritoneal dialysis (the infusion of fluid into the abdominal cavity at home to remove toxins), or they will need a kidney transplant from a recently deceased or live donor. Eventually, nearly all patients on dialysis will require a kidney transplant to avoid death.

When patients have hemodialysis, they go to a dialysis center three times a week for three to four hours to have a machine filter their blood. Patients can have peritoneal dialysis at home, where fluid is placed in the abdominal cavity and then drained. This can be done continuously or overnight.

Risks of ESRD for People with Diabetes

People with both Type 1 and Type 2 diabetes have a greater risk for developing ESRD than nondiabetics although the risk is higher for patients with Type 1 diabetes. An estimated 40 percent of patients with Type 1 diabetes develop either severe nephropathy or ESRD by the time they are age 50.

Interestingly, there are indications that in the United States, the rate of development of ESRD in patients with Type 1 diabetes may be slowly declining, perhaps due to better control of blood glucose and blood pressure levels.

People with Type 2 diabetes are at greater risk for ESRD than nondiabetics, especially when the illness is not in control. Kidney failure is seen in about 5–15 percent of patients with Type 2 diabetes, although it is an even greater problem among some ethnic groups, such as AFRICAN AMERICANS and HISPANICS.

ESRD is increasing among people with Type 2 diabetes As contrasted to Type 1 diabetes, the rate of ESRD among patients with Type 2 diabetes may be increasing. Experts at the National Institutes of Health stated in 2000 that there was a "worrisome increase in the number of new cases of kidney failure" from 1987 to 1997. The rate of 142 cases per million population in the United States in 1987 increased to 296 per million by 1997 and up further to 311 per million by 1998. Experts believe that one key reason for the rise in end-stage renal disease cases is the rise in diabetes patients, particularly patients with Type 2 diabetes.

Other risks for ESRD   Some genetic studies on ESRD link the disease to abnormalities with the body's ability to transport small molecules in and out of cells (abnormal sodium-lithium countertransport). Certain families have varying levels of the angiotensin-converting enzyme, and this may increase or decrease their risk of developing ESRD. When researchers are better able to determine these genetic markers, medical experts may be able to decide who will need the most aggressive therapy at the earliest point.

Ethnic risks for ESRD   As mentioned, risks for ESRD are higher among some ethnic groups, often due to the fact that non-whites are more likely to have both Type 2 diabetes and hypertension, although these two factors don't fully explain the discrepancy.

African Americans have about four times as many new cases of end-stage renal disease as Caucasians. In 1996, African Americans represented about 13 percent of the population in the United States, but they were 30 percent of all ESRD patients. African Americans also develop the disease much earlier in their lives than Caucasians. For example, the average white person who develops kidney failure is about 62 years old; the average black person, about 56 years old.

TABLE 1 AGE AND INCIDENCE OF ESRD

Total Population, 1997	New Cases of End-Stage Renal Disease (rate per million)
Under 20 years	13
20 to 44 years	109
45 to 64 years	545
65 to 74 years	1,296
75 years and older	1,292

Source: "Chronic Kidney Disease," in *Healthy People 2010*, National Institutes of Health, 2000.

Native Americans and Alaska Natives are also at higher risk for ESRD than Caucasians and develop end-stage renal disease at about one and a half times the rate for Caucasians. Experts believe that one tribe in two communities in the US has the highest rate of end-stage renal disease in the world: the Zuni Pueblo tribe in New Mexico and in Arizona. Their rates are 13.6 and 14.0 times the average rate for the United States.

Age and ESRD   The kidneys can fail at any age, but the failure risk generally increases with age. In looking at new cases of ESRD in 1997, the highest rates are seen among people over age 65. (See Table 1.)

Gender and ESRD   In looking at people with diabetes who suffer from ESRD, men have a slightly higher rate of the disease than WOMEN WITH DIABETES. (See Table 2.)

TABLE 2 PEOPLE WITH DIABETES AND INCIDENCE OF ESRD

Persons with Diabetes, 1996	New Cases of ESRD (rate per million)
Total	113
Race and Ethnicity	
Native American or Alaska Native	482
Asian or Pacific Islander	156
African American	329
White	79
Gender	
Men	112
Women	103
Age Groups	
Under 20 years	0
20 to 44 years	35
45 to 64 years	276
65 to 74 years	514
≥75 years	263

Source: "Chronic Kidney Disease," in *Healthy People 2010*, National Institutes of Health, 2000.

Cardiovascular disease kills most people with ESRD   People who are ill with ESRD are more likely to die from CARDIOVASCULAR DISEASE (CVD) than they are to die from actual kidney failure. CVD death among people with ESRD is estimated at 30 times the rate for the general population. Patients with ESRD often already have diabetes and/or hypertension. In addition, many have a lipid disorder and the toxins that are present due to their renal failure lead to a more aggressive form of atherosclerosis.

Preventing or Delaying ESRD

It may not be possible to avoid ESRD altogether, but it is certainly possible for many people with diabetes to delay the disease by maintaining excellent GLYCEMIC CONTROL, keeping their blood pressure as close to normal as possible and being careful with their diet, especially avoiding a high intake of protein.

Glycemic control can prevent/delay kidney failure   Studies such as the DIABETES CONTROL AND COMPLICATIONS TRIAL (DCCT) and the UNITED KINGDOM PROSPECTIVE DIABETES STUDY (UKPDS) have definitively demonstrated that tight glycemic control can prevent or delay kidney failure among people with Type 1 diabetes and Type 2 diabetes.

People with Type 1 diabetes who followed a tight glucose control regimen (HgbA1c at 7.0 percent) experienced a drop of 39–50 percent in both the development and the advancement of Stages I and II kidney disease. The UKPDS performed on individuals with Type 2 diabetes (HgbA1c 7.9 percent) showed a 34 percent reduction in the development of microalbuminuria, which over time will translate to fewer cases of ESRD.

Tight blood pressure control   Blood pressure lowering is the most important factor when trying to save kidney function in patients with diabetes. The degree of blood pressure lowering is more important than the specific medication utilized, although ACE drugs remain the preferred class of medication to use first, unless there is a specific contraindication.

Importance of diet   If a patient with diabetes eats a diet with an excessively high protein content, he or she is more likely to develop kidney abnormalities. Several studies have shown that restriction of protein and phosphate in the diet can slow the decline in renal function. Currently, patients are taught to eat no more than 0.8 g/kg/day of protein. Lowering protein intake to less than 0.6 g/kg/day may place less strain on their kidneys and may slow the development of kidney disease. However, many patients find these dietary changes very difficult to maintain.

Kidney Transplants

When a person's kidney fails or it is expected to fail imminently, the individual must be placed on kidney dialysis, so that the impurities in the blood will be cleaned out mechanically. Another alternative is a kidney transplant. Physicians use kidneys from recently deceased people and sometimes from live donors. (A person needs only one kidney to live and most people have two kidneys.) Transplants from live donors have a better success rate.

In 1997, there were 12,445 kidney transplants performed in the United States. Survival rates have steadily increased for kidney transplant patients.

American Diabetes Association, "Diabetic Nephropathy," *Diabetes Care* 24, Supp. 1 (2001): S69–S72.

"End-Stage Renal Disease Attributed to Diabetes Among American Indians/Alaska Natives with Diabetes—United States, 1990–1999," *Morbidity and Mortality Weekly Report* 49, no. 42 (October 27, 2000): 959–962.

S. Kobrin, "Diabetic Nephropathy," *Disease-A-Month* 44 (1998): 214–234.

A. Krowlewski, M. Canessa, and J. Warram, et al., "Predisposition to Hypertension and Susceptibility to Renal Disease in Insulin-dependent Diabetes Mellitus," *New England Journal of Medicine* 318, no. 3 (1988): 140–145.

National Institutes of Health, "Chronic Kidney Disease," in *Healthy People 2010,* National Institutes of Health, 2000.

National Institutes of Health, National Institute of Diabetes and Digestive and Kidney Diseases, *2000 Annual Data Report: Atlas of End-Stage Renal Disease in the United States,* 2001.

Eberhard Ritz, M.D., et al., "How Can We Improve Prognosis I Diabetic Patients with End-Stage Renal Disease," *Diabetes Care* 22, Supp. 2 (March 1999): B80–B83.

K. Zeller, E. Whittaker, and L. Sullivan, et al. "Effect of Restricting Dietary Protein on the Progression of Renal Failure in Patients with Insulin-dependent

Diabetes Mellitus," *New England Journal of Medicine* 324, no. 2 (1991): 78–84.

epinephrine   A substance secreted by the adrenal gland and the sympathetic nervous system. Also known as adrenaline. Epinephrine stimulates the liver to break down glycogen and to increase glucose levels. Epinephrine also impairs the action of insulin in the muscles and, thus, causes increase in insulin resistance, i.e., glucose is less able to get inside the cell, and, thus, the level of glucose in the blood is higher.

Epinephrine also speeds up the heart rate and raises blood pressure. It is the "fight/flight" hormone, which is generally activated in times of heightened physical and emotional stress. Increased levels of epinephrine are also found with illness or HYPOGLYCEMIA. It is, in fact, the physiological effects of epinephrine that lead to the typical symptoms of hypoglycemia.

Erb's palsy   Tremors and weaknesses that have occurred as the result of an injury to a newborn infant as the consequence of a birthing crisis. This medical problem may be found in infants who are very large (macrosomic) at the time of delivery. Women with diabetes diagnosed prior to pregnancy or who have GESTATIONAL DIABETES have a greater risk of delivering very large babies, particularly when their glucose levels are not under control.

Erb's palsy is the result of harm to the fourth and fifth nerve roots in the baby, which usually occurs because the baby cannot move its arm and shoulder correctly while being delivered. SHOULDER DYSTOCIA is a common cause of the problem but it can also occur without shoulder dystocia.

According to author Barbara Apgar in an article for *American Family Physician,* 80 percent of the cases of Erb's palsy resolve within three to six months and only 1–5 percent are unresolved after a one-year period. In a two-year study, 126 incidents of shoulder dystocia were found among 9,071 children born of vaginal deliveries.

Of these, 40 children had Erb's palsy and it is estimated that the risk of the infant having Erb's palsy with shoulder dystocia is 18.3 percent.

When children with Erb's palsy did *not* have shoulder dystocia, they were generally not as large as the babies that did have shoulder dystocia and were within the normal range of birth weights. The babies that did not have shoulder dystocia were more likely to have experienced fractures of the clavicle. These children generally took longer to recover. (See also PREGNANCY.)

Barbara Apgar, "Spontaneous Vaginal Delivery and Risk of Erb's Palsy," *American Family Physician* 58, no. 4 (1998): 973–976.

erectile dysfunction (ED)   An inability to attain or maintain an erection that is satisfactory for sexual intercourse. Also commonly referred to as IMPOTENCE. Men with diabetes have a greater risk for ED than nondiabetic men.

Erectile dysfunction does *not* refer to an occasional inability to attain or maintain an erection, nor does it include diminished libido (sex drive), premature ejaculation, or the inability to ejaculate or reach orgasm. Many men have intermittent sexual difficulties, and this is normal. It is when the problem becomes frequent or constant that the diagnosis may be one of erectile dysfunction. Erectile dysfunction is usually not a sudden problem but is rather a more gradual one. That is, the man may have some difficulty maintaining an erection but it is still possible. Then the instances of difficulty gradually increase to a point where he may not be able to attain an erection at all.

Who Has Erectile Dysfunction

Erectile dysfunction is a common problem for an estimated 10–15 million men in the United States, and the rate of ED increases with age. About 5 percent of all men who are age 40 have problems with impotence. This percentage rises to about 15–25 percent of men at the age of 65.

It is estimated that 50–60 percent of men with diabetes who are over age 50 have problems with erectile dysfunction. In addition, ED becomes a problem for men with diabetes about 10 to 15 years earlier than when it becomes a problem for nondiabetic males.

Major Causes of ED

In general, erectile dysfunction may be caused by diseases or injuries or may be due to a side effect of other medications that the man is taking. Any problem that affects the blood flow or nerve connections to the penis can cause ED.

Smoking can cause ED because it can affect the blood flow to the arteries and veins.

Hormonal causes may also be a factor in causing erectile dysfunction, such as a low amount of the male hormone, testosterone. Sometimes replacement therapy with supplemental testosterone can resolve the problem; however, this is rarely the cause of ED. Instead, low testosterone levels generally cause men to have low libido with intact erectile function.

Many medications can cause a temporary problem with erectile dysfunction and experts estimate that up to 25 percent of all cases of ED are related to medications. Some examples of particular categories of drugs which have such a side effect are: hypertension medications (especially beta-blockers and diuretics), antihistamines, tranquilizers, and most antidepressants. Even a common over-the-counter drug such as Tagamet, taken for stomach upset or heartburn, can impair the ability to have an erection. Illegal drugs such as anabolic steroids that are taken for weightlifting and marijuana, cocaine, heroin, or any narcotic may also cause or contribute to ED.

Surgery on the prostate gland or in the pelvis or genitourinary tract in general may also cause ED. In most cases, if the entire prostate gland is removed (usually because of cancer), the man will develop ED. However, some specialty urologists seek to maintain the nerve connections, even with removal of the entire gland, so that the man can still achieve erections.

Diabetes and Erectile Dysfunction

ED in men with diabetes is often multifactorial. Poor glycemic control will damage both nerves (DIABETIC NEUROPATHY) and blood vessels (ATHEROSCLEROSIS). Medications used to treat HYPERTENSION or DIABETIC NEPHROPATHY also can lead to ED.

When men with diabetes are heavy consumers of ALCOHOL (two to three drinks per day or more), they increase their risk of ED. ALCOHOL ABUSE can also subvert sexual relationships.

Emotional Issues Related to Erectile Dysfunction

Sometimes emotional or psychological concerns can be involved in ED. Interestingly, as recently as 20 to 30 years ago, it was thought that the majority of ED cases were caused by psychological or emotional problems. At that time, most experts believed that only in a minority of cases was there an underlying physical cause for the ED. Now it is known that the reverse is true and that most ED actually stems from physical problems rather than psychological ones.

Despite this, it is undeniable that an inability to achieve or sustain an erection may cause great anxiety in a man and that anxiety can further contribute to his difficulties with erection. Ironically, he may become so worried about whether or not he can achieve an erection that the very worry itself contributes or causes him to be unable to have one. It is also true that the man may not be worried about his sexuality but instead be very stressed about other problems such as at work or with other issues. Stress definitely contributes to ED.

Diagnosing Erectile Dysfunction

Most cases of ED in the United States are first evaluated by the patient's primary care provider, internist or family practitioner, or endocrinologist. The patient may also be referred to a urologist for further evaluation and treatment. Often the urologist will wish to question both the man and his sexual partner, to obtain an understanding of the full extent of the problem. The physician will make a diagnosis based on the man's medical history, a physical examination, and a limited number of laboratory tests. Some laboratory tests that the doctor may order for a man with diabetes are:

- HbA1C
- free testosterone
- thyroid function
- prolactin levels
- kidney function
- liver function

Important areas of the physical exam are an assessment of the following:

- secondary sexual characteristics (scalp, axillary, pubic hair, muscle mass, pitch of voice)
- arterial pulses
- size and shape of the penis and testicles

The doctor will also examine the penis itself for any abnormalities and will often order a urinalysis to determine if there may be an infection that is contributing to the problem.

Treating Erectile Dysfunction

There are a variety of different treatments for ED, including medications, devices, and surgery. The most commonly known remedy is sildenafil (Viagra).

Viagra and erectile dysfunction   Viagra (sildenafil) was approved by the FDA in 1998 and was immediately a very popular drug. It raises the nitric oxide in the blood vessels in the penis, allowing them to stay distended and trapping the blood in place in order to maintain the erection. Viagra has proven successful in about 56 percent of men with diabetes who have erectile dysfunction. (The success rate for nondiabetic men is about 70 percent.) Viagra is taken an hour or two before intercourse is planned. Viagra must be absorbed and delivered by the bloodstream to the appropriate blood vessels. The standard starting dosage is 50 mg.

Sexual stimulation is still necessary to attain an erection when taking Viagra. According to an article by Doctors Chu and Edelman in the Winter 2001 issue of *Clinical Diabetes,* a patient complained to physicians that Viagra did not work at all for him. Doctors later learned that the man took the pill and then he sat on the couch and read a book about how to grow tomatoes. This did not sexually stimulate him; hence, Viagra had no effect.

Viagra should only be prescribed for men who have problems with ED since it has no effect on sexual desire or the ability to ejaculate/come to orgasm. Men who note that Viagra greatly improves their sex lives almost always had erectile dysfunction problems. Viagra is not intended to be used by men with normal erectile function because it will not improve their erectile function to a significant degree. If a man says that Viagra dramatically improved his sexual performance, then he may have had ED prior to taking Viagra.

Most doctors suggest that their patients use the 50 mg dose a minimum of three times with limited or no success before increasing the medication to the 100 mg dose. Many managed care plans will now cover a limited number of Viagra tablets monthly, generally between five and 10.

Side effects of Viagra   There are side effects to using Viagra, for some men. Facial or body flushing (reddening) is a common side effect. About 10–15 percent of men experience headaches, and nasal congestion is seen in 5–10 percent of men. One side effect reported by some men is having a transient change in color vision, so that they feel like they are wearing blue sunglasses for several hours. This is because the drug affects enzyme levels in the retina.

Viagra must never be used by a man who is taking any form of nitroglycerin, whether it is an oral tablet, sublingual tablet, spray, topical patch or paste. The combination of Viagra and nitrates can cause the blood pressure to drop suddenly and cause fatal hypotension (low blood pressure). For men with underlying cardiac disorders who are not on nitrates, Viagra has been found safe as of this writing.

If a man with ED uses Viagra and then he develops chest pain (angina) during or within 24–48 hours after intercourse occurs, then he *absolutely* cannot use nitrates. He must also immediately proceed to the nearest hospital facility to obtain relief of symptoms with another type of analgesic such as morphine. Of course, he must also inform the ER staff that he has taken Viagra.

Other drugs   Viagra is not the only medication for erectile dysfunction. Other drugs can be injected directly into the penis in order to dilate the blood vessels. Caverject (alprostadil) and Genabid (papaverine) have been used in this manner, with a success rate of over 70 percent. The patient is trained to self-inject the drug about 10–15 minutes prior to planned intercourse. Patients have reported that the injection is not painful.

An insertable pellet is another drug that may succeed. Muse (alprostadil) is a pellet, inserted into the urethra, and used 5–10 minutes before intercourse. It should not be used to have intercourse with a pregnant woman because it could be dangerous to the woman and/or the fetus.

Nondrug treatments   Other nondrug treatments for erectile dysfunction are also available. For example, there are mechanical vacuum devices that force blood into the penis and they are reported to succeed for about 67 percent of men with erectile dysfunction.

Surgical solutions   Surgery may be the answer for some men. The doctor may implant a device called a prosthesis, which can restore erection. The prosthesis may be an implant or a rod that is inserted into the penis and which the man can manually adjust. There are also inflatable implants. According to experts, the primary problem with surgery is postoperative infection, which may be difficult to treat because of the location of the infection. Also, if the patient does have surgery, the other options, such as oral medications or vacuum devices, will no longer work.

The problem that is causing impotence is rarely an internal blockage; however, if a blockage is present, it can be surgically corrected.

For more information on erectile dysfunction, contact the following organizations:

Impotence Institute of America (IIA)
Impotence World Association
119 South Ruth Street
Maryville, TN 337803
(865) 379-2154 or (800) 669-1603 (Toll-free)
www.impotenceworld.org

Sexual Function Health Council
American Foundation for Urologic Disease
300 West Pratt Street, Suite 401
Baltimore, MD 21201
(800) 242-2383

(See also SEXUALITY.)

Neelima V. Chu, M.D., and Steven V. Edelman, M.D., "Diabetes and Erectile Function," *Clinical Diabetes* 19, no. 1 (Winter 2001): 45–47.

estrogen replacent therapy   See HORMONE REPLACEMENT THERAPY.

euglycemia/normoglycemia   A level of blood glucose that is within the normal range. This level can vary, depending on whether the blood is measured from a finger stick (capillary) or a venipuncture (vein), or it is taken arterially. Normalcy also depends on whether the blood test is taken when a person is fasting or after a meal. Typically, the normal fasting range is 65–109 mg/dL.

The person with diabetes (both Type 1 and Type 2 diabetes) uses HOME BLOOD GLUCOSE MONITORING to try to reach or approach this goal of glycemic normalcy or to be as close as possible to the normal glucose levels. By doing so successfully, he or she greatly reduces the risk of serious medical COMPLICATIONS in the future, as proven by clinical studies, most notably the DIABETES CONTROL AND COMPLICATIONS TRIAL (DCCT) on people with Type 1 diabetes and also the UNITED KINGDOM PROSPECTIVE DIABETES STUDY on people with Type 2 diabetes. (See also GLYCEMIC CONTROL.)

exchange list/plan A nutrition plan that may be used by a person with diabetes and which will help keep glycemic levels as close to normal as possible. A food serving in one group may be replaced by an equivalent food serving within the same group in a predetermined amount. Each food serving has similar amounts of carbohydrates, proteins, fats, and calories. The exchange list used by the American Diabetes Association includes seven basic groups:

1. Starch
2. Other carbohydrates
3. Meat and meat substitutes
4. Vegetables
5. Fruits
6. Milks
7. Fats

(See also CARBOHYDRATES, CARBOHYDRATE COUNTING, NUTRITION.)

exercise Planned and often repetitive physical activity with the goal of improving physical fitness and overall health. Regular exercise is very important for people who have diabetes because it reduces the risk of HYPERTENSION, OBESITY, DEPRESSION, joint disorders, and other ailments. At the same time, people with Type 1 diabetes need to carefully monitor their glucose levels as a routine part of their exercise regimens, because they could become either hyperglycemic or hypoglycemic as a result of exercise. Monitoring their blood levels will let them know, for example, if a glucose snack is indicated or if more insulin is needed.

People with Type 2 diabetes usually have fewer problems with exercise causing hypoglycemia and it often will improve their glucose levels, moving them toward the normal range.

Exercise need not be complicated or intense, and moderate exercise can reap very large rewards for people with diabetes. For example, researchers of one study that was reported in the *Archives of Internal Medicine* evaluated about 5,000 British men with Type 2 diabetes who were between the ages of 40–59 years. These men had no family history of cardiac problems. The study found a direct and inverse relationship between exercise and cardiac problems: the more physical activity that the men engaged in, the less their risk for a heart attack.

It can also be risky to pursue extremely active physical activities after living a sedentary life. According to the 1996 Surgeon General's report, physical activity should not be excessive because it

can sometimes cause persons with diabetes (particularly those who take insulin for blood glucose control) to experience detrimental effects, such as worsening of hyperglycemia and ketosis from poorly controlled diabetes, hypoglycemia (insulin-reaction) either during vigorous physical activity or—more commonly— several hours after prolonged physical activity, complications from proliferative retinopathy (e.g. detached retina), complications from superficial foot injuries, and a risk of myocardial infarction and sudden death, particularly among older people with NIDDM [Type 2 diabetes] and advanced, but silent, coronary atherosclerosis. These risks can be minimized by a pre-exercise medical evaluation and by taking proper precautions.

This does not, however, mean that people with diabetes must always restrict themselves to only moderate exercise. If the physician agrees, individuals with diabetes can engage in very active exercise. Swimmer Gary Hall, Jr. has diabetes and it did not hold him back from winning an Olympic gold medal in Australia in 2000.

Exercise Can Prevent or Delay Diabetes

Regular exercise among people who do not have diabetes generally decreases the probability that they will later develop Type 2 diabetes, particularly when the primary problem is INSULIN RESISTANCE, or the body's inability to effectively use all the insulin that is produced.

In a study of male physicians who were at high risk for later developing Type 2 diabetes (due to a family history of diabetes, their own HYPERTENSION, and other factors), researchers found an inverse relationship between physical activity and the onset of diabetes. The more that the men exercised, the less likely they were to develop diabetes.

Regular exercise also decreases the risks for developing STROKE, OSTEOPOROSIS, and other serious medical problems that are more commonly found among sedentary individuals, including some forms of cancer, such as colon cancer.

Exercise Precautions for People with Diabetes

Any person with diabetes who plans to engage in an exercise program after an inactive period should have a physical examination. They should be sure to have their eyes, kidneys, heart, and nervous system checked by the doctor and should also discuss the type of exercise they plan to engage in, so that the doctor can offer advice.

Some people with diabetes should also have an exercise stress test before undergoing a moderate or intensive exercise program in order to rule out CARDIOVASCULAR DISEASE. According to the American Diabetes Association in their 2001 Position Statement on exercise, people who fit the following categories are most likely to need a stress test before undertaking moderate or high intensity exercise. Those who:

- are over age 35
- have had Type 2 diabetes for more than 10 years
- have had Type 1 diabetes for more than 15 years
- have any microvascular diseases, such as nephropathy (kidney disease) or proliferative retinopathy
- have peripheral vascular disease
- have autonomic neuropathy
- have any other risk factors for coronary artery disease (hypertension, hyperlipidemia, family history)

Precautions on Types of Exercise

The type of exercise they choose to perform is also very important for people with diabetes, particularly if they have any diabetic complications. For example, according to the American Diabetes Association, a person with diabetic retinopathy should avoid weight lifting, jogging, racquet sports, and high impact aerobic exercise, because such types of exercise could worsen their condition. Instead, better choices would be low-impact activities such as walking, swimming, and stationary cycling.

A person with some loss of sensations, such as neuropathy that affects the feet, should avoid jogging, using the treadmill or prolonged walking. Instead, swimming, bicycling, and other nonweight-bearing exercises would be preferable. Of course, whatever exercise the person chooses should be performed wearing well-fitted and well-made athletic shoes and socks. Shoes and socks should be changed after exercising.

How Much Exercise Is Enough?

According to the Surgeon General's 1996 report on physical activity, individuals over the age of two years should engage in 30 minutes of endurance-type physical activity that is moderately intense on all or most days of the week—with the warning that people with diabetes, cardiovascular diseases, and other chronic health problems would first consult with their doctor before starting an exercise program. In addition, all previously inactive men who are over age 40 or previously inactive women over age 50 should discuss their new fitness plans with their doctor first.

Older Individuals and Exercise

People who are over age 65 and have diabetes as well as other ailments can still benefit from exercise but they also need to make adaptations. For example, if they lift weights, older individuals should lift lighter weights than younger individuals. They also will probably do fewer repetitions of exercises and may need special shoes and other items. Dr. Robert Petrella said in his 1999 article for *Physician & Sportsmedicine:*

> Exercise is an effective adjunctive treatment for patients who have type 2 diabetes, especially for those who are older. Patients should be instructed on how to integrate diet and hydration management with workouts and glucose monitoring, use of proper footwear, and adequate warm-up and cool-down routines. Patients may want to consult a podiatrist or athletic trainer with expertise in footwear. Timing high-energy snacks with workouts and balanced fluids should facilitate a euglycemic exercise.

For further information, contact the following organizations:

International Diabetic Athletes Association
1647 West Bethany Home Road #B
Phoenix, AZ 85015-2507
(800) 898-IDAA
www.getnet.com/~idaa/

President's Council on Physical Fitness and Sports
701 Pennsylvania Avenue NW
Suite 250
Washington, DC 20004
(202) 272-3421

(See also OBESITY, WALKING.)

American Diabetes Association, "Diabetes Mellitus and Exercise," *Diabetes Care* 24, Suppl. 1 (2001): S51–S55.

Robert J. Petrella, M.D., Ph.D., "Exercise for Older Patients with Chronic Disease," *Physician & Sportsmedicine* 27, no. 11 (October 15, 1999). (www.physsports.med.comissues/1999/10_15_99/petrella.htm.

U.S. Department of Health and Human Services, *Physical Activity and Health: A Report of the Surgeon General,* Atlanta, Ga.: U.S. Department of Health and Human Services, Centers for Disease Control and Prevention, National Center for Chronic Disease Prevention and Health Promotion, 1996.

S. Goya Wannamethee, Ph.D., et al., "Physical Activity, Metabolic Factors, and the Incidence of Coronary Heart Disease and Type 2 Diabetes," *Archives of Internal Medicine* 160, no. 14 (2000): 2108–2116.

eye diseases Illnesses that occur to the eye. Individuals with diabetes are more likely to develop eye diseases such as CATARACTS, DIABETIC RETINOPATHY, GLAUCOMA, and MACULAR EDEMA. If undiagnosed and untreated, diseases that stem from diabetes can lead to BLINDNESS, although annual checkups can usually detect problems in the early stages. In those cases, effective treatment can be initiated well before the complete loss of sight.

Often there are no symptoms in the early stages of eye diseases, although eye disease can usually be detected in an eye examination. Individuals who know that they have diabetes should be sure to have at least annual examinations of their eyes so that an eye care professional can detect and treat any early changes before symptoms of the disease start to occur.

Because many people with diabetes fail to obtain eye examinations, and this failure can lead to BLINDNESS, national organizations of ophthalmologists and optometrists teamed with the federal Centers for Medicare and Medicaid Services (CMS), formerly the Health Care Financing Administration (HCFA), in 2001 to create the NATIONAL DIABETES EYE EXAMINATION PROGRAM. This is a plan for some patients with diabetes who are on MEDICARE. In this program, if a patient over age 65 has not had a dilated eye examination for three or more years, then he or she may be matched with an opthalmologist or optometrist in the area to receive a comprehensive eye examination and a year of follow-up care for conditions diagnosed during that examination. The only cost may be the Medicare co-pay, which may be waived if there is a financial need. (See also BLURRED VISION.)

family, the impact of diabetes on   The effect of family members on a person with diabetes and his or her effect on them. The family of the person with diabetes has a major role in his or her life and can provide enormous care and support. Children and adolescents with diabetes need their parents and other family members to assist them in monitoring and controlling their symptoms. Adults with diabetes should educate other family members, including children, on their needs and possible dangerous symptoms, such as indicators of possible HYPOGLYCEMIA. Family members will also need to know how to inject GLUCAGON for severe hypoglycemia, if needed. (See also FAMILY AND MEDICAL LEAVE ACT.)

Lawrence Fisher, Ph.D., et al., "The Family and Disease Management in Hispanic and European-American Patients with Type 2 Diabetes," *Diabetes Care* 23, no. 3 (2000): 267–272.

Family and Medical Leave Act (FMLA)   A law in the United States that allows leave from work in relation to the illness of an employee or family members.

Enacted by the U.S. Congress in 1993, the Family and Medical Leave Act went into effect on August 5, 1993 and the final regulations took effect on April 6, 1995. The law requires most employers in the United States to allow employees who have worked for them for at least a year (and have met other provisions of the law) to take up to 12 weeks of *unpaid* leave per year.

There are two primary reasons for leave: a serious health condition in oneself or in another family member who needs an employee's care and assistance. A serious health condition is de-fined as "an illness, injury, impairment, or physical or mental condition that involves inpatient care or continuing treatment by a health care provider." As a result, if a person was hospitalized and then needed to recuperate at home for some period, the FMLA would generally apply.

The FMLA specifically lists diabetes under the law in 29 C.F.R. § 825.114 (a)(1), (2), where it is one of five situations under "continuing treatment by a health care provider." That situation is defined as follows: "any period of incapacity or treatment due to a chronic serious health condition requiring periodic visits for treatment, including episodic conditions such as asthma, diabetes, and epilepsy."

Thus, if a person with diabetes becomes seriously ill or a family member becomes seriously ill with complications from diabetes or other illnesses that fit the parameters, then the provisions of the FMLA could be used.

The person may also take time off under the FMLA to take care of a new baby or newly adopted child (whether ill or not) or to care for a parent with a serious health condition.

The leave can be taken for 12 consecutive weeks or may be split up into smaller increments, according to the Department of Labor. The Department of Labor enforces violations of the FMLA.

Many people do not use the entire 12 weeks because the leave is unpaid and most people can only afford to take a few unpaid weeks off. The person may also combine paid sick leave from work with FMLA leave.

The employee has certain responsibilities under the law. For example, the employer must be notified about what the serious health condition is, although this can be done confidentially.

While on leave under the provisions of the FMLA, any health insurance benefits that the employee previously held before the leave will continue, as long as the employee pays the premium expense. When the leave is over, the employer must allow the worker to come back to the same job or to a comparable job.

To learn more about the FMLA, the employer's human resources office should be able to provide needed information. For background information on the FMLA and the Americans with Disabilities Act, the following website is useful: www.eeoc.gov/docs/fmlaada.html. (See also AMERICANS WITH DISABILITIES ACT, EMPLOYMENT.)

fasting plasma glucose (FPG) test   A simple blood test taken to diagnose diabetes. The blood is drawn after eight to 12 hours of fasting. Many doctors in the United States prefer this test. If the FPG level is 126 mg/dL or higher, then the person may be diagnosed with diabetes, usually subsequent to a test that later confirms the diagnosis.

Physicians in other countries may prefer the ORAL GLUCOSE TOLERANCE TEST (OGTT), a test taken after the individual drinks a glucose-containing liquid. Plasma glucose levels are approximately 10–15 percent higher than whole blood levels, although now most meters convert their readouts to plasma concentrations.

fatigue   Extreme tiredness. Diabetes can lead to severe fatigue, although extreme fatigue is not normal for people with diabetes and could be a sign of an individual entering a state of HYPOGLYCEMIA or even DIABETIC KETOACIDOSIS. It may also be an indication of kidney disease (DIABETIC NEPHROPATHY), or CARDIOVASCULAR DISEASE. Typically, glucose levels must be very uncontrolled (250–500 mg/dL) to contribute to ongoing fatigue.

fats   See CHOLESTEROL, HDL, LDL, TRIGYLCERIDE.

federal government   See GOVERNMENT, FEDERAL.

fertility   The ability to create a pregnancy. There are some indications that fertility may be impaired among people who have Type 2 diabetes.

In 2000, scientists reporting their results in *Nature* revealed that insulin receptor substrate-2 (IRS-2), a special cellular protein that is needed for a normal response to insulin, was also needed by mice to avoid obesity and infertility. Apparently, the lack of IRS-2 caused the mice to develop Type 2 diabetes and also to become infertile and obese. Scientists speculate that if IRS-2 should act in the same way in humans, then its lack could be the reason for Type 2 diabetes, as well as excessive eating and problems with fertility.

Because of the increasingly prevalent problem of OBESITY that is found in people in the United States as well as in other Western countries, this research finding may have profound implications, particularly if scientists can find a way to correct the genetic deficiency. Women with insulin resistance syndrome/polycystic ovarian syndrome often have irregular periods and anovulation leading to infertility that can be treated with METFORMIN, rosiglitazone, or pioglitazone (all non-FDA-approved for this indication.)

D.J. Burks et al., "IRS-2 Pathways Integrate Female Reproduction and Energy Homeostasis," *Nature* 407 (September 2000): 377–382.

fiber   Material from plant cell walls that cannot be digested by the stomach but which the body can use to aid in the healthy functioning of the gastrointestinal tract. Many physicians recommend a diet that is high in fiber as a preventive to a broad array of medical problems. A high fiber diet has also been proven to benefit many people with diabetes. There are some indications that individuals with diabetes may consume even less fiber than the average American. Some studies have also indicated that eating WHOLE GRAIN foods may act as a factor to prevent the development of Type 2 diabetes.

Note: people with diabetes who also suffer from GASTROPARESIS (slow stomach emptying) or from colon dysmotility should consult with their physicians before increasing their fiber levels, because fiber can make these conditions worse.

Water insoluble fiber comes from wheat, wheat bran, and some fruits and vegetables. Water soluble fiber is found in oats, beans, peas, and some fruits and vegetables, and it may help lower blood lipid levels.

Some researchers believe that diets that are high in natural dietary fiber are very beneficial for individuals with both Type 1 and Type 2 diabetes because such a diet has the effect of both improving GLYCEMIC CONTROL and lowering CHOLESTEROL levels. High fiber diets that are recommended by experts include many servings of fruits and vegetables, generally far more helpings than are consumed by the average American. Some individuals increase their fiber intake by ingesting fiber powder that is mixed with water or by eating high fiber wafers.

In a 2000 article in the *New England Journal of Medicine,* researchers studied 12 men and one woman with Type 2 diabetes who had greatly increased their consumption of fiber to about 50 grams per week. This is roughly triple what the average American consumes in fiber every week and is approximately double what is recommended by the American Diabetes Association, as of this writing.

Subjects were placed on either a high fiber diet for six weeks or the American Diabetes Association (ADA) diet for six weeks. At the end of the six weeks, subjects switched to the other diet.

The results: the glucose levels for the high fiber group improved significantly. Other improvements were also found. For example, the high fiber diet lowered the subjects' total cholesterol concentrations by nearly 7 percent. In addition, this diet resulted in cutting back tri-glyceride concentration by about 10 percent and also in reducing very low-density lipoprotein cholesterol concentrations ("bad" cholesterol) by 12.5 percent.

The researchers concluded that dietary guidelines for individuals with Type 2 diabetes "should emphasize an overall increase in dietary fiber through the consumption of unfortified foods, rather than the use of fiber supplements."

The researchers said their subjects had excellent compliance with the high fiber diet. However, others have stated that they would have great difficulty in convincing patients that they should eat twice as much fiber as the level recommended by the American Diabetes Association. The researchers themselves speculated that it would be difficult to convince most patients to increase their fiber intake so greatly.

In another study of 63 patients with Type 1 diabetes, 32 subjects were placed on a high fiber diet (about 30 grams per day) and 31 on a low fiber diet for 24 weeks. It should be noted that the percentage of fiber given to these subjects was lower in this study than in the *New England Journal of Medicine* study.

Researchers reported that about 83 percent of the subjects were compliant with the high fiber diet. Of those who did comply, individuals on the high fiber diet significantly improved their glucose control and they had less incidences of hypoglycemia. The high fiber diet group experienced more incidents of mild gastrointestinal complaints.

Fruits that are especially high in fiber content are: apples, blueberries, avocados, blackberries, oranges, and pears. Vegetables that are high in fiber content are: peas, Brussels sprouts, carrots, green beans, and tomatoes.

In the EURODIAB IDDM Complications Study, an increased fiber intake led to lower LDL and increased HDL in men and women with Type 1 diabetes. (See also NUTRITION.)

Manisha Chandalia, M.D., et al., "Beneficial Effects of High Dietary Fiber Intake in Patients with Type 2 Diabetes Mellitus," *The New England Journal of Medicine* 342 (May 11, 2000): 1392–1398.

Rosalba Giacco, M.D., et al., "Long-Term Dietary Treatment with Increased Amounts of Fiber-Rich Low-Glycemic Index Natural Foods Improves Blood Glucose Control and Reduces the Number of Hypoglycemic Events in Type 1 Diabetic Patients," *Diabetes Care* 23, no. 10 (October 2000): 1461–1466.

M. Toeller et al., "Fiber Intake, Serum Cholesterol Levels, and Cardiovascular Disease in European Individuals with Type 1 Diabetes: The EURODIAB IDDM Complication Study Group," *Diabetes Care* 22 (1999): B21–B28.

finger prick Tiny hole made on the finger in order to extract a droplet of blood to be tested. Individuals with diabetes must test their blood glucose levels at least once daily and some must test their blood four to 10 or more times per day. To make the hole, people usually use a LANCET to prick the finger and they then use special meters to test the blood.

Newer devices enable people with diabetes to extract the blood from their forearm, which is less painful because there are fewer nerve endings in the arm than in the fingertip. As of this writing, researchers are working on BLOODLESS TESTING, such as the "Glucowatch," offered by Cygnus Therapeutics, that can sense glucose levels through the skin, thus avoiding the invasiveness and pain of a blood test. (See also GLYCEMIC CONTROL.)

flu See IMMUNIZATIONS.

foot care Attention to and care of the feet, including at least annual examinations of the feet by a physician as well as regular cleaning and drying of the feet and careful trimming of toenails. The feet should also be examined for any sores, cuts, or other damage. People with diabetes should check their own feet every day, and they should never go barefoot (even in the home). They should always wear shoes that are chosen more for comfort than for stylishness.

According to the American College of Foot and Ankle Surgeons (ACFAS), 15 percent of all diabetic patients will experience a serious foot problem at some point in their lifetime. More than 20 percent of the hospitalizations of people with diabetes result from ulcers of the feet. ACFAS says that more than 86,000 lower extremity amputations are performed each year on patients with diabetes.

The majority of these problems are related to foot ulcerations and most of these conditions are avoidable with the regular inspection of their feet. This suggests that attentive foot care can mean the difference between keeping or losing a limb for many people with diabetes.

Although everyone with diabetes should examine their feet, it is particularly important for those with Type 1 diabetes or DIABETIC NEUROPATHY, which causes limited or no feeling in their feet. Yet according to the CENTERS FOR DISEASE CONTROL AND PREVENTION (CDC) in 1997, only about 55 percent of people with diabetes in 41 states reported receiving a foot examination in the past year. Males were more likely than females to have a foot examination, as were people over age 65 years.

There are three primary types of feet problems that people with diabetes may experience: peripheral neuropathy, peripheral vascular disease, and infection.

Peripheral neuropathy of the foot When a person has peripheral sensory neuropathy, this means that they still may feel some pain but the pain is not always a reliable indicator of the severity of a foot injury. Typically, loss of sensation is the most worrisome type of neuropathy because it can mask a significant acute injury or repetitive minor traumas that can lead to ulceration. This loss of sensation of feedback from the feet can also mask problems caused by poorly fitting footwear. Thus, people with diabetes need to visually inspect their feet every day.

The person diagnosed with PERIPHERAL NEUROPATHY needs to realize that shoes that fit well are more important than stylish shoes. They also need to realize they should never go barefoot, even inside their own home. They should also wear socks to protect the feet.

Peripheral vascular disease in the foot
Another form of foot damage is peripheral vascular disease (PVD), a circulation disorder that can cause severe cramping and that may cause the affected foot to become very red. People with diabetes who are diagnosed with peripheral vascular disease risk infection and even gangrene. They may need special shoes. If they cannot examine the bottoms of their own feet, they need someone else to check them or they will need to use mirrors to check their feet for injuries or damage. PVD leads to intermittent claudication, which is pain in the buttocks, thighs, calves, or the feet. It indicates a poor blood flow to the affected area.

Foot infections   Any infection of the foot can contribute to foot damage. When such infections are also combined with hyperglycemia, a foot injury takes longer to heal and the infection could spread to the bone and even lead to the necessity for amputation of limbs.

Foot ulcers   Individuals with diabetes are more likely to suffer from foot ulcers than non-diabetics. In one study of 91 patients who had heel wounds that did not heal after one to 12 months, reported in a June 2000 issue of the *Journal of Vascular Surgery,* 70 percent of the patients had diabetes. Several patients had to have amputations of their legs below the knee.

Foot ulcers and amputation   Studies have revealed disturbing statistics surrounding problems with foot ulceration among people with diabetes. In a large study of 8,905 people with Type 1 and Type 2 diabetes, reported in a 1999 issue of *Diabetes Care,* researchers found that 514 patients developed foot ulcers over a three-year period. Of these patients, 16 percent had lost a limb.

Foot ulcers and survival   A significant number of patients who have had foot ulcers died earlier than did people with diabetes who did not have foot ulcers. Researchers have also found that the survival rate after three years for patients with diabetes who did not have foot ulcers was about 88 percent but for the patients who did have foot ulcers, the survival rate was

much lower, at 72 percent. Clearly, it is very important for people with diabetes to prevent foot ulcers. Identifying them in the first place is the first step toward attaining that control.

The study also revealed that the foot ulcer patients required much more medical care than others with diabetes, averaging about five additional days in the hospital per year and needing 22 more outpatient visits than patients with diabetes who did not have foot ulcers.

Patients at greatest risk for foot ulcers   In a study of 248 patients at three United States diabetes clinics, reported in a 2000 issue of *Diabetes Care,* researchers found that some patients who have diabetes are at greater risk for developing foot ulcers than others. Men were more likely to develop the problem, particularly men who had had diabetes for many years. The most clear-cut factors indicating a high predictability of the development of foot ulcers were high scores on a neuropathy disability scale (NDS) and also a poor ability to sense feeling on a specific test administered by specialists: the Semmes-Winstein monofilaments (SWFs) test.

Patients with END-STAGE RENAL DISEASE (ESRD) also have a very high incidence of foot ulcers.

Foot Deformities Caused by Diabetes

Charcot's foot (also called Charcot's joint or Charcot's arthropathy) is another serious medical problem experienced by people with diabetes. It is also one that should be treated immediately because joints can self-destruct within weeks of the onset of the disease. Charcot's foot is due to a loss of sensation in the joint and bones, which causes bone destruction and drastic changes in the shape of the feet. If patients develop warm and swollen joints in their feet, they should seek immediate medical attention. Often there is only slight pain, so pain is not an indicator of the severity of the problem. Charcot's foot is often misdiagnosed as an infection. Bone scans and an MRI may be needed for diagnosis.

Other foot deformities experienced by people with diabetes are bunions, corns, calluses, and blisters. Of course, people who do not have diabetes may also experience these foot problems; however, when the person also has a lack of feeling in the foot, they go untreated. As a result, these foot problems, which start out as minor medical problems can escalate rapidly to serious and even life-threatening conditions.

Important General Aspects of Foot Care

In her article on avoiding foot problems, published in a 2000 issue of *Clinical Diabetes*, podiatrist Ingrid Kruse made several suggestions for individuals with diabetes to follow. Some of the tips advanced by Kruse were:

- Make a foot inspection part of the daily routine, along with brushing the teeth.

- Wear comfortable shoes that were purchased at the end of the day when feet are usually most swollen.

- Avoid sandals with thongs because they can cut gashes into the toes.

- Always wear socks. Consider purchasing socks with extra padding under the ball and heel of the foot.

- Always check shoes before putting them on. Slide a hand inside them first, in order to check for any small sharp objects that might have fallen inside and that could harm the feet.

- Do not walk barefoot, in or out of the house.

- Avoid scalding feet at bath time by checking the temperature of bath water with the hand first or, if hand sensations are impaired, by using a thermometer.

- Wash feet daily and dry them carefully, especially between the toes.

Periodic changing of shoes   Daniel Porte, Jr., M.D. and Robert S. Sherwin, M.D., the editors of *Ellenberg & Rifkin's Diabetes Mellitus* (Appleton &

Lange, 1997) recommend that people with diabetes should change their shoes about every five hours. According to this book,

> This involves keeping a pair of shoes at the office or factory. The patient wears one pair of shoes to go to work and at work until lunchtime. At lunch, he or she changes shoes and leaves the morning shoes in the locker. The second pair is worn until he or she gets home in the evening, when he or she changes into house shoes or slippers until going to bed.
>
> Thus, each pair of shoes is worn about 5 hours, for example, 7 A.M. to noon; noon to 5 P.M.; and 5 P.M. to 10 P.M. If this habit is developed, the patient will never be in danger of an ischemic pressure ulcer, because even if one pair of shoes is tight, it will not cause necrosis [tissue death] in 5 hours, and the next pair will either not be tight or may be tight in a different place.

Other issues   Some patients with diabetes will need specially made shoes. If they are receiving Medicare, they may qualify for such shoes under the Medicare Therapeutic Shoe Act. They can receive a prescription for therapeutic shoes from their medical doctors.

It is also important for people with diabetes to make lifestyle changes that might seem disassociated from their feet. For example, giving up smoking is an important way to limit complications of vascular diseases that can lead to DIABETIC NEUROPATHY and loss of sensation in the feet. They will need to adjust their patterns of EXERCISE, for example, going on shorter walks or exercising using stationary equipment rather than taking mile-long hikes. Individuals with diabetes should consult with their physicians for the best approach to preserve the health of their feet.

According to the American Diabetes Association, individuals with impaired or lost sensations in the feet should avoid exercise that involves the treadmill, step exercises, jogging, and extended walking. Instead, preferred exercise activities are swimming, bicycling, and rowing.

(See also AMPUTATION, MEDICARE THERAPEUTIC SHOE ACT, DIABETIC NEUROPATHY, PODIATRIST.)

For more information, contact:

The American College of Foot and Ankle Surgeons (ACFAS)
515 Busse Highway
Park Ridge, IL 60068
(847) 292-2237
www.acfas.org

Pedorthic Footwear Association
9861 Broken Land Parkway
Suite 255
Columbia, MD 21046-1151
(410) 381-7278 or (800) 673-8447 (Toll-free)

American College of Foot and Ankle Surgeons, "Diabetic Foot Problems and Treatment," 2001. www.acfas.org/brdiabfp.html.
American Diabetes Association, "Preventive Foot Care in People with Diabetes," *Diabetes Care* 24, Supp. 1 (January 2001): S56–S57.
John L. Culleton, M.D., "Preventing Diabetic Foot Complications," *Postgraduate Medicine* 106, no. 1 (July 1999): 74–78, 83.
Ingrid Kruse, D.P.M., "How to Avoid Foot Problems If You Have Neuropathy," *Clinical Diabetes* 18, no. 3 (Summer 2000): 119–121.
Jennifer A. Mayfield, M.D., M.P.H., "Preventive Foot Care in People with Diabetes," *Diabetes Care* 21, no. 12 (December 1998): 2161–2177.
Hau Pham, D.P.M., et al., "Screening Techniques to Identify People at High Risk for Diabetic Foot Ulceration," *Diabetes Care* 23, no. 5 (May 2000): 606–611.
Scott D. Ramsey, M.D., Ph.D., et al., "Incidence, Outcomes, and Cost of Foot Ulcers in Patients with Diabetes," *Diabetes Care* 22, no. 3 (1999): 382–387.
Gerald S. Treiman et al., "Management of Ischemic Heel Ulceration and Gangrene: An Evaluation of Factors Associated with Successful Healing," *Journal of Vascular Surgery* 31, no. 6 (June 2000): 1110–1118.

fructosamine The name for glycosylated albumin. A measure of the average glucose level in the blood over two to three weeks. Measurement of fructosamine is mainly done during pregnancy to corroborate blood glucose records over the past two to three weeks. This test is now available as a finger stick tabletop measurement via meter and it can be done at home. The strips, however, cost about $8 to $12. (See also CARBOHYDRATE COUNTING.)

fructose A monosaccharide or fruit sugar. It contains 4 kcal/g and causes a smaller increase in blood glucose then glucose or sucrose (table sugar). Studies have shown that substituting fructose for other sugars can improve postmeal glucose levels. Conversely, if patients with diabetes increase their fructose consumption excessively (for example, to 75 percent of total calories), then the LDL and triglyceride levels may increase as well.

J. Bantle et al., "Metabolic Effects of Dietary Fructose and Sucrose in Type I and II Diabetic Subjects," *JAMA* 2556 (1986): 3241–3246.
K. N. Frayn et al., "Dietary Sugar and Lipid Metabolism in Humans," *American Journal of Clinical Nutrition* 62 (1997): 250S–263S.

fundraisers for diabetes Special events designed to raise money for diabetes. A variety of organizations periodically work to raise money for diabetes research that will lead to more information as well as a cure for both Type 1 and Type 2 diabetes. The most prominent diabetes fundraising organization in the United States is the AMERICAN DIABETES ASSOCIATION (ADA). It is the only organization in the country that raises money for research, patient care and education; provides services to patients, their families, and medical professionals; and publishes the world's leading research journals and educational magazines for patients. In fiscal year 2000, the fundraising of the ADA led to the funding of $22.4 million in diabetes research.

Another important organization, which centers on Type 1 diabetes and concentrates on raising money for research is the JUVENILE DIA-

BETES RESEARCH FOUNDATION INTERNATIONAL (JDRF). Both the ADA and the JDRF are good fundraisers.

Whenever donating money to a medical charity, it is always important to check that the bulk (about 80 percent) of the money that is raised will be going to help the people or cause that the donor provides funds for, and that 20 percent or less is spent on administrative and fundraising costs, as with the ADA and the JDRF.

gabapentin   See NEURONTIN.

gangrene   Death of body tissues that is usually caused by inadequate or no blood supply, followed by or accompanied with a very severe infection. This condition will lead to a loss of life if the affected body part is not amputated. People with diabetes are far more prone to developing gangrene because of their greater tendency to have circulatory difficulties (ATHEROSCLEROSIS) and nerve problems (DIABETIC NEUROPATHY), both of which can be exacerbated by poor glycemic control.

Around 1921 in North America (and before the discovery of insulin), many physicians did not treat gangrene with amputation because they felt that people with diabetes would not heal after the surgery. As a result, individuals who were affected had to suffer as the gangrene spread and wait until they died from the infection.

Amputation is still the common therapy for gangrene today, although physicians seek to prevent this infection by encouraging appropriate FOOT CARE. On occasion, an area of gangrene such as a toe is left to "auto-amputate" (essentially dries up and falls off due to complete lack of blood flow) but most of the time, the surgeon amputates the dead tissue and will save as much living tissue as possible.

Diabetes is not the only cause of gangrene. Injuries sustained during wartime were also responsible for cases of gangrene. For example, many people became aware of gangrene during the Civil War in the United States, when many soldiers were severely wounded in the leg or arm. Because of the lack of sanitation or antibiotics, infection and gangrene quickly set in. Doctors amputated the limb to save the soldier's life. An estimated 60,000 soldiers had limbs amputated during the Civil War, and few if any of them had diabetes.

gastroesophageal reflux disease (GERD) Chronic disease in which gastric acid backs up from the stomach into the esophagus. Also known as "acid reflux" disease or "heartburn." People with diabetes have a greater risk for developing GERD than nondiabetics.

Causes of GERD

According to a 1997 issue of *Diabetes Forecast,* as many as 75 percent of people with diabetes have problems with "motility," or the movement of the food along the esophagus. This problem can lead to GERD, in which acid "refluxes" or backs up, sometimes leading to regurgitation. This illness may be more common among individuals with diabetes, in part because of the presence of GASTROPARESIS, or a slower rate of stomach emptying than normal. Gastroparesis occurs largely because of nerve damage.

Some medications can lead to the development of GERD; for example, some medications prescribed for the treatment of hypertension can slow the action of the stomach and, subsequently, cause acid reflux. The primary medication culprits are aspirin and nonsteroidal anti-inflammatory drugs (NSAIDs). Medications known as COX-2 inhibitors are less likely to cause GERD or esophagitis, but may still do so.

Other illnesses contribute to or are associated with GERD; for example, OBESITY and untreated hypothyroidism are associated with acid reflux disease.

People Most at Risk for GERD

In addition to diabetes being a risk factor for GERD, other associated risk factors are smoking, alcohol consumption, an overall sedentary life, and obesity.

Elderly people, particularly those residing in skilled nursing facilities (SNFs, formerly known as "nursing homes"), are at high risk for developing GERD, largely because of two factors. SNF patients who must lie down most of the time and who get very little exercise are at risk for GERD. In addition, acid reflux may also be found in elderly individuals who have had acid reflux problems for years but symptoms were not recognized and the illness was not treated. The elderly person may complain less of heartburn than about the more atypical symptoms, which can in turn inhibit proper diagnosis.

Symptoms of GERD

The symptoms vary, but in general they include: heartburn, chronic cough, hoarseness, and difficulty swallowing. The individual with GERD may also have chest pains that are not cardiac in nature (if a heart attack has been ruled out). Some less common symptoms of GERD are: GINGIVITIS (gum disease), a constant sore throat, and the frequent clearing of the throat. GERD is also associated with asthma, although medical experts disagree on whether GERD results from asthma or GERD causes asthma. Many experts also believe that GERD causes a chronic cough and vocal cord dysfunction that may mimic asthma.

GERD symptoms are frequently ignored and the disease may go undiagnosed because it is not brought to a physician's attention until the individual has difficulty swallowing due to narrowing of the esophagus (stricture) or heartburn symptoms have become extremely severe, leading to esophagitis (erosion of the esophagus) and other ailments. Untreated GERD can lead to a precancerous condition known as "Barrett's esophagus."

Another symptom is the constant consumption of over-the-counter antacids. Some patients take as many as 20 or more antacids per day before asking a physician for help.

Treatment of GERD

This illness may need to be treated by a gastroenterologist, a physician who is an expert in gastrointestinal diseases, but it is usually treated by internists and other primary care physicians.

Medications known as "proton pump inhibitors" or "H2 blockers" (histamine-2 blockers), usually taken as pills, are given to many people diagnosed with acid reflux disease. These medications can suppress the production of acid and enable the esophagus to heal. Some individuals may also need a prescribed dose of an antacid medication, because of a problem known as "nocturnal breakthrough" of GERD that can occur in the evening. In severe cases, surgery may be necessary.

Lifestyle changes recommended Physicians generally recommend lifestyle changes for people who have been diagnosed with GERD, such as raising the head of the bed, taking smaller and more frequent meals (five small meals as opposed to three large ones), and avoiding eating a large meal at night. Some activities aggravate GERD, such as weightlifting, extensive bicycling, and jogging.

People with GERD should avoid SMOKING, which can exacerbate the illness. They should also restrict their consumption of ALCOHOL, caffeine, and fatty foods.

Obese individuals should lose weight because excessive weight can exacerbate heartburn symptoms. (See also DIGESTIVE DISORDERS, EXERCISE, GASTROPARESIS, OBESITY.)

A. Minocha, M.D., and Christine Adamec, *How to Stop Heartburn: Simple Ways to Heal Heartburn & Acid Reflux* (New York: John Wiley & Sons, 2001).

gastroparesis diabeticorum Refers to a delayed emptying of the stomach, due to nerve damage (AUTONOMIC NEUROPATHY) caused by diabetes. Gastroparesis may also be a consequence of medications that the patient takes that have a side effect of slowing down digestion, such as some antidepressants, tranquilizers, calcium channel–blocker medications, and other drugs.

As many as half of all patients with Type 1 and Type 2 diabetes have some level of gastroparesis. In some patients, the problem is so severe that the patient may require gastric surgery. Smoking is known to exacerbate gastroparesis and smokers are urged to stop immediately before the problem gets worse. (Even if the smoker does not yet have a problem with gastroparesis, it is advisable to quit smoking before the condition develops.)

In the earlier stages of gastroparesis, the individual has a problem with the stomach's delay in digesting solids. If the condition deteriorates, then there is also a delay in the emptying of liquids as well. Patients with gastroparesis need to monitor their glucose levels to avoid hypoglycemia, especially if they are taking insulin. A new diagnosis of gastroparesis warrants referral to a diabetes care team.

Gastroparesis can make it very difficult for the person with diabetes to control glucose levels, including controlling them through both dietary and medication controls. Gastroparesis also often leads to GASTROESOPHAGEAL REFLUX DISEASE (GERD).

Symptoms of Gastroparesis

Some individuals who have gastroparesis have no symptoms while others have problems with nausea, vomiting, anorexia, early satiety (feeling full very quickly), bloating, and abdominal pain. Acid reflux commonly accompanies gastroparesis.

Treatment for Gastroparesis

Lifestyle changes are usually recommended for patients who have mild-to-moderate cases of gastroparesis, including a *low* fiber diet (because fiber may exacerbate the condition), and five or six small meals per day rather than three large meals. Some patients are placed on a liquid diet.

As of this writing, few medications are considered effective at treating gastroparesis. In the United States, metoclopramide is the only drug that is specifically approved for treatment of this condition; however, metoclopramide has serious potential side effects because of its action on the central nervous system, causing tremors and Parkinsonian effects. Some physicians have also used erythromycin to treat gastroparesis. Cisapride was an effective medication for gastroparesis but because of its side effects, the Food and Drug Administration (FDA) decreed that it be prescribed on an individual basis only in the United States.

Medical procedures may be required in very severe cases. Some physicians have reported success with the endoscopic insertion of a percutaneous endoscopic jejunostomy (PEJ), although this procedure would not be used except in advanced cases. In this procedure, a tube is placed into the small bowel, bypassing the stomach. (See also DIGESTIVE DISORDERS, GASTROESOPHAGEAL REFLUX DISEASE (GERD).)

Marie-France Kong, M.B.Ch.B., M.R.C.P. (U.K.), et al., "Natural History of Diabetic Gastroparesis," *Diabetes Care* 22, no. 2 (February 1999): 503–507.

genetic manipulation/gene therapy Changing genetic material to achieve a desired result. Based on genetic mapping information, medical researchers hope that in the future, they will be able to interfere with genetic processes that lead to diseases such as diabetes. For example, gene therapy could theoretically interrupt the process that leads to the damage and death of beta cells in the pancreas and that ultimately causes Type 1 diabetes. As of this writing, this genetic research is in its early stages.

Several genes that lead to a predisposition to diabetes for both Type 1 and 2 diabetes have been identified by researchers. Perhaps as these findings become clearer, physicians will be better able to ascertain a patient's risk for developing diabetes. Those patients could then be approached more aggressively in terms of nutrition, exercise, and medications.

Concerns about Genetic Manipulation

As attractive as it is to think that diabetes could be eliminated through genetic manipulation, there are several potential disadvantages of having this individual genetic information. Some people may not want to know that they are at a serious risk for a medical illness, especially if they have a low risk. Other people worry that genetic information in the wrong hands could lead to profiling (being singled out in a negative way), larger insurance premiums, and other forms of social and business prejudice. They worry about being turned down for jobs, promotions, insurance, or other opportunities.

It is also true that a genetic predisposition does not mean that the person will always develop the disease. It usually means that the probability is higher for the person to develop the disease than for others without the genetic predisposition. But it rarely means that it is a certainty.

Another issue to consider with regard to genetic manipulation is that people react differently to the news of genetic predispositions. For example, some people who learn that they have a genetic risk for diabetes (or cancer or another disease) may take appropriate actions to decrease the risk. The person at risk for diabetes might exercise, eat a healthy diet, and avoid drinking and smoking. If genetic manipulation is available as an option, they will take advantage of it.

However, there are some people who think more fatalistically and mistakenly assume that they are doomed to develop a disease. Such people are less likely to take appropriate actions, because they wrongly assume that there is no point in doing so. They are also less likely to accept genetic manipulation. Some people may fear that it is wrong or even sinful to do so.

Appropriate genetic study and manipulation may lead to new therapies, including vaccines.

However, it also remains a complex social, religious, and scientific area that is yet unresolved.

genetic risks Inherited predispositions to develop diseases. One genetic risk is the possibility that people may carry a gene predisposing them to develop diabetes; for example, children born to parents with Type 2 diabetes are more likely to develop Type 2 diabetes, as are the siblings of those who have Type 2 diabetes. Often, however, the genetic predisposition alone is not enough to cause the development of diabetes. An environmental trigger is also necessary. Thus, without an environmental or other trigger, a person may not develop diabetes but could pass on the predisposition to develop the disease to their biological children.

Some researchers have found that the gene, calpain 10, is significantly linked to the development of Type 2 diabetes among the PIMA INDIANS, Mexican Americans, and people from a Northern European lineage. Not all Pima Indians, however, develop diabetes. The Pima Indians in Mexico have a markedly reduced rate of diabetes compared to the Pima Indians in the United States.

In a study for genetic markers for Type 2 diabetes, described in a 2000 issue of the *American Journal of Human Genetics,* researchers looked for actual genetic markers for diabetes among 835 whites, 591 Mexican Americans, 229 blacks, and 128 Japanese Americans. They found such markers, although they were in different chromosomal places, depending on race and ethnicity. Thus, there is not just one gene that makes people develop diabetes but a group of genes that lead to a predisposition or susceptibility. Research must continue before scientists can provide more predictability of diabetes than exists at present.

Ongoing research since 1946 by Dr. Elliott Joslin, founder of the JOSLIN DIABETES CENTER, and other physicians who have followed him, have determined some general genetic risks. For example, if a parent or sibling has Type 1 diabetes, the risk for other individuals in the immediate family is greater than the risk of other families. The risk is higher for a child if the father rather than the mother has Type 1 diabetes.

In general, Type 2 diabetes is more highly heritable than Type 1 diabetes. For example, in identical twin studies, where the twins are raised in the same environment, if one twin develops Type 1 diabetes, then the other twin has a risk of 30–50 percent of also developing Type 1 diabetes. However, when twins who are raised together have one member with Type 2 diabetes, the risk for the other twin developing Type 2 diabetes is 60–80 percent.

The HLA DR3 and DR4 genes are highly linked with Type 1 diabetes. For Type 2 diabetes, researchers have also located a gene for a protein called PL-1, which affects the insulin receptor and causes insulin resistance. (See also GENETIC SYNDROMES, HUMAN GENOME PROJECT.)

Margaret Gelder Ehm et al., "Genomewide Search for Type 2 Diabetes Susceptibility Genes in Four American Populations," *American Journal of Human Genetics* 66 (2000): 1871–1881.

Deborah Josefson, "New Gene Implicated in Type 2 Diabetes," *British Medical Journal* 321 (2000): 321.

genetic syndromes Diseases that are largely genetically based. Individuals who have inherited some genetic syndromes are also at risk for developing diabetes. Examples of such syndromes that carry an additional risk for diabetes are:

- Down's syndrome
- myotonic dystrophy
- Klinefelter's syndrome
- Turner's syndrome
- Wolfram's syndrome
- Friedreich's ataxia
- Huntington's chorea
- porphyria
- Prader-Willi syndrome
- Lawrence-Moon-Bardet-Biedel syndrome

gestational diabetes mellitus (GDM) Diabetes that has its onset during pregnancy and which usually ends after childbirth; however, women with gestational diabetes are more likely to experience the problem again with subsequent pregnancies. When treated by competent specialist physicians and when patients closely follow medical advice, most women and their babies can do well.

Women who have had gestational diabetes are also at high risk for developing diabetes later in life. Forty to 60 percent of the women who have had gestational diabetes will ultimately develop Type 2 diabetes about 15 to 20 years later. It is suspected that the genes for susceptibility to gestational diabetes are similar to those for Type 2 diabetes. The risk of later developing diabetes is highest among women of Hispanic, Native American, and African-American origin.

Possible Causes and Risks of GDM

The exact cause of gestational diabetes is unknown; however, experts theorize that the development of the placenta and the growth of the fetus are both factors. However, the major influences appear to be the hormonal changes that the mother experiences during pregnancy, which may create an increasing strain upon her system.

In women with gestational diabetes, this strain is too great and the woman's pancreas is unable to make sufficient insulin, usually during the third trimester. As a result, she becomes hyperglycemic. Researchers have also found some damage to the beta (insulin-producing) cells of some women who have had gestational diabetes, which is another reason why diabetes may occur later in life.

In addition to the physical strain of pregnancy, some women may face a genetic predisposition to developing gestational diabetes.

A study of 498 women in Norway, who had experienced gestational diabetes, reported in a 2000 issue of the *British Medical Journal* by Egeland et al., looked at the characteristics of these women when they were infants. The researchers found that women born to mothers who had GDM during their pregnancies were in turn more likely to themselves have GDM when they later became pregnant. They also found that women who were born at a low birth weight were more likely to develop GDM when they became pregnant.

The researchers found other factors relating to gestational diabetes; for example, the prevalence of the disease increased with the age of the mother, with the lowest risk to women ages 20 and under and the highest risk to women age 30 and over. "Parity," or the number of children the women had borne, was another significant factor and the risk of having gestational diabetes increased with each pregnancy.

Some experts believe that a thiamine vitamin deficiency (Vitamin B_1) may lead to gestational diabetes, although further study on this issue is needed. This is the contention of Bakker et al., in their article in a 2000 issue of *Medical Hypotheses*. These researchers contend that the average non-pregnant woman is barely at an adequate level of thiamine and that a thiamine deficiency resulting from the additional strain on the body caused by pregnancy could trigger hyperglycemia in some women.

In some cases that are diagnosed as gestational diabetes, the women actually had undiagnosed diabetes prior to their pregnancy. An estimated 10–15 percent of the women who are diagnosed with gestational diabetes had Type 2 diabetes before their pregnancies. However, the majority of women diagnosed with GDM were nondiabetic before pregnancy and become nondiabetic again after delivery for years unless or until another pregnancy or a later onset of diabetes occurs.

Characteristics of women with GDM Pregnant women are more prone to developing gestational diabetes if they have a problem with OBESITY (particularly if they weigh more than 200 pounds), although the problem can occur in slender women. Other women prone to gestational diabetes are women who:

- have a family history of diabetes

- are over age 25

- had gestational diabetes with previous pregnancies

- previously gave birth to very large infants

- previously had problem pregnancies (stillbirths or miscarriages)

- are Native American, African-American, Hispanic, Indigenous Australian, Southeast Asian, or Pacific Islander

Screening for GDM

The pregnant woman should be screened for risk factors in her first prenatal visit, according to the American Diabetes Association. Physicians should consider if risk factors such as obesity, a previous history of GDM, or a family history of the disease are present. At a minimum, the urine should also be checked for GLYCOSURIA (glucose in the urine). The physician will also usually test the glucose level and order a two-hour oral glucose tolerance test in high-risk women. If the high-risk woman does not have GDM at that early point, she should still be screened again later, between the 24th and 28th week of pregnancy.

All pregnant women, whether previously screened or tested or not, should be screened for GDM between the 24th and 28th week of pregnancy, although a minority of doctors exclude diabetes screening for very low risk women who are under age 25 and had a normal pre-pregnancy weight.

Many doctors test all pregnant women for GDM in the third trimester as a precaution. Some studies have revealed small numbers of cases of women who fit no criteria for developing GDM and yet, when tested, they do have gestational diabetes. For example, in one study of nearly 3,000 pregnant Australian women who were screened in their third trimester, 573 were considered low-risk for GDM. Of these women, about 3 percent tested positive for GDM. Since the consequences of untreated

GDM can be very dire, testing seems like a reasonable precaution.

Not all physicians are in favor of screening all pregnant women and these doctors were described in a February 2000 issue of the British medical journal *The Lancet*, which stated:

> The opponents of screening are commonly epidemiologists and public-health physicians who live their life according to the credo of evidence-based medicine, and as a group, are rarely left holding the macrosomic [very large] baby or dealing with a difficult shoulder delivery. Those in favour are more likely to be obstetric physicians with a wealth of anecdotal experience of dealing with the emotional aftermath of stillbirth and birth trauma, which, rightly or wrongly, have been attributed to gestational diabetes. For these obstetricians, not to screen is tantamount to negligence.

How testing is performed Laboratory screening for GDM is often accomplished through a FASTING PLASMA GLUCOSE (FPG) test or an ORAL GLUCOSE TOLERANCE TEST (OGTT) and requires no special preparation and no fasting.

Studies indicate there are about 30 percent false positives with the fasting plasma glucose test, requiring women who test positive to undergo the lengthier (three hours) oral glucose tolerance test.

OGTT is used after the screening fasting plasma glucose test. The patient should have unrestricted activities and at least 100 g of carbohydrate daily on the three days prior to the test. The woman must also fast for about eight to 14 hours before the test. These requirements may be difficult for the woman in her third trimester. Typically, a 75 g load is given. If a woman fails the screening and if the fasting plasma glucose level is greater than 95 mg/dL OR the one-hour glucose is greater than 180 mg/dL OR the two-hour glucose is greater than 155 mg/dL, then gestational diabetes mellitus is formally diagnosed. The three-hour cutoff value is 140 mg/dL.

However, many women with glucose levels lower than these may be treated with diet and insulin at the discretion of their physician to attempt to minimize the risks to the mother and the baby.

In their chapter on gestational diabetes, Ratner and Passaro state,

> Studies suggest that lowering the glucose values to a fasting value of 90 mg/dL and a two hour value of 140 mg/dL, closer to the current World Health Organization criteria, should be considered to reduce significantly the rate of large-for-gestational-age infants and obstetric interventions.

If GDM Is Untreated

Women with untreated gestational diabetes also face the risk of severe HYPOGLYCEMIA that could lead to COMA. Other risks are HYPERTENSION, DYSLIPIDEMIA, and DIABETIC RETINOPATHY. According to Catherine Davis et al., in a 1999 article for the *Journal of Diabetes Complications,* women who have had gestational diabetes are also at increased risk for the later development of coronary heart disease and atherosclerosis.

Gestational diabetes occurs frequently enough to concern both the public and medical practitioners. According to the American Diabetes Association, in their position statement on gestational diabetes published in *Diabetes Care* in 2001, GDM is a problem for about 7 percent of all pregnant women in the United States, or about 200,000 cases per year.

Women with gestational diabetes may also have a higher risk of requiring cesarean sections to deliver their babies, primarily because of the very large size of the infant and the consequent difficulty of a vaginal delivery. About 30 percent of the infants delivered to women with GDM in the United States in 2000 were macrosomic (very large).

It is not inevitable, however, that GDM leads to cesarean births. A study performed in Australia by Moses et al., (described by Kripke in a 1999 issue of *American Family Physician*) compared 216 women with GDM to 216 women without GDM. The researchers found no significant differences in the rate of cesarean sections in the two groups.

Risks to the Infant

The most severe risks to the child of the woman with gestational diabetes are being under- or oversized (although babies of gestational pregnancies are much more likely to be oversized) and experiencing respiratory distress, congenital malformations, and miscarriage or stillbirth. Some studies have found that the risk of perinatal mortality (fetal death) is four times greater in cases of untreated GDM versus the rate found among pregnant women with normal glucose levels.

Other risks to the child are SHOULDER DYSTOCIA and ERB'S PALSY, conditions that result from a difficult birth of a large infant. Hypoglycemia may be a major problem for the newborn, and the child may need glucose intravenously after delivery. Rare medical problems include hypocalcemia (low calcium levels), jaundice, and abnormal Apgar scores for the newborn. The child may also be at risk for childhood obesity and for diabetes in adulthood, although some experts dispute this contention. (See CHILDREN OF DIABETIC MOTHERS.)

To determine the periodic status of the fetus, physicians may monitor the 28+-week fetus with "kick counts," or the number of times the fetus kicks when the mother lies on her side about an hour after a meal. About ten kicks are considered normal. Ultrasound and other tests may also help monitor the status as well as the size of the fetus.

Glycemic Control Is Crucial

Most experts recommend that the woman with gestational diabetes should test her blood at least four times per day. The woman will need a thorough education on how to test her blood and on what actions she will need to take, based on these daily findings. For example, she may need to adjust her diet or the timing of meals. As soon as a pregnant woman is diagnosed with GDM,

she should be referred to the diabetes care team within 48 hours.

Insulin may be needed Sometimes women with GDM may need to take INSULIN if diet and exercise cannot control the diabetes. About 30–60 percent of women with GDM will need insulin. If insulin is required, human insulin is recommended during pregnancy. As the pregnancy progresses, women may need higher doses of insulin, particularly in the case of obese women. Some women who have not previously required insulin at all will need it as their pregnancies progress.

Some experts say that measurements may be used to determine if insulin therapy should be initiated. According to Langer in his 2000 article in *Clinical Obstetrics and Gynecology,* some physicians have used amniotic fluid taken at the 28th week of pregnancy to test for maternal hyperglycemia, fetal hyperinsulinemia, and the risk for fetal death. This is however, an invasive test and most medical doctors rely instead on glucose measurements and the size of the fetus.

There are indications that some women may be able to take oral glyburide medication to control their diabetes rather than insulin. Apparently only low amounts of glyburide cross the human placenta, in contrast to other oral medications for diabetes. According to a study in a 2000 issue of the *New England Journal of Medicine,* researchers studied 404 women with gestational diabetes who were divided into glyburide or insulin groups.

The women in the glyburide group appeared to fare as well or better than the insulin group; for example, they had fewer incidents of hypoglycemia. The two groups did not differ significantly in the outcome of their pregnancies. Further analysis is clearly needed before considering glyburide as a therapy in GDM. In some foreign countries, metformin is also used. However, in the United States, *only* insulin is approved for use in GDM.

Diet and Exercise in GDM

If gestational diabetes is diagnosed, treatment usually includes an emphasis on very careful monitoring of the woman's diet. In general, women are encouraged to eat three meals and three snacks per day, eating a small breakfast in order to avoid midmorning hyperglycemia. Some physicians recommend the complete avoidance of carbohydrates at breakfast because a person's glucose tolerance is lower upon arising. The woman with GDM should be advised to consult with a diabetes care team. Although obese patients are not advised to lose weight, any weight gain is very carefully monitored.

The physician may also prescribe a regular exercise plan with such nonweight-bearing exercise as walking or bicycling. Contraindications to exercise are a risk of premature labor or the existence of cardiac, pulmonary, or thyroid disease, among other risk factors. Each woman should consult with her own obstetrician and diabetes care team about what exercise is appropriate in her case.

Delivery of the Baby

Physicians may recommend the induction of labor if the child is full-term when there are no indications that labor is starting. The reason for induction is to avert delivery of a very large infant. Sometimes pediatricians and neonatologists are on "standby" or are in the delivery room, should the newborn experience any distress. The newborn baby is carefully checked, especially for indications of hypoglycemia and respiratory distress. If the baby weighs more than nine pounds at delivery, calcium and magnesium levels are also checked to determine if the infant needs supplemental calcium or magnesium.

After Delivery

Only about 10–15 percent of women with GDM have overt diabetes immediately after the birth. After the child is born and the placenta is delivered, if the mother was receiving insulin during her pregnancy, her doctor may decide to cut the mother's insulin dose by as much as half or stop it altogether; however, medical experts warn that women who have just had gestational diabetes should continue to monitor their blood glucose levels for at least several weeks after being discharged from the hospital.

Breastfeeding After GDM

BREASTFEEDING is generally encouraged for the woman who had GDM. In addition to the many known benefits of breastfeeding to both the mother and child, breastfeeding may also improve the mother's insulin status. In addition, it may help her to lose weight and further decrease her susceptibility to developing Type 2 diabetes.

Attitudes of Pregnant Women Diagnosed with GDM

Women who have been notified of their gestational diabetes may find it difficult to accept and may even deny the condition. The woman may experience no symptoms of diabetes, thus increasing the difficulty of acceptance. It is important for women with gestational diabetes to understand the potentially dire consequences of ignoring the illness.

Home glucose monitoring is essential not only to verify the problem to newly diagnosed women with gestational diabetes but also to provide them with a feeling of some control and a realization that their own actions are important. Blood glucose monitoring provides immediate feedback to the mother and clearly shows her the role of specific items in changing her blood levels.

Some mothers have very positive attitudes. Lorraine Fascione named her infant Hannah Joslin Fascione, with the middle name given in honor of the JOSLIN DIABETES CENTER at New Britain General Hospital in New Britain, Connecticut. According to the March 10, 2000 edition of the *Hartford Courant,* Fascione needed four insulin injections daily and very close monitoring by her physicians. She attributed her ability to tolerate the difficult pregnancy and the successful delivery of her child to her diabetes care team at the Joslin Center. (See also CHILDREN OF DIABETIC MOTHERS, PREGNANCY.)

American Diabetes Association, "Gestational Diabetes Mellitus," *Diabetes Care* 24, Supp. 1 (January 2001): S77–S79.

S. J. L. Bakker et al., "Thiamine Supplementation to Prevent Induction of Low Birth Weight by Conventional Therapy for Gestational Diabetes Mellitus," *Medical Hypotheses* (July 2000): 88–90.

Catherine L. Davis et al., "History of Gestational Diabetes, Insulin Resistance and Coronary Risk," *Journal of Diabetes Complications* 13, no. 4 (July–August 1999): 216–223.

Anne Dornhorst and Gary Frost, "Jelly-Beans, Only a Colourful Distraction from Gestational Glucose-Challenge Tests," *Lancet* 355, no. 9205 (February 2000): 674.

J. L. Ecker et al., "Gestational Diabetes," *New England Journal of Medicine* 342, no. 12 (March 23, 2000): 896–897.

Grace M. Egeland et al., "Birth Characteristics of Women Who Develop Gestational Diabetes: Population Based Study," *British Medical Journal* 321, no. 7250 (September 2000): 546–547.

D. M. Jensen et al., "Maternal and Perinatal Outcomes in 143 Danish Women with Gestational Diabetes Mellitus and 143 Controls with a Similar Risk Profile," *Diabetes Medicine* 17, no. 4 (April 2000): 281–286.

Marion W. Jones and Lisa C. Stone, "Management of the Woman with Gestational Diabetes Mellitus," *Journal of Perinatal & Neonatal Nursing* (March 1, 1998): 13–24.

O. Langer, "A Comparison of Glyburide and Insulin in Women with Gestational Diabetes," *New England Journal of Medicine* 343, no. 16 (October 19, 2000): 1134–1138, 1178–1179.

O. Langer, "Management of Gestational Diabetes," *Clinical Obstetrics & Gynecology* 43, no. 1 (March 2000): 106–115.

Robert G. Moses, F.R.A.C.P., "Gestational Diabetes: Is A Higher Cesarean Section Rate Inevitable?," *Diabetes Care* 23, no. 1 (January 2000): 15–17.

William Petit, Jr., M.D., "Management of Diabetes Mellitus During Pregnancy," in *Self-Assessment Profile in Endocrinology and Metabolism,* Palumbo, Pasquale J., M.D., M.A.C.E., Chair (Washington, D.C.: The American Association of Clinical Endocrinologists and The American College of Endocrinology) 2001: 102–107.

Robert E. Ratner and Maureen D. Passaro, "Gestational Diabetes," in *Diabetes Mellitus: A Fundamental and Clinical Text,* eds., LeRouth, Taylor, and Olefsky (Philadelphia, Pa.: Lippincott Williams & Wilkins 2000).

Ralph Roberts, M.B., B.Ch., M.R.C.P., M.R.C.O.G., M.D., "Hypertension in Women with Gestational Diabetes," *Diabetes Care* 21, Supp. 2 (1998): B27–B32.

Deborah Thomas-Dobersen, R.D., M.S., C.D.E., "Nutritional Management of Gestational Diabetes and Nutritional Management of Women with a History of Gestational Diabetes: Two Different Therapies or the Same?," *Clinical Diabetes* 17, no. 4 (1999): http://www.findarticles.com/cf_0/m0682/4_17/57562557/print.jhtml

Jennifer Uvena-Celebrezze, M.D., and Patrick M. Catalano, M.D., "The Infant of the Woman with Gestational Diabetes Mellitus," *Clinical Obstetrics and Gynecology* 43, no. 1 (March 2000): 127–139.

gingivitis Serious gum inflammation and infection. Gingivitis is an early stage of PERIODONTAL DISEASE and people with diabetes have a higher risk of gingivitis than nondiabetics. If left untreated, it may lead to periodontitis, which can cause bone and tooth loss. All cases of periodontitis start out as gingivitis, although not all cases of gingivitis deteriorate to the point of periodontitis. The key symptom of gingivitis is painful bleeding gums, although symptoms are often minor and unnoticeable to the average person.

Gingivitis is easily diagnosed by a dentist, who will then recommend treatment for the problem. Usually, regular tooth brushing, flossing, and dental checkups will resolve the problem. If the disease progresses to periodontitis, then gum surgery may be needed.

Gingivitis is very common. In 1999, health experts estimated that nearly half (48 percent) of Americans in the 35–44 age group had gingivitis. The disease also occurs frequently among people with diabetes of all ages. Another risk factor for gingivitis, whether individuals have diabetes or not, is SMOKING. This is yet another good reason for smokers to end their smoking.

Diabetes and Gingivitis

There are a variety of reasons why people with diabetes are more likely to develop gingivitis.

One reason is that poor blood sugar control increases the risk of getting gingivitis, and many people with diabetes do not maintain good GLYCEMIC CONTROL.

Medications may be another cause; for example, many medications have a side effect of creating chronic dry mouth (xerostomia), which can increase the risk for gingivitis. A final reason why people with diabetes may be more likely to have dental problems is that they do not go to the dentist frequently enough.

A study reported in a 2000 issue of *Diabetes Care* compared "dentate adults" (people with at least some teeth of their own) with and without diabetes. The researchers found that people with diabetes were less likely to have seen a dentist than nondiabetics. About 66 percent had seen a dentist in the past year, compared to 73 percent of those who did not have diabetes.

There were also racial differences between people with diabetes who had seen a dentist and those who had not. For example, only about half of Hispanics with diabetes saw a dentist, versus 58 percent of African Americans and 70 percent of Caucasians with diabetes.

In addition, those with more education were more likely to see a dentist. Only about 48 percent of subjects with diabetes who had less than a high school diploma had seen a dentist in the past year. The percentage increased dramatically to 66 percent of high school graduates and further to 73 percent of those with some education beyond high school.

People with diabetes who had more education may have seen a dentist more often because they had enough money to afford to pay the dentist or they had dental insurance. This likelihood is further underlined by the fact that when looking at income alone, the percentage that saw a dentist increased as income increased.

Only about 41 percent of people with diabetes earning $10,000 or less per year saw a dentist. This figure steadily increased with income with 55 percent of people with diabetes earning $15,000–$19,999 and 68 percent earning $25,000–$34,999 seeing dentists. Those who earned $50,000 or more per year had a rate of 82 percent for seeing a dentist in the past year.

However, when asked why they had not seen a dentist in the past year, the main reason respondents gave was that they believed there was no need for them to see the dentist. Other reasons for not seeing a dentist were cost, followed by fear and anxiety about seeing a dentist. The researchers said,

> The lower use of dental services among people with diabetes suggests a need for promotion of appropriate dental preventive and treatment services in that group. However, the finding that the leading reason for not seeing a dentist within the preceding 12 months was a lack of a perceived need, regardless of diabetic status, suggests the need for the general promotion of regular preventive dental visits. Adults may not yet appreciate the interrelationship between oral health and general health.

Dental recommendations for people with diabetes   People with diabetes should have a dental cleaning every six months. They should brush their teeth twice each day and floss once daily. A dentist should be called if any of the following is observed:

- bleeding gums
- puffy, swollen, tender gums
- persistent bad breath
- gums appear to recess from teeth
- a change in the fit of dentures

National Institutes of Health, "21: Oral Health," in *Healthy People 2010,* National Institutes of Health, 2000.
Scott L. Tomar, D.M.D., Dr.P.H., and Arlene Lester, D.D.S., M.P.H., "Dental and Other Health Care Visits Among U.S. Adults with Diabetes," *Diabetes Care* 23, no. 10 (October 2000): 1505–1510.

glaucoma   Eye disease in which the fluid pressure inside the eye increases and may damage the optic nerve of the eye. People with diabetes have nearly twice the risk for developing glaucoma as those with normal glucose tolerance. Glaucoma is highly treatable when diagnosed in an annual eye examination. As of January 2002, Medicare covers an annual dilated-eye examination for people with diabetes. Check with Medicare or an OPHTHALMOLOGIST for details.

There are few or no symptoms of glaucoma in the early stages, although an eye professional such as an ophthalmologist or an OPTOMETRIST could detect the disease with special equipment used in an annual eye examination. The diagnosis of glaucoma involves both the measurement of intraocular pressure as well as a determination of visual fields.

Unfortunately, many people with diabetes do not have these examinations. The consequences of not diagnosing and treating glaucoma can be very grim. The increased pressure in the eye from glaucoma can cause damage to the optic nerve and result in vision impairment, abnormal visual fields, and even BLINDNESS.

About 3 million people in the United States have glaucoma and an estimated 120,000 have become blind from the disease. Glaucoma is also the biggest cause of blindness among African Americans. Glaucoma becomes increasingly likely to occur with aging and is most common among African Americans, those over age 60, and people with a history of glaucoma in their family.

There are two types of glaucoma: closed angle and open angle glaucoma. Open angle glaucoma is more common and people with diabetes are also more likely to have open angle glaucoma. Open angle glaucoma leads to painless progressive visual loss. Because it does not hurt the patient, it is easily ignored.

Closed angle glaucoma refers to a narrowing of the angle of the eye such that the aqueous fluid does not flow properly. It is painful to the patient and it must be treated immediately.

Symptoms of Glaucoma

In the early stages of glaucoma, there may be no symptoms at all. As the disease progresses, the person may notice a worsening of peripheral (side) vision. Some other symptoms of open angle glaucoma may be difficulty seeing well enough to drive at night and difficulty seeing in the dark. Some symptoms of closed angle glaucoma are pain, headache, and nausea/vomiting.

Diagnosis and Treatment

An annual dilated eye examination is recommended for people with diabetes to determine the presence of glaucoma, CATARACTS, DIABETIC RETINOPATHY, macular edema/degeneration, or other eye diseases. If the patient has diabetes, he or she should be sure to tell the ophthalmologist or an optometrist, so that the eye professional can be even more aware of potential problems to look for.

If open angle glaucoma is diagnosed, the treatment is usually prescribed eye drops. For closed angle glaucoma, the pain is likely to require surgery or laser treatment of the afflicted eye.

One class of medications used to treat glaucoma, the beta-blockers, can sometimes have an effect on a patient's diabetes. When applied to the eye in the form of eye drops, if there is any significant systemic absorption through the tear duct, then there can be systemic effects that should be taken into consideration.

Beta-blockers can also blunt the perception of symptoms of HYPOGLYCEMIA because they block the binding of catecholamines (adrenaline/noradrenaline) and, consequently, decrease warning symtoms of hypoglycemia such as rapid heart rate, nervousness, tremulousness, etc. This does not mean these medications cannot be used in patients with diabetes, merely that the patient must be aware of the potential effect and occlude the tear duct after applying the drops.

For further information, contact the following organization:

The Glaucoma Foundation
116 John Street
Suite 1605
New York, NY 10038

(800) GLAUCOMA (Toll-free) or (212) 651-1900
www.glaucoma-foundation.org

(See also CATARACTS, EYE DISEASE, DIABETIC RETINOPATHY.)

glomerular filtration rate (GFR) The rate at which the kidneys filter and remove waste products. A problem in the rate indicates probable kidney disease. It is difficult to measure the filtration rate directly, so instead, physicians use the blood CREATININE levels or, better still, the 24-hour urine collection to estimate the GFR.

The normal creatinine clearance as an estimate of GFR is approximately 100–120 cc/min in 20-year-old men and slightly lower in women due to differences in muscle mass. There may be an approximately 1 percent decline per year independent of the presence of diabetes.

glomerulopathy Kidney difficulty in which one or both kidneys cannot perform the function of filtering and removing wastes.

This is a general term that refers to a kidney problem caused by damage to the glomerulus (the essential filtering units of the kidney that can be damaged by diabetes, hypertension, drugs, toxins, etc.). The roots of the word can be broken down into "glom" which means "ball" (the glomerulus looks like a small ball when looked at under a microscope) and "pathos," which means suffering or disease.

glucagon A polypeptide (protein) hormone that is secreted by the alpha cells of the pancreas. The hormone is administered to a person with diabetes in the event of severe HYPOGLYCEMIA and an inability to eat or drink. These cells lie within the ISLETS OF LANGERHANS of the pancreas. Glucagon acts to increase the glucose level of the blood by stimulating glycogen that is stored in the liver to break down (glycogenolysis). Thus, if a person has no stored glucose, the glucagon cannot work, for example, in the cases of severe alcoholism or starvation.

Interestingly, after five years of Type 1 diabetes, although glucagon remains present in the alpha cells, it can no longer be secreted in response to hypoglycemia. This response is a counterregulatory mechanism that the body has made in an attempt to maintain the glucose level within the normal range.

Glucagon is also available in an emergency kit to be injected intramuscularly into a patient with severe hypoglycemia who is unable to correct the low blood glucose level by eating and drinking. Someone must do this injection other than the patient, because they are often incoherent or unconscious when their glucose is low enough to require an injection of glucagon. The injection will work within 10–20 minutes to increase blood glucose level. The most common side effect is nausea. Adults are generally given 1 mg and children 0.25 mg–1.0 mg.

The standard procedure away from the hospital when someone is thought to be experiencing severe hypoglycemia would be to: 1) call 911; 2) mix the diluent provided in the kit with the glucagon that is kept in a separate vial as a powder; 3) draw the mixed glucagon into the syringe to be used for injection; 4) inject the glucagon intramuscularly into a large muscle group such as the thigh or shoulder. Thus, when a person has episodes of severe hypoglycemia it is critical for them to have access to glucagon and, more importantly, for their spouse, parent, child, friend, or roommate to be capable of injecting it properly. If glucagon is premixed it is only stable for about 48 hours. When the diluent and the glucagon powder are kept separate they are stable for about two years. Patients should check the expiration date.

Glucophage See METFORMIN.

glucose A simple (monosaccharide) sugar that is found in the blood and that is required for energy. It is the only fuel used by the brain during usual living conditions. People with diabetes should carefully monitor their own blood glucose levels because the body is unable to do so, either because of low or no insulin (Type 1 diabetes) or because of INSULIN RESISTANCE (Type 2 diabetes). If levels are high or low, changes to diet and medication are needed.

Other forms of sugar are dextrose, fructose (fruit sugar), lactose (milk sugar), galactose, sucrose (table sugar), sorghum, corn syrup, maple syrup, and carob powder.

Many people mistakenly believe that people with diabetes must or should forego consumption of all sugar forever, but this is not true. Instead, most experts recommend moderation in the consumption of sugar and advise people with diabetes to practice CARBOHYDRATE COUNTING. (See also GLYCEMIC CONTROL.)

glucose intolerance The physiological phase between normal glucose levels and diabetes mellitus. It is formally defined by the two-hour ORAL GLUCOSE TOLERANCE TEST (OGTT), in which the one- and two-hour glucoses are greater than 140 but less than 199 or more mg/dL. It is typically associated with the insulin resistance syndrome and thus these patients often have OBESITY, HYPERTENSION, DYSLIPIDEMIA, polycystic ovarian syndrome, and premature coronary artery disease.

Many patients are relieved to find that they do not have diabetes, but it is a mistake for them or for their medical doctors to believe that IMPAIRED GLUCOSE TOLERANCE is a benign syndrome.

It is important to note that not all patients with impaired glucose tolerance (IGT) progress to diabetes, although it is a risk factor. The risk varies with ethnic groups; for example, Pima Indians with IGT have a higher risk of developing diabetes.

In the Paris Police Study, individuals with IGT and impaired fasting glucose levels had the highest risk of developing diabetes.

A variety of studies have shown that IGT is associated with a greatly increased risk of cardiovascular disease. It is likely that it is not only the level of glycemia but also concomitant risk factors that greatly increase the risk (obesity, hyperlipidemia, hypertension, etc.). Some people have multiple risk factors. The seven-and-a-half-year risk of cardiovascular death was double among those with IGT in the Whitehall Study. (See also CARDIOVASCULAR DISEASE, IMPAIRED GLUCOSE TOLERANCE.)

J. H. Fuller et al., "Coronary Heart Disease Risk and Impaired Glucose Tolerance: The Whitehall Study," *The Lancet* 1373 (1980): 1.

M. F. Saad et al., "The Natural History of Impaired Glucose Tolerance in the Pima Indians," *New England Journal of Medicine* 1500 (1988): 319.

glucose toxicity/glucotoxicity Refers to the action of glucose on the islets of Langerhans and, specifically, on the beta cells that produce insulin. The largely irreversible damage to the pancreatic beta cells is caused by exposure to excessively high levels of glucose. This leads to changes in insulin production.

L. Rossetti et al., "Glucose Toxicity," *Diabetes Care* 13 (1990): 610–630.

GLUT transporters A family of membrane glycoproteins that are involved in transporting glucose into the cells. To date, five types of GLUT transporters have been studied. GLUT-4 transporters are responsive to insulin and are distributed in muscle, heart, and fat cells. GLUT-2 transporters are present in the brain and changes in brain levels or activity are likely contributors to HYPOGLYCEMIC UNAWARENESS.

In animal models, excessive GLUT-4 transporters in muscle tissue decrease hyperglycemia and insulin resistance. As a result, many researchers are considering ways to manipulate the gene responsible for GLUT transporters.

glycemic control A description of overall blood glucose control. A favorable level of glycemic control depends on the ability of a person with diabetes (or others who provide care, when the person with diabetes needs help) to keep glucose levels as close to normal as possible. Attaining good or excellent glycemic control is the critical goal to attain and the key concept to grasp for every person who has diabetes.

Tight glycemic control is the key to decreasing risks for many severe short-term and long-term complications, which experts believe are avoidable. It may also increase an individual's life span, adding years to the person's life compared to inadequate glycemic control.

It is not mere speculation that glycemic control enhances the lives of people with diabetes. Studies such as the DIABETES CONTROL AND COMPLICATIONS TRIAL, on individuals with Type 1 diabetes and the UNITED KINGDOM PROSPECTIVE DIABETES STUDY, on individuals with Type 2 diabetes, have clearly and definitively illustrated that tight glycemic control can greatly reduce the risk of serious complications from diabetes.

Some medical problems/complications of diabetes that can be prevented or delayed with good glycemic control include:

- diabetic neuropathy
- diabetic retinopathy
- diabetic ketoacidosis/hyperosmolar state
- diabetic nephropathy/kidney failure
- amputation of limbs
- erectile dysfunction
- cardiovascular disease
- problem pregnancies/large babies
- periodontal disease
- yeast (Candida) vaginitis/balanitis

Key Elements of Glycemic Control

Glycemic control is maintained through a combination of medication, good nutrition, exercise, and frequent blood glucose testing with an appropriate response to those test results (modification of diet, exercise, oral medication, and/or the insulin dose). This requires education and involvement with a diabetes care team. Yet sadly, many people with diabetes do not attend to each of these key proponents of glycemic control—and some people ignore all of them, to their physical and emotional detriment as well as their families'.

The problem may lie in their denial of the existence of their illness and its severity. It may also be due to a lack of education. A third cause of poor glycemic control is fear or dislike of pain, including the brief pain of blood testing and the pain of injecting medication. Some people may also dislike the additional burden of time and money that their illness brings.

Improvements in Blood Testing and Monitoring

Until the latter part of the 20th century, it was difficult or impossible for most people with diabetes to monitor their glucose blood levels. The creation of glucose meters that can be easily used at home resolved this issue. Still, many people dislike having to pierce their skin to extract a drop of blood for evaluation.

As a result, less painful micro-lancet equipment such as PEN DEVICES were developed, as well as devices which could extract the blood from the forearm or other body parts with less sensitive nerve endings than the fingertip.

In 2001, the "Glucowatch" was introduced by Cygnus. This is a device to which users attach special sensors to gauge glucose levels through the skin, thus avoiding the need for a puncture. (As of this writing, experts recommend that some blood testing through the skin must still be done, especially if the watch shows a dramatic change in levels.)

Another aspect of glycemic control disliked by most people with diabetes is the injection of medication, which is a must for all those with Type 1 diabetes and for some people with Type 2 diabetes. Since they don't want to give themselves shots, they may skip testing their blood altogether and ignore their illness. New breakthroughs may make the taking of medication painless and thus, more people will work on glycemic control.

For example, inhaled insulin is another emerging 21st century option for people with Type 1 diabetes. Experts report that early results on this painless product are very promising. Other methods of medication delivery are being researched.

Several companies are teaming together to work on insulin that can be given under the tongue much like a nitroglycerin tablet.

Glycemic Control Is Spotty or Inadequate among Many Groups

According to 1998 statistics provided by the Centers for Disease Control and Prevention (CDC), only 42 percent of individuals with diabetes in the United States test their blood at least once a day. Native American and Alaska Natives were the most likely (53 percent) to perform daily glucose testing, followed by Caucasians (43 percent), African Americans (40 percent), Hispanics or Latinos (36 percent), and Asian or Pacific Islanders (30 percent).

This finding appears to be backed up by another study reported by Maureen Harris in a 2001 issue of *Diabetes Care*. This study looked at the self-monitoring of patients with Type 2 diabetes, some of whom used oral agents while others used insulin. According to this study, 29 percent of those who treated their diabetes with insulin had either never monitored their blood glucose or they monitored it only once a month or less. Among those who treated their diabetes with oral medications, 65 percent never or only once a month or less had monitored their blood levels. Among patients who treated their diabetes with diet only, 80 percent had never or only once a month or less monitored their blood glucose levels.

These are discouraging findings because most physicians expect patients to perform daily blood monitoring so that they can make adjustments to their diet and medication and report extreme changes to their physician.

Dietary control   Few people enjoy having to think critically about what they should or should not eat and how and why it may affect their blood glucose levels. Yet this is another essential aspect of good glycemic control for people with both Type 1 and Type 2 diabetes. Thus nutritional education is critical as well as support from family and friends.

Lifestyle changes   Another aspect of good glycemic control is for the person with diabetes to make basic lifestyle changes in order to avoid behaviors that can worsen glucose levels. For example, SMOKING is known to cause many severe problems for people with diabetes. However, since people with diabetes have a higher risk than the general population without diabetes for developing HYPERTENSION, STROKE, CARDIOVASCULAR DISEASE, and many other blood vessel–related diseases that are aggravated by smoking, it is critical and lifesaving for anyone who has diabetes to stop smoking as soon as possible.

OBESITY is a risk factor for the development of Type 2 diabetes and after diagnosis will increase insulin resistance and thus worsen overall glycemic control. Most people with IMPAIRED GLUCOSE TOLERANCE or Type 2 diabetes or HYPERTENSION or HYPERLIPIDEMIA (or any combination of those problems) will improve their condition by losing weight.

Regular daily exercise is another way for people with diabetes to maintain healthy glycemic control. (See also BLOOD GLUCOSE MONITORING, NUTRITION.)

Maureen I. Harris, Ph.D., M.P.H., "Frequency of Blood Glucose Monitoring in Relation to Glycemic Control in Patients with Type 2 Diabetes," *Diabetes Care* 24, no. 6 (June 2001): 979–982.

Linda M. Hunt et al., "How Patients Adapt Diabetes Self-Care Recommendations to Everyday Life," *Journal of Family Practice* 46, no. 3 (March 1998): 207–216.

glycogen   Stored glucose within the body, found primarily in the liver and the muscles. When needed by the body, it is transformed through glycogenolysis, back into glucose. Conversely, glycogenesis is the process by which glucose is converted into glycogen.

Glycogen can be thought of as stored glucose. It is comprised of strands that are bound end to end in a branching form, much like the branches on a Christmas tree. Two enzymes are important in this process. Glycogen synthase controls synthesis and glycogen phosphorylase controls breakdown of glycogen. Working together, these enzymes control the glucose balance.

During times between meals when glucose is needed, the body breaks down stored glycogen to normalize the blood glucose level. At one time, it was thought that an excessive breakdown of liver glycogen was the major determinant of the fasting blood glucose level in patients with Type 2 diabetes. However, special liver studies (in vivo nuclear magnetic resonance spectroscopy) have determined that the predominant contributor to the increase in fasting glucose is due to gluconeogenesis; that is the formation of new glucose.

The average person has about 18 hours of glycogen stores in the liver before the body needs to begin making new glucose or burning fat (i.e., ketosis).

glycosuria/glucosuria Glucose in the urine, which is an abnormal sign, and an indicator of diabetes. People with undiagnosed diabetes have a typically sweet taste to their urine, attractive to insects and which has been noted since ancient times.

Generally, glucose will "spill over" into the urine in this condition, if the glucose blood levels are greater than 180 mg/dL. In people who have diabetes, their kidneys adapt and glucose may not show up in the urine until levels are greater than 250–300 mg/dL. As a result relying on urine testing only is an inadequate method of screening for and monitoring diabetes.

Occasionally, people without diabetes have a lower than normal renal glucose threshold and it will spill glucose into the urine even when the person has normal blood glucose levels.

glycosylated albumin Another name for FRUC-TOSAMINE.

government, federal The U.S. government and its role in diabetes research, treatment, and payment.

The federal government performs or pays for research on diabetes, primarily through the NATIONAL INSTITUTES OF HEALTH and based on

funds that are provided by Congress. Federal agencies also provide information to individuals with diabetes and their families.

The key federal organizations involved in diabetes are the CENTERS FOR DISEASE CONTROL AND PREVENTION, the NATIONAL DIABETES INFORMATION CLEARINGHOUSE and the NATIONAL INSTITUTE OF DIABETES AND DIGESTIVE AND KIDNEY DISEASES (NIDDK).

There are also several programs important to many people with diabetes, including MEDICARE and MEDICAID. Medicare is a federal medical program that is primarily oriented to people over age 65 and that also includes many younger disabled people. Medicaid is a program that receives some federal funds but that is managed by the states. It provides medical care to indigent people of all ages.

As of this writing, Medicare does not cover medications but Medicaid does provide such coverage. Medicare does provide coverage for IMMUNIZATIONS for flu and pneumonia, which are important for people with diabetes. Medicare recipients also receive coverage of syringes and related material that are needed by individuals with diabetes. (Insulin is not covered.) Medicare also covers some limited HOME HEALTH CARE services and very limited (30 days after hospitalization, as of this writing) SKILLED NURSING CARE services. Medicare also pays for therapeutic shoes for patients who need them.

For further information, go to the following website: www.niddk.nih.gov/health/diabetes/diabetes.htm.

government, state Governments at the state level and their role in research, treatment, and payment for diabetes programs.

All state governments have an agency that is dedicated in part or solely to the subject of diabetes. Some states place this responsibility within their state health department while others place it under other offices. Some states have more active programs than others and this may also vary from year to year.

State governments administer the MEDICAID program, receiving some federal money as well. Medicaid is a program for indigent people who are eligible for assistance because of old age, disability, or other reasons.

growth hormone   A substance that is naturally produced by the anterior pituitary gland in response to stimulation by growth hormone-releasing hormone (GHRH) produced by the hypothalamus. In growing children, growth hormone is released in a pulsatile fashion mainly at night, and it stimulates growth and development via an array of intermediary hormones.

Growth hormone is also released in response to HYPOGLYCEMIA, although its metabolic effects are slow and most people's recovery from hypoglycemia is mainly mediated via adrenaline and noradrenaline.

Natural levels of growth hormone tend to be slightly higher in overweight patients with Type 2 diabetes. Excessive growth hormone production in children can cause GIGANTISM and excessive levels of growth hormone in adults can result in ACROMEGALY.

Growth Hormone as Treatment

Growth hormone that was created from recombinant processes is administered to children with documented growth hormone deficiency due to pituitary tumor or trauma. Females with Turner's syndrome may also be given growth hormone to help them grow taller.

Growth hormone may be administered to adults to increase their lean body mass, increase strength, and improve their quality of life. Typically, growth hormone is given only to adults with documented growth hormone deficiency. When they are stronger and have less fat, most people feel better. They are also less likely to fall and become injured and more likely to be able to lift and exercise. Currently ongoing studies are looking at whether or not the use of an oral GHRH, which will increase endogenous growth hormone secretion, will benefit the "pre-frail elderly."

A disadvantage to administered growth hormone is that it may induce diabetes or impaired glucose tolerance in susceptible children, especially if the dose is excessive. Experts recommend that before administering any growth hormone to children (or adults), their blood glucose levels should be checked first to verify that they are within the normal range.

According to an article in a 2000 issue of *The Lancet* by Cutfield et al., the researchers found that although the risk was very low, children who were given growth hormone had a six times greater rate of developing Type 2 diabetes than children who did not receive the hormone. It is possible that the children would have developed diabetes anyway without receiving the growth hormone. Further research is needed on this topic before conclusions can be drawn.

It was also interesting to note that the children who received growth hormone and, subsequently, developed Type 2 diabetes were *not* obese, in contrast to the majority of children and adolescents with Type 2 diabetes, 80 percent of whom are obese. It is not clear why this was true.

Wayne S. Cutfield et al., "Incidence of Diabetes Mellitus and Impaired Glucose Tolerance in Children and Adolescents Receiving Growth-Hormone Treatment," *The Lancet* 355, no. 9204 (February 2000): 610–613.

Michiaki Fukui et al., "Growth-Hormone Treatment and Risk of Diabetes," *The Lancet* 355, no. 9218 (May 2000): 1912–1913.

gum disease   Generally refers to GINGIVITIS, an inflammation and infection of gum disease and the first stage of PERIODONTAL DISEASE or to periodontitis, a more advanced stage of periodontal disease which may lead to bone and teeth loss. Individuals with diabetes are more likely to have infections and diseases of the gum than are nondiabetics.

HDL   A fatty lipid protein that circulates in the blood and is found throughout the body. High density lipoprotein (HDL) cholesterol, is often referred to as "good" cholesterol because high levels of HDL decrease a person's risk for having a heart attack or stroke. HDL is responsible for removing cholesterol from blood vessels and back to the liver, a process also known as "reverse cholesterol transport."

If a person has a low level of HDL, it is possible to increase the levels by as much as 10 percent through exercise, weight loss, and smoking cessation.

Because people with diabetes have a higher risk than nondiabetics for both heart attack and stroke, it's important for physicians to run periodic testing on blood levels of HDL and LDL. (Low density lipoproteins are considered "bad" cholesterol and high levels of LDL increase the risk for heart attack or stroke because the LDL stays within the arteries and builds up.) (See also ARTHEROSCLEROSIS/ARTERIOSCLEROSIS, CHOLESTEROL, LDL, TRIGYLCERIDES.)

hepatitis C virus (HCV)   A type of hepatitis virus, an infectious agent. There is an apparent association between the hepatitis C virus and Type 2 diabetes, based on a study reported in a 2000 issue of the *Annals of Internal Medicine.*

Researchers studied 9,841 people with HCV infection and noted that 8.4 percent of the subjects had Type 2 diabetes. They also found that subjects who were age 40 or older were more than three times more likely to have Type 2 diabetes. Type 2 diabetes was also found more frequently among subjects who were nonwhite, had low socioeconomic status, and had high BODY MASS INDEX ratings. It is not clear if HCV may in some way cause or trigger Type 2 diabetes.

Shruti H. Mehta, M.P.H., et al., "Prevalence of Type 2 Diabetes Mellitus among Persons with Hepatitis C Virus Infection in the United States," *Annals of Internal Medicine* 133 (2000): 592–599.

HHNS   See HYPEROSMOLAR COMA.

Hispanics/Latinos   People of Latin origin, including Mexican Americans, Puerto Ricans, Central and South Americans, and Cuban Americans, as well as individuals of mixed ethnicities of one or more of these groups. Hispanics in the United States, particularly those who are Mexican American, have a higher risk of developing Type 2 diabetes than do non-Hispanic whites, although they appear to have a lower risk of developing Type 1 diabetes.

Hispanics represent a rapidly growing group in the US. In 2000, about 12 percent of the population were people of Hispanic origin, according to the U.S. Census Bureau. It is estimated that Hispanics will represent about 25 percent of the total population of the United States by 2050. As a result, the overall problem of diabetes will accelerate because of the greater numbers of this group in the general population.

According to the National Diabetes Information Clearinghouse (NDIC), 1.2 million of 30 million Hispanic Americans have been diagnosed with diabetes and an additional 675,000 have diabetes but have not yet been diagnosed.

Most of these cases of diabetes (90–95 percent) were Type 2 diabetes. Among Hispanics over age 50, 25 to 30 percent have diagnosed or undiagnosed diabetes.

Hispanics and Latinos in other countries do not have this high rate, possibly because of differences in diet and activity levels. In general, people in the United States consume more calories than do individuals in other countries and lead more sedentary lives than non-Americans.

According to the National Institute of Diabetes and Digestive and Kidney Diseases, diabetes among Hispanics is the most common among both Mexican Americans and Puerto Ricans, who have a rate that is twice as high as the rate found among non-Hispanic whites. Cuban Americans also experience a rate of diabetes that is higher than non-Hispanic whites, although it is lower than the rate found among Mexican Americans and Puerto Ricans. Experts at NIDDK report that one in four Mexican Americans and one in four Puerto Ricans over age 45 have diabetes, versus one in six Cuban Americans over age 45 who have diabetes. (See Table 1 for a comparison of the rate of diabetes among different ethnic groups and ages of Hispanics.)

The rates of diabetes for Hispanics are not as high as found among African Americans. According to information released by the U.S. Department of Health and Human Services in their "Healthy People 2010" report, released in 2000, the rates for diagnosed diabetes in 1997 are shown in Table 2.

TABLE 2 RATES OF DIABETES PER 1000 PEOPLE

Total population in United States	40
African Americans	74
Caucasians	36
Hispanic/Latinos	61

Hispanics at Risk for Complications

Groups identified as Hispanic Americans are more at risk than non-Hispanic whites to develop the complications of diabetes such as kidney disease, eye disease, and other medical problems that stem from long-term and serious cases of diabetes. For example, several studies on diabetic retinopathy indicated that Mexican Americans suffered twice the rate of retinopathy than that experienced by non-Hispanic whites.

GESTATIONAL DIABETES may be a greater problem for Hispanics than it is for non-Hispanic whites. One study in California found that 12 percent of Mexican American women who became pregnant developed gestational diabetes. The generally accepted rate of gestational diabetes is 3–5 percent among all pregnant women. Some women diagnosed with gestational diabetes actually had undiagnosed Type 2 diabetes prior to pregnancy. This may account for some, but not all, of this discrepancy.

Risk Factors for Hispanics

The primary risk factors for Hispanic Americans to develop diabetes are as follows:

- a family history of diabetes
- gestational diabetes

TABLE 1   HISPANIC AMERICAN POPULATION IN THE UNITED STATES AND PERCENTAGE WITH DIABETES

Hispanic American Population	% of Total Hispanic Population	% with Diabetes Ages 20–44	% with Diabetes Ages 45–74
Mexican Americans	64.3	3.8	26.2
Central/South Americans	13.4	unknown	unknown
Puerto Ricans	10.6	4.1	26.1
Cuban Americans	4.7	2.4	15.8
Others	7.0	unknown	unknown

Source: "Diabetes in Hispanic Americans," National Diabetes Information Clearinghouse, National Institute of Diabetes and Digestive and Kidney Diseases, National Institutes of Health, 1999.

- insulin resistance
- physical inactivity
- obesity
- hyperinsulinemia

Some positive findings The news for Hispanics is not all bad. One study indicated a positive finding for Mexican Americans. They lived longer on kidney dialysis than did non-Hispanic whites. Several studies also found that Mexican Americans with diabetes in Texas and Colorado had lower rates of heart attacks than non-Hispanic whites had experienced.

Study on self-reported diagnosed diabetes Some studies have indicated that 10 percent or more of all Mexican Americans over age 20 have diabetes. According to a report published in *Morbidity and Mortality Weekly Report* in 1999, their research information was derived from a telephone survey conducted in all 50 states, the District of Columbia, Puerto Rico, and U.S. territories.

The researchers found that the rate of diabetes was higher among those without a high school education, regardless of ethnicity. The rate of diabetes was 9.8 percent for Hispanic adults without a high school education versus 6.5 percent for those with at least a high school education. Among non-Hispanic whites without a high school education, the rate of diabetes was 5.9 percent versus 3.6 percent of those with at least a high school education. Generally, individuals with more education have a better diet, get more exercise, and have a lower risk of OBESITY than individuals with less education.

The rates for diabetes also varied by region. For example, the highest rates for diabetes were found in Puerto Rico, where the overall adult rate was 10.9 percent. (Probably because most of the population is Hispanic and any risk for Hispanics would then be magnified.)

Within the United States, the highest rates of diabetes for Hispanics (8.5 percent for Hispanics versus 3.7 percent for non-Hispanic whites) were found in the West/Southwest region, again probably because of the high concentration of Hispanic individuals who were living in this area.

Age was another factor affecting diagnosed cases of diabetes. For example, the percentage of diabetes for people ages 18–44 was 2.3 percent for Hispanics and 1.2 percent for non-Hispanic whites. The rate increased greatly as the population aged. See the table below for more information.

PERCENTAGE OF SELF-REPORTED DIABETES BY AGE, 1994–1997		
Age	**Hispanics**	**Non-Hispanic Whites**
18–44 years	2.3%	1.2%
45–64 years	12.0%	6.0%
Over 65 years	21.4%	10.4%

Source: "Self-Reported Prevalence of Diabetes Among Hispanic—United States, 1994–1997," *Morbidity and Mortality Weekly Report,* 1999.

Many Hispanics Are Undiagnosed

It's important to keep in mind that the above-described research was based on individuals who said that they had been diagnosed with diabetes; however, many individuals have diabetes but have not yet been diagnosed. This may be particularly true for those under age 45, who may not have received screening for Type 2 diabetes, despite risk factors such as family members with diabetes, obesity, inactive lifestyle, and racial and ethnic risk factors. Early symptoms and possible indicators of diabetes are sometimes ignored in younger or even middle-aged individuals.

As a result, the rates for both Hispanics and non-Hispanic whites were almost undoubtedly higher than was reported, albeit in about the same proportions of about two to one, based on previous studies.

Depression among Older Mexican Americans with Diabetes

In a study reported in 1999 in *Diabetes Care,* researchers sought to compare the rate of depression among Mexican Americans with diabetes and who were over age 65 in Texas, California, New Mexico, Arizona, and Colorado versus nondiabetic older Mexican Americans in the same areas and same age groups. The research was based on 636 Mexican Americans with diabetes and 2,196 nondiabetic Mexican Americans.

Nearly one-third (31.1 percent) of Mexican Americans with diabetes reported depressive symptoms. This rate was significantly higher than the rate of 24.1 percent found among the nondiabetic older Mexican Americans.

Women with diabetes were found to be much more prone to depression than were men with diabetes. The rate of depression for older Mexican American women with diabetes was 37.9 percent versus the rate of 22.6 percent for older men with diabetes.

In addition, adults with higher levels of education had significantly lower levels of depression. (See also ALCOHOL ABUSE, COMPLICATIONS, DEATH, DEPRESSION, OBESITY, RACE/ETHNICITY, RETINOPATHY.)

Sandra A. Black, Ph.D., "Increased Health Burden Associated with Comorbid Depression in Older Diabetic Mexican Americans: Results from the Hispanic Established Population for the Epidemiologic Study of the Elderly Survey," *Diabetes Care* 22, no. 1 (January 1999): 56–64.

"Diabetes in Hispanic Americans," National Diabetes Information Clearinghouse, NIH Publication 99–3265, April 1999.

Healthy People 2010, Conference Edition. U.S. Department of Health and Human Services, January 2000.

"Self-Reported Prevalence of Diabetes among Hispanics—United States, 1994–1997," *Morbidity and Mortality Weekly Report* 48, no. 1 (January 15, 1999): 8–12.

HLA antigens   Proteins that aid the body in fighting illness and which vary from person to person. Some research indicates that certain types of HLA genes, and thus, the protein that they code for, make some people more genetically susceptible to developing Type 1 diabetes.

HMOs/managed care   Refers to health maintenance organizations (HMOs), preferred provider organizations (PPOs), and other entities that limit and control medical benefits available to groups of individuals. The individuals receiving health insurance coverage may be employees of an organization and their families or they may be recipients of MEDICAID or MEDICARE government plans. Health insurance is an important issue for people who have diabetes because they are more likely to need to see their physicians, and as they age, they are also increasingly more likely to require medical treatment.

Prior to the 1980s, much of healthcare was based on a "fee for service" model. This meant that individuals with health insurance could seek medical treatment from virtually any physician they chose and, in most cases, the health insurance carrier would pay all or most of the bill. Those who did not have health insurance would forgo treatment, pay the bill themselves or limit their treatment to emergency room care, paid for with public funds.

To put the situation in perspective, consider that in 1960, the patient paid for 20 percent of all hospital charges. By 1996, 97 percent of hospital payments came through third parties such as HMOs. Some experts estimate that the administrative expense needed to comply with a variety of HMOs represents at least 20 percent of all costs.

Many controls and constraints were set up by corporate employers and health insurance companies, who directly contracted with physicians, hospitals, and clinics to create agreements on conditions and fee schedules for health insurance coverage.

The HMO/managed care system also provides disincentives for patients to see physicians "out of network," or not on a preapproved list of physicians. If the patient sees an out-of-network doctor, the insurance company may pay a small part or none of the medical fee, depending on the particular plan. The HMO may also have a provision for the primary care physician who oversees the patient's case to make a "referral" to an out-of-network physician, if his or her expertise is not available within the plan.

Control over patients has also increased because many organizations under managed care insisted that all patients must go to one physician who manages the care of that individual. In order to see another doctor, the individual needs permission in the form of a referral from the "primary care" physician. Specific treatments, particularly surgeries or expensive diagnostic tools (such as magnetic resonance imaging or other diagnostic tests), would require advance authorization from the insurance company.

As of this writing, however, many large corporations have abandoned their complex authorization systems, seeing them as not cost-effective. Analysis by some companies has revealed that in the broad majority of cases, the insurance company had been approving the procedures the doctors recommended. They also analyzed the cost of managing preauthorizations, which was found to be extremely high. As a result, in the interests of saving money (and perhaps also an interest in alleviating some patient and physician unhappiness with preauthorizations), some HMOs have eliminated the requirement for preapproval to see specialists or have procedures.

For example, according to a report on managed care in a 2000 *Bulletin of the World Health Organization,* when United Healthcare required preauthorizations for services, they issued denials in only 1 percent of the cases. The utilization review staff cost the company millions of dollars per year. As a result, the corporation eliminated preauthorization requirements.

Managed Care as a Research Tool

It is possible to use HMOs as a management tool to help patients as well as cut costs. In a study described in a 1999 issue of *Diabetes Care,* patients who had both Type 1 and Type 2 diabetes and received treatment at the Kaiser Permanente clinic in Pleasanton, California, were divided into two groups. One group, the "inter-

vention" group, received comprehensive care from a team including a physician, a diabetes nurse educator, a psychologist, a nutritionist, and a pharmacist for about six months. The other group did not receive the team services.

The researchers found that HbA1C levels declined by 1.3 percent among members of the intervention group versus a decline of 0.2 percent in the control group members. Self-care and self-sufficiency improved among the intervention group members, who were reportedly pleased with the program.

The subjects were followed up and it was found that subjects in the intervention group experienced 80 percent fewer hospitalizations than those in the control group. The researchers' findings stated,

> Because of the poor outcomes and high cost of care for patients with diabetes, managed care organizations are actively developing new approaches to care for this large group of members. This study suggests that innovative approaches may be cost neutral in the short term, an observation that, if replicated, would remove a key barrier in adopting and implementing these effective innovations in treatment.

Problems with Managed Care

Along with some benefits to managed care, there are also many problems. As of this writing, Congress is debating a patient's bill of rights to enable patients to sue managed care companies for a variety of reasons.

Managed medications With regard to medication, some HMOs and other organizations that provided medication benefits set up "formularies," in which only the medications on their list are paid for and the individual is responsible for the entire cost of medicines not on the list.

Complicated for doctors Managed care has become difficult for U.S. physicians because they may be coping with many different health plans and a broad array of what is and is not payable, insofar as tests, treatments, or medications. The payment to the physician can also vary drastically, with some health plans paying most or all of what the doctor feels is fair for his or her services and with some radically undercharging the physician.

Whatever the type of managed care system, doctors must also spend greater amounts on administration than in the past. In 1960, an estimated 20 percent of a hospital's payment came directly from the consumer. In contrast, in 1996, only about 3 percent of hospital payment came from the consumer. The insurance companies who paid 97 percent of the hospital fees provided considerable oversight to the process that was absent a generation ago.

Eroded consumer confidence   In the late 1990s and early 21st century, some individuals and groups complained that they were prevented by managed care systems from obtaining good medical care. Some states passed laws mandating that certain types of services must be covered or that patients must be allowed to stay in a hospital for a certain number of days. Many states, as well as the federal government, began considering a "patient bill of rights" for the type of care that should be covered by insurance.

As of this writing, the managed care experience continues in the United States and is likely to continue for the foreseeable future. It appears to have contained medical costs for the present but it remains to be seen, with the rapidly aging population, if managed care companies can continue to hold costs down or if employers will continue to agree to bear the brunt of medical insurance premium increases.

Questions patients should ask about insurance coverage   Patients with diabetes should ask their health insurance company the following questions:

- Are there limits on the number of physician visits? If so, what are they?
- Is there a patient copayment? If so, what is it?
- Is diabetes education covered?

- Does the insurance plan cover seeing an endocrinologist, podiatrist, ophthalmologist, and other specialists that may be needed?
- Does the insurance cover supplies and medications?
- Is home care included in coverage?

(See also HOSPITALIZATION, INSURANCE.)

Craig N. Sadur, M.D., et al., "Diabetes Management in a Health Maintenance Organization: Efficacy of Care Management Using Cluster Visits," *Diabetes Care* 22, no. 12 (December 1999): 2011–2017.

Neelam K. Sekhri, "Managed Care: the U.S. Experience," *Bulletin of the World Health Organization* 78, no. 6 (June 2000): 830–844.

home blood glucose monitoring/self-blood glucose monitoring   Testing of the levels of the blood, performed by an individual at home, and subsequent actions based on the results of the test. (Such as taking medication, consuming a snack for low levels of glucose, etc.) Home blood glucose monitoring is critically important for all individuals with diabetes because it is not possible for physicians or other medical professionals to provide daily testing.

People diagnosed with both Type 1 and Type 2 diabetes need to keep track of their blood glucose level and watch themselves for any signs of a surge or sudden drop. This is referred to as maintaining GLYCEMIC CONTROL.

Very large scale studies, such as the DIABETES CONTROL AND COMPLICATIONS TRIAL (DCCT), a 10-year, federally funded study of individuals in North America with Type 1 diabetes, have validated the importance of self-monitoring and maintaining tight glucose levels in limiting the risk of severe future complications of diabetes, such as AMPUTATION, END-STAGE RENAL DISEASE, and other complications including an earlier than necessary death.

In addition, a large-scale study on individuals with Type 2 diabetes, the UNITED KINGDOM PROSPECTIVE DIABETES STUDY (UKPDS), also revealed the importance of tight glucose monitoring in aiding patients with Type 2 diabetes to avoid severe complications in the future.

A plunge in blood glucose level is an indication of HYPOGLYCEMIA, while elevated levels indicate HYPERGLYCEMIA. Many patients believe that they can tell what their glucose level is without performing any monitoring, but this is generally unreliable except when glucose levels are exceedingly high or low.

Although most people with diabetes are well aware of the need to monitor blood, sometimes compliance is lax because the person is ill or tired or distracted by other activities.

Most individuals with Type 1 diabetes must test their blood at least several times a day and if they are complying with an intensive testing regimen, at least four times per day is considered best. To achieve tight glycemic control, most people with Type 1 diabetes need to monitor their blood four times a day (three times before meals and one time at bedtime). People on insulin pumps often monitor themselves seven times a day, including three times a day pre-meal, three times post meal and once at bedtime. Patients should do extra tests when they are ill or they suspect they are hypoglycemic or hyperglycemic. They should also perform extra tests if they change their diet, exercise, or activity levels.

Patients with Type 2 diabetes and who do not require injections of insulin, may test their blood as infrequently as several times per month or 3–4 times per day. Each patient should consult with his or her physician and diabetes team to determine how much monitoring will help to optimize the individual's glycemic control.

Based on the glucose level readings, the individual can adjust his or her diet or exercise plan. The person with Type 1 diabetes can also adjust his or her insulin intake as well as adjust diet and exercise programs. Some people with Type 2 diabetes also require insulin and must make adjustments to their intake based on the results of their blood glucose test.

Excellent glycemic control levels are as follows:

pre-meal: 80–120
pre-bedtime: 100–140
(See also GLYCEMIC CONTROL.)

home health care   Health care that is provided to people within their homes, rather than in hospitals, clinics, or other settings. This may include injections, special treatments, or any other medical care that is indicated for a home-bound individual. Some people with diabetes need to receive home health care due to severe kidney disease or other ailments that are directly or indirectly related to their diabetes. They may need home health care aides or may need visits from nurses or other medically trained individuals.

MEDICARE has strict rules on what services may be paid for in home health care.

Medicare and Home Health Care

According to the Centers for Medicare and Medicaid Services, formerly the Health Care Financing Administration (HCFA), the organization that determines Medicare payments, there are four conditions that must *all* be met in order for Medicare to approve home health care. They are:

- A physician has determined that home health care is needed and has written a plan for care. This plan must be updated about every two months.

- The patient needs one or more of the following: skilled nursing care, or intermittent nursing care, or physical or speech therapy.

- The patient cannot leave the house except with extreme difficulty and is essentially considered "housebound."

- The home health care agency is approved by the Medicare program.

If the above conditions have been met, Medicare will pay (as of this writing) for the following types of services:

- skilled nursing care that is part time or intermittent and is provided by either a licensed practical nurse or registered nurse (for example, help with taking medications or injections)
- home health aide services provided on a part-time or intermittent basis. Examples of services are help with dressing, bathing, toileting, etc.
- physical therapy
- speech language pathology services
- occupational therapy
- medical social services such as counseling or assistance in locating resources in the patient's area
- assistance with blood glucose monitoring at home and reviews of medications
- some medical supplies such as bandages but not to include prescribed medications
- some medical equipment, which Medicare may pay 80 percent towards, such as a walker or a wheelchair.

Medicaid and Home Health Care

For patients who are indigent and receiving Medicaid services, home health care may be available. In some cases, Medicaid will cover services not paid by Medicare, such as homecare services, and personal care. (See also MEDICAID, MEDICARE.)

homocysteine An amino acid found in the bloodstream. Epidemiological studies indicate that patients with the highest levels of homocysteine have the highest risk of coronary heart disease and death from coronary heart disease. People with diabetes are at high risk for coronary heart disease. Homocysteine levels can theoretically provide an early indication of early or ongoing problems so that treatment can begin.

A combination of folic acid, Vitamin B_6, and Vitamin B_{12} may help lower the homocysteine level.

honeymoon phase A time that may occur early after a person with Type 1 diabetes has been diagnosed with the disease. By definition, people with Type 1 diabetes make no insulin and they are thus dependent upon insulin to live. However, early in the disease process, the patient's body may actually still make small amounts of insulin.

The person with new diabetes may also begin to have hypoglycemic episodes that lead the patient and physician to appropriately decrease the insulin dose. Sometimes insulin can be discontinued for a short period, which is generally no more than weeks. However, many endocrinologists prefer to maintain patients on small doses of insulin to avoid giving the patient false hope that the diabetes is cured. Also, some endocrinologists argue that stopping and starting insulin therapy may induce antibody formation and could cause the body to become more resistant to insulin. This could then result in the injected dose to become less effective in the future. In that event, a larger injected dose of insulin would be needed.

HOPE Study Refers to the Heart Outcomes Prevention Evaluation (HOPE) study in Canada, which was performed with subjects who had a high risk for developing cardiovascular disease. The subjects were about 9,000 patients over age 55 who were also at very high risk for developing cardiac ailments. Of these patients, 1,808 were men and women with diabetes. The average age of the patients studied was 65 years and 58 percent of them had a previous history of HYPERTENSION. Two thirds of the subjects also had a problem with high CHOLESTEROL.

The purpose of the study, which was completed in 1999, was to determine if the administration of a specific angiotensin-converting enzyme (ACE) inhibitor medication (ramipril) would reduce the risk of heart disease. The researchers found that treatment with the medication was successful at reducing the overall death rates, dropping the risk for heart attack by

20 percent, and decreasing the incidence of complications related to diabetes by 16 percent. Overall, the risk of death was reduced by 16 percent. The study was ended early because the findings were so promising for the patients receiving the medication. Researchers wanted those patients taking the placebo to have the chance to take an ACE inhibitor drug and gain from its benefits.

Among the diabetic subjects, the researchers found that the medication effectively decreased the risk of serious cardiovascular problems, whether the patients were also taking oral hypoglycemic medications or they were injecting insulin and even if patients had a prior history of cardiovascular ailments. The study also revealed that ramipril decreased the risk of DIABETIC NEPHROPATHY (kidney disease) in patients by about 24 percent.

Tonny Jensen, et al., "The HOPE Study and Diabetes," *The Lancet* 355, no. 9210 (April 2000): 1181.

Anne Peters, M.D., "Landmark Studies: Hope for the Diabetic Heart," *Clinical Diabetes* 18, no. 3 (Summer 2000): 130–131.

hormone replacement therapy (HRT)/estrogen replacement therapy (ERT)   Hormones prescribed for women, with and without diabetes, after the onset of menopause or in the transitional period known as the "perimenopause." This entry covers both estrogen-only therapy and combination therapy (estrogen and progestogen), and umbrellas both therapies under "hormone replacement therapy." It should be noted that most doctors consider only combination therapy as HRT and they call estrogen therapy alone "ERT."

Many physicians recommend medications to replace the hormones that are no longer produced or are produced in diminished quantities by the woman's own body. Doctors may recommend estrogen replacement therapy (ERT) if patients have had a hysterectomy. If the woman still has her uterus, physicians may recommend a combination therapy of estrogen and a progestational agent such as medroxyprogesterone

acetate, which will allow the lining of the uterus [endometrium] to cycle and minimize the risk of endometrial cancer. These medications are offered to women with and without diabetes.

Pros and Cons of HRT

As of this writing there are mixed findings on the pros and cons of administering hormone replacement therapy to menopausal women, including women with diabetes. In general, HRT may provide some protection against heart disease, STROKE, ALZHEIMER'S DISEASE, colorectal cancer, tooth loss, age-related macular degeneration, and OSTEOPOROSIS/fractures. These problems are also experienced by many women with diabetes. HRT may also give the woman relief from sleep disorders, improving the quality and duration of sleep. HRT may also improve cognitive function. In addition, women who take HRT may find relief from many other problems such as atrophy of the genitourinary track and vasomotor symptoms, such as hot flashes and temperature intolerance. HRT may also bring relief from emotional problems such as DEPRESSION. Many women with diabetes have high risks for the aforementioned problems.

There are also some negative aspects to taking female hormones. Women who use HRT are more prone to developing gallbladder disease, blood clots (phlebitis, phlebothrombosis, and pulmonary embolism-blood clots from the legs or pelvis that can break off and travel to the lungs). Breast cancer is another risk of HRT, particularly in women with a family history for the disease. In addition, if the woman still has her uterus, HRT may present a greater risk than the woman not taking hormones for causing the development of endometrial (uterine lining) cancer. Added estrogen may also cause breast tenderness, precipitate migraine headaches, and also cause fluid retention and mild weight gain. It can create depression in some women.

Studies on HRT and Heart Disease

There are currently 35 observational studies that show a 50 percent decrease in heart disease in women on HRT. This makes sense given what we know of the effects of estrogen; improved lipid profile, decreased INSULIN RESISTANCE, decreased stickiness of platelets, increased blood flow, as well as an improved ability of the coronary arteries to dilate, better pumping of heart muscle, and decreased plaque formation in blood vessels.

Much of the controversy over HRT in recent years has come up in studies that looked at the potential benefits of HRT in women with known HEART DISEASE (which includes many women with diabetes mellitus). For example, the Heart and Estrogen/Progestin Replacement Study (HERS), was a study of 2,763 women with an average age of 66.7 years. The subjects were treated with both 0.625 mg of estrogen and 2.5 mg of medroxyprogesterone acetate for 5 years. A control group received a placebo.

At the end of the study, researchers concluded that there were no major differences between the treated and untreated groups. Of greatest concern, however, was the observation that there was actually an *increased* incidence of heart problems in the first eight months in the women who were treated with HRT. Paradoxically, however, as the study carried on, this trend reversed itself. The women who continued in the study were found to have a greater protection from heart events.

It may be that the initial effects of estrogen tend to lead to an increased risk of clotting and, thus, blockages that are already present in women taking HRT become a problem. Over time, however, as the multiple positive metabolic effects kick in, HRT may offer greater protection and overcome the impact of the clotting effects.

Similar results were reported in the Women's Health Initiative (WHI) study. In the first two years of the study, about 1 percent of the women had heart attacks, strokes, and blood clots in their legs and lungs whether they were on estrogen therapy, combination therapy, or placebo. Again, as in the HERS study, the situation changed after two years and the hormones were shown to be protective.

As a result of these studies, current recommendations are that hormone replacement drugs should not be considered as therapy for secondary prevention for women who already have known heart disease. But in women who do not have heart disease but who are at risk for disease, HRT may be beneficial.

To be effective and safe, it appears that women who use HRT need to start taking hormones prior to the development of problems in the blood vessels in order to allow the medication to continue to protect women. If a woman already has heart problems, it's best to avoid these drugs unless further evidence indicates this group should take them.

Women with Diabetes and HRT

It had long been thought that administering HRT to women with diabetes would worsen their control of glucose levels; however, recent studies have shown that this is generally not the case. All parameters of glucose metabolism, especially insulin resistance and lipid profiles, appear to improve with HRT.

Note: HRT is not the same situation as is found with oral contraceptives (which also have female hormones) prescribed for birth control. The reason for this is that birth control pills may contain a larger dose of estrogen than found in hormone replacement therapy. Consequently, birth control pills are more likely to increase insulin resistance (probably because of the progestational component) than HRT. Thus, women with normal glucose tolerance and with risk factors for diabetes who are taking birth control pills may find that their condition worsens to IMPAIRED GLUCOSE TOLERANCE (IGT), with higher than normal glucose levels but not high enough to be diagnosed with diabetes. Women who already have IGT and who take oral contraceptives may progress to overt diabetes. Women who already have diabetes may require an adjustment in their medication in order to continue to maintain their usual level of glycemic control.

Consulting with gynecologists Because the issue is so complex and so individual for each woman, and because there are many types of medications and dosages, it's best for menopausal women with diabetes who are considering HRT to consult with their own gynecologists on what course of action to take. If the woman is under age 50, it's probably a good idea to request a blood test of estrogen levels (generally, FSH), to avoid unnecessary medication.

Multiple medical professional organizations such as the American Association of Clinical Endocrinologists (AACE), the American College of Obstetricians and Gynecologists (ACOG), and the Association of Professors of Gynecology and Obstetrics (APGO), have published evidence-based guidelines on HRT/ERT that attempt to weigh the benefits and risks of this therapy.

For further information on the Internet, go to the National Women's Health Information Center at www.4woman.gov/faq/hormone.htm. The National Institute on Aging also offers information on the pros and cons of HRT on the following website: www.aoa.dhhs.gov/aoa/pages/agepages/hormone.html.

"AACE Medical Guidelines for Clinical Practice for Management of Menopause," *Endocrine Practice* 5 (1999): 355–366.

"Hormone Replacement Therapy," *ACOG Educational Bulletin,* no. 247 (1998).

S. Hulley, D. Grady, T. Bush, et al., "Randomized Trial of Estrogen Plus Progestin for Secondary Prevention of Coronary Heart Disease in Postmenopausal Women. Heart and Estrogen/Progestin Replacement Study (HERS) Research Group," *JAMA* 280, no. 7 (1998): 605–613.

N. F. Col Santoro, M. H. Eckman, et al., "Therapeutic Controversy: Hormone Replacement—Where Are We Going," *Journal of Clinical Endocrinology and Metabolism* 84, no. 6 (1999): 1798–1812.

hospitalization Admission to a hospital for treatment of a serious disease. Individuals with diabetes may need hospitalization for a variety of problems, including severe foot problems, extreme HYPOGLYCEMIA or HYPERGLYCEMIA, DIA-BETIC KETOACIDOSIS (DKA), HYPERTENSION, COMA, and an array of other medical problems. According to the Centers for Disease Control and Prevention (CDC), diabetes was the first diagnosis in 503,000 hospital discharges in 1996. Diabetes was also a factor in thousands of other cases in which it was not the first diagnosis.

Diabetic individuals are also more likely than nondiabetics to need hospitalization; for example, studies indicate that people with diabetes are four times more likely to be hospitalized than nondiabetics, or 24 percent to 6 percent, respectively. People with diabetes in the United States are hospitalized over 3 million days per year and also make over 15 million visits to their physicians on an outpatient basis.

This high rate of hospitalization may be due in part to the fact that 51 percent of the population with diabetes is in fair or poor physical health versus 9 percent of nondiabetics who are in fair to poor health. An estimated 80,000 former workers are permanently disabled because of their diabetes.

In one study of the risks for hospitalization among people with diabetes, reported in a 1999 issue of the *Archives of Internal Medicine,* the researchers found that people with Type 1 diabetes had a greater risk for hospitalization when they had high glycosylated hemoglobin levels or they had hypertension. Among those with Type 2 diabetes, the key factor that predicted hospitalization was high glycosylated hemoglobin levels. As a result, good GLYCEMIC CONTROL was a factor in keeping both Type 1 and Type 2 diabetes patients out of the hospital. (See also EMERGENCY CARE.)

S. E. Moss et al., "Risk Factors for Hospitalization in People with Diabetes," *Archives of Internal Medicine* 159 (1999): 2053–2057.

National Academy on an Aging Society, "Diabetes: A Drain on U.S. Resources," *Challenges for the 21st Century: Chronic and Disabling Conditions* 1, no. 6 (April 2000): 1–6.

HS-CRP test High sensitivity C-reactive protein test, a test that measures the inflammation in the blood vessels of the body. If results are elevated, they can be lowered with aspirin and HMG CoA reductase inhibitor medications. The test is inaccurate if the patient has any other cause of inflammation such as infection.

Patients with diabetes are at high risk for ATHEROSCLEROSIS, and thus, this test is of great interest to them because if identified at an early stage, it may enable some patients to obtain treatment to prevent the disease or delay a further progression of existing atherosclerosis.

Humalog   A form of insulin lispro trademarked by Eli Lilly & Company and approved by the Food and Drug Administration (FDA) in the United States in 1996. Humalog is made from manipulated DNA material rather than from beef or pork insulin. Such forms are generally better tolerated by people with diabetes than are forms derived from animal insulin. Humalog is a rapid-acting insulin that starts working within five to 15 minutes from injection. The bulk of its action ends within three to four hours, as opposed to five to eight hours with regular insulin. Humalog is less likely to cause HYPOGLYCEMIA.

Because of the change in the amino acids, Humalog is more rapidly absorbed from subcutaneous fat sites after absorption. It peaks in one hour, which is typically when the body's glucose level peaks, thus creating a good match. Humalog is more convenient and effective than traditional regular insulin. (See also INSULIN.)

hyperglycemia   An excessive level of glucose in the bloodstream of an individual and the hallmark feature of diabetes.

The key symptoms of hyperglycemia (and diabetes) are:

- increased urination
- increased thirst
- unexplained weight loss
- blurred vision

Individuals diagnosed with TYPE 1 DIABETES should self-test their blood three to four times per day, and should also use INSULIN as prescribed by their physicians in order to control the hyperglycemia. Individuals with TYPE 2 DIABETES should also do daily blood testing and use oral medications, diet, and exercise to control hyperglycemia. Those with Type 1 and Type 2 diabetes need to monitor their diet carefully and also exercise on a regular basis in order to better control the symptoms and the moderate-to-severe complications that can come with diabetes. (See also GLYCEMIC CONTROL.)

hyperinsulinism/hyperinsulinemia   Excessive amounts of insulin in the body. This condition may occur when the body creates large amounts of insulin in an attempt to overcome INSULIN RESISTANCE (the inability to properly use the insulin). Hyperinsulinism results in a lowered blood level of HDL cholesterol ("good" cholesterol) and is also associated with increased levels of TRIGLYCERIDES. This condition may lead to the development of Type 2 diabetes, although it is not inevitable that diabetes will occur. The likelihood of developing diabetes is increased, however, if there are other family members who have a medical history of diabetes.

If a person has HYPERTENSION in addition to hyperinsulinism, this condition can cause DIABETIC NEPHROPATHY, or kidney damage. When hyperinsulinism is associated with hypertension, obesity, DYSLIPIDEMIA, polycystic ovarian syndrome, or premature cardiovascular disease, it is known as SYNDROME X. Other names for Syndrome X are Cardiac Dysmetabolic Syndrome and Insulin Resistance Syndrome.

G. M. Reaven, "Role of Insulin Resistance in Human Disease," *Diabetes* 37 (1998): 1495.

hyperlipidemia   Excessive levels of blood lipids (fats), such as LDL cholesterol and trigylcerides. This is a dangerous condition that can lead to serious medical consequences, such as heart attack, STROKE, and other problems. A physician will almost invariably recommend dietary changes and, if the patient is overweight as well, will also recommend weight loss. The doctor may also prescribe medications to lower cholesterol levels. (See CHOLESTEROL, DYSLIPIDEMIA, HDL, LDL, LIPIDS, TRIGYLCERIDES.)

hyperosmolar coma   A very serious condition of unconsciousness that occurs in patients with Type 2 diabetes. Also known as Hyperosmolar Hyperglycemic Nonketotic Coma (HHNC). Daily blood testing will generally alert a person with diabetes to increasing glucose levels before they reach the stage of hyperosmolar coma. In about 33 percent of the cases, a hyperosmolar coma is the presenting sign of diabetes: the person was previously undiagnosed.

This condition is more common among elderly individuals with other coexisting (intercurrent) serious illnesses. The individual is hyperglycemic and severely dehydrated and requires immediate medical attention. Blood glucose levels may be 500–1,000 mg/dL. Generally, there is less vomiting and nausea than seen in DIABETIC KETOACIDOSIS (DKA) and the syndrome may develop over days to a week.

Symptoms of Hyperosmolar Coma

The primary symptoms are:

- Thirst and dry mouth
- Decreased sweating
- Increased urination initially and then decreased urination
- Confusion or increased sleepiness
- Glucose levels that are greater than 500 mg/dL
- Sunken eyes and rapid pulse
- Weakness and leg cramps

Causes

Hyperosmolar coma can be precipitated by infection (urinary tract infection, pneumonia, etc.),

dehydration (poor oral intake, diarrhea, bleeding), alcohol abuse, or other co-occurring medical illness.

Treatment of Hyperosmolar Coma

The person needs to be hospitalized. Primary treatment at the hospital is aimed at rehydration with intravenous fluids and correction of the underlying cause.

hypertension   Excessively high levels of blood pressure. Also known as "high blood pressure."

Global Definition of Hypertension

In 1997, the National Committee on Prevention, Detection, Evaluation, and Treatment of High Blood Pressure defined hypertension in adults age 18 and over in their 1997 report. The World Health Organization adopted essentially the same definitions in their 1999 report on hypertension.

According to these experts, optimal SYSTOLIC PRESSURE (the upper number in the measurement of blood pressure) is less than 120 mm Hg and optimal DIASTOLIC PRESSURE (the lower number) is less than 80 mm Hg. (See the chart in this essay on levels of blood pressure).

Hypertension is a serious medical condition experienced by many people with (and without) diabetes throughout the world. It can lead to severe complications such as heart disease, kidney disease, BLINDNESS, and many other complications, up to and including death.

In addition, the combination of diabetes and hypertension is very dangerous; for example, people with both diabetes and high blood pressure have two to four times the risk of stroke than is experienced by others.

An estimated 42 percent of patients with hypertension who will ultimately need kidney dialysis or require kidney transplantation also have diabetes, according to the authors of a 2000 article in the *American Journal of Kidney Diseases.*

An estimated 60–65 percent of all those who have diabetes suffer from hypertension. In general, people with Type 1 diabetes have hypertension at about the same level as those in the general population, although it is often diagnosed subsequent to renal impairment. In contrast, hypertension is a common problem for people with Type 2 diabetes and is frequently associated with obesity. The diagnosis of hypertension may also pre-date the diagnosis of diabetes or it may be diagnosed at the same time as diabetes. Many patients with essential hypertension have insulin resistance and may manifest other signs and symptoms of SYNDROME X.

This does not mean that people who have both diabetes and hypertension should despair. Study after study has proven a direct correlation between reducing blood pressure and greatly reducing the risk of heart attack, stroke, and death.

The solution lies in both lifestyle changes and medications, which can reduce blood pressure and also greatly diminish the risk of medical complications that may come from the combination of diabetes and hypertension. A key problem, however, is that many people with hypertension do not make needed lifestyle changes nor do they take prescribed medications. Instead, sadly, the majority of the people in the world who have hypertension are not receiving adequate treatment.

About 50 million people in the United States have hypertension and about 75 percent of adults with hypertension are not controlling their blood pressure to below 135/85 mm Hg, thus, unnecessarily increasing their risks for medical complications. Globally, an estimated 600 million people have hypertension, according to the World Health Organization (WHO). Some countries have a very severe problem: over 100 million people in China suffer from hypertension.

Most people with hypertension (95 percent) have "essential hypertension," which is high blood pressure with no clear-cut cause. Five percent of those with hypertension have "secondary hypertension," which is high blood pressure that is brought on by other identifiable causes.

Causes of Hypertension

High blood pressure may be caused by genetic risk, combined with OBESITY, a stressful lifestyle, and other factors. Sometimes medication is the cause of hypertension. For example, oral contraceptives may raise blood pressure. The risk factor is further exacerbated among women who also smoke.

Demographics of Hypertension

Although people of any age, even children, can be hypertensive, most people with hypertension are middle-aged or older and the risk for developing hypertension increases with age.

Ethnic factors   Another key factor associated with hypertension is ethnicity: African Americans, New Zealand Maoris, and some Native American tribes in the United States, such as the PIMA INDIANS, have higher rates of hypertension and greater risks for cardiovascular diseases than do individuals of other ethnicities.

Age   The gap between blacks and whites who have hypertension in the United States is greatest for those between the ages of 55–64, when hypertension among blacks is twice that experienced by whites. But even at older ages, blacks have higher rates of hypertension; for example, 54 percent of blacks over age 75 have hypertension versus 38 percent of whites in the same age group.

Elderly people and hypertension   Older people are at a greater risk for developing hypertension or experiencing a worsening of already-existing high blood pressure. In the Systolic Hypertension in the Elderly Program (SHEP) study in 1996, researchers studied 4,736 men and women over age 60. Of these, 584 of the subjects had Type 2 diabetes. The "active" group received a diuretic medication (chlorthalidone) and when needed, a beta-blocker drug such as atenolol was used, or another drug, such as resperine, was added. The placebo group received any medication that their own doctor prescribed.

The results clearly demonstrated the benefits of active treatment. Jennifer Marks said in her article for a 1999 issue of *Clinical Diabetes,*

The results from the active treatment diabetic group demonstrated reductions in rates for all major cardiovascular events (34%), for nonfatal and fatal stroke (22%), for nonfatal and fatal myocardial infarction (MI) (56%), and for all-cause mortality (26%).

Another study, the Systolic Hypertension in Europe study (Syst-Eur) also clearly indicated that patients with diabetes who were intensively treated had reduced death rates, reduced rates of stroke, and much lower rates of heart disease.

Gender and hypertension In considering gender, both women and men suffer from hypertension, although WOMEN WITH DIABETES have higher rates of hypertension than either nondiabetic individuals or diabetic men. African American women are particularly at risk for high blood pressure.

Costs for Hypertension Are High

The American Heart Association estimated that the total cost of hypertension in the United States was $37 billion in 1999, including $26 billion in direct costs and $11 million in lost wages. This does not include other costs, such as caregiving expenses, emotional constraints, and other "hard" and "soft" costs accruing to the costs of hypertension.

Regular medical and self-monitoring of blood pressure is essential The UNITED KINGDOM PROSPECTIVE DIABETES STUDY (UKPDS) clearly demonstrated that tight control of hypertension significantly reduces the risk of later complications among people who have diabetes. In fact, hypertension control was actually found to be a greater factor than glycemic control for reducing the risks of certain complications among people who have both hypertension and diabetes.

The National High Blood Pressure Education Program Working Group and Joint National Committee on Prevention, Detection, Evaluation, and Treatment of High Blood Pressure has recommended that blood pressure be lowered to less than 130/85 or lower. Studies have also revealed clinical improvements and fewer complications for people with diabetes who have lowered their diastolic pressure to less than 80—even though 80 is considered a "normal" reading.

Hypertension Is a Chronic Condition

People with hypertension and their families need to realize that this is a chronic and lifelong condition. Although lifestyle changes and medication can vastly improve blood pressure measurements, it is still necessary to continue to monitor the condition. Many patients make a classic mistake of taking their medicine and noting their improved blood pressure readings. They may decide they are "cured" and stop taking their medication. The blood pressure will typically go up again and serious medical complications can ensue.

It may be possible to "step down" on medications, taking a lower dose, but only upon the advice of the treating doctor. It may also be advisable to change or add medications, should the physician believe it becomes necessary.

Diabetes and Hypertension: A Dangerous Combination

According to Dr. George Bakris and his colleague physicians of the National Kidney Foundation Hypertension and Diabetes Executive Committees Working Group, in their article in a 2000 issue of *American Journal of Kidney Diseases,* "Hypertension exacerbates all of the vascular complications of diabetes, including renal disease, coronary heart disease, stroke, peripheral vascular disease, lower extremity amputations, and retinopathy. Moreover, people with both diabetes and hypertension have a 5- to 6-fold greater risk of developing ESRD [end stage renal disease] compared with people with hypertension and no evidence of diabetes."

Cardiovascular Risk Factors and Hypertension

When combined with hypertension, diabetes is a major risk factor for the development of cardiovascular diseases. Other risk factors that further exacerbate the risk of cardiovascular diseases among all people with hypertension include:

- smoking
- dyslipidemia (abnormal cholesterol levels: increased levels of LDL and triglycerides and decreased levels of HDL)
- age: over 60 years
- family history of cardiovascular disease in females over age 65 and in males over age 55

There are also particular organs within the body that are most prone to damage from hypertension. The major types of damage that may occur are:

- heart disease (left ventricular hypertrophy [thickening of heart muscle]/angina/myocardial infarction [heart attack]/heart failure)
- stroke or transient ischemic attack (TIA)
- renal (kidney) disease, up to and including end-stage renal disease that requires dialysis and kidney transplant
- erectile dysfunction
- peripheral arterial disease/claudication
- diabetic retinopathy

The existence of risk factors are important considerations because, when taken together, they provide a different picture. For example, according to the WHO-ISH study in 1999,

> Among patients with mild hypertension, differences in the risks of cardiovascular disease are determined not only by the level of blood pressure, but also by the presence or levels of other risk factors.
>
> For example, a man aged 65 years with diabetes, a history of TIA, and a blood pressure of 145/90 mm Hg will have an annual risk of a major cardiovascular event that is more than **20 times greater** [boldface and italics per original text] than that in a man aged 40 years with the same blood pressure but without either diabetes or a history of cardiovascular disease.

Major Studies on Hypertension

Several major studies on individuals with hypertension are often cited by experts and re-searchers. These studies placed subjects in groups with different medications that reduced blood pressure. The researchers worked to intensively reduce blood pressure in one group and achieve a more moderate blood pressure goal in the other group. The researchers then compared the two groups to each other. Invariably, the group who brought their blood pressure down lower fared much better and had far lower rates of later developing serious complications in most categories.

CLASSIFICATION OF BLOOD PRESSURE FOR ADULTS AGE 18 AND OLDER*

Category	Systolic (mm Hg)		Diastolic (mm Hg)
Optimal†	<120	and	<80
Normal	<130	and	<85
High-normal	130–139	or	85–89
Hypertension‡			
Stage 1	140–159	or	90–99
Stage 2	160–179	or	100–109
Stage 3	≥180	or	≥110

* Not taking antihypertensive drugs and not acutely ill. When systolic and diastolic blood pressure fall into different categories, the higher category should be selected to classify the individual's blood pressure status. For example, 160/92 mm Hg should be classified as stage 2 hypertension and 174/120 mm Hg should be classified as stage 3 hypertension. Isolated systolic hypertension is defined as SBP of 140 mm Hg or greater and DBP below 90 mm Hg and staged appropriately (for example, 170/82 mm Hg is defined as stage 2 isolated systolic hypertension). In addition to classifying stage of hypertension on the basis of average blood pressure levels, clinicians should specify presence of absence of target organ disease and additional risk factors.

† Optimal blood pressure with respect to cardiovascular risk is below 120/80 mm Hg. However, unusually low readings should be evaluated for clinical significance.

‡ Based on the average of two or more readings taken at each of two or more visits after an initial screening.

Source: "The Sixth Report of the Joint National Committee on Prevention, Detection, Evaluation, and Treatment of High Blood Pressure, National Heart, Lung, and Blood Institute, National Institutes of Health, NIH Publication, No. 98-4080, November 1997.

The Hypertension Optimal Treatment (HOT) trial studied 1,501 patients with both diabetes and hypertension. Study results, reported in 1998, clearly revealed that the patients who achieved the lowest blood pressure were also the patients with the least number of cardiovascular problems.

The United Kingdom Prospective Diabetes Study (UKPDS) looked at 1,148 patients with diabetes, comparing the results of the "intensively treated" group to the "conventional" group and then following them for more than eight years. Results: the intensively treated group had 32 percent fewer deaths and 44 percent fewer strokes and also accrued other health benefits. This was true even though the intensively treated group averaged a still-high blood pressure of 144/82 mm Hg versus the control group's average blood pressure of 154/87 mm Hg. Thus, the improvement was only a very small 10/5 and yet it meant the difference between life and death for some.

Experts now know, however, that when a person has both diabetes and hypertension, even those with high/normal blood pressures of between 130–139/85–89 will benefit from lifestyle changes as well as medication therapy. One reason for this is that many people with diabetes ("non-dippers") do not experience a nocturnal decrease in their blood pressure, as do nondiabetics. As a result, the continued higher level of pressure at a "24/7" level, along with the harm that diabetes alone can bring, can be very damaging.

Diagnosis of Hypertension

Physicians, nurses, staff members, and even a patient can determine blood pressure levels with a cuff device. Experts say that devices that take the blood pressure by insertion of a finger in a cuff are generally not as accurate as the devices that determine the blood pressure taken in the arm.

Before the blood pressure is taken, the person should avoid caffeine for several hours and also should not smoke. Just before the reading is taken, the person should rest for about five minutes and his or her arm should be supported. It's also important to use the right cuff size. It may be difficult to obtain an accurate measure on a very obese or extremely thin per-son. Large or small devices may work better, depending on the size of the person.

Laboratory tests may be taken to look for an underlying cause of the hypertension or to determine if any complications already exist. Doctors generally order urinalysis and blood tests that measure hematocrit, serum electrolytes (especially sodium and potassium), BUN, creatinine and glucose levels, and plasma lipid levels. The patient's urine may be checked for albumin excretion and an electrocardiogram may also be ordered. A 24-hour urinary protein excretion level can provide important diagnostic information; for example, the normal range of urinary albumin excertion rate is less than 150 mg/day. Any amount above that level may be indicative of diabetic nephropathy and other complications.

Spot urine levels can also be taken. Levels of 0–30 mg of albumin/grams creatinine are normal. If albumin levels are between 30 and 300, the person has microalbuminuria and needs to be treated. If the levels are greater than 300, then this is a sign of overt PROTEINURIA and a problem that must be treated.

Treatment of Hypertension: Lifestyle Changes

Hypertension can be treated with lifestyle changes, such as improvements in diet, weight loss, and increased exercise. Individuals who smoke should immediately stop smoking. According to the World Health Organization and the International Society of Hypertension, in their WHO-ISH guidelines, "Smoking cessation is the single most powerful lifestyle measure for the prevention of both cardiovascular and noncardiovascular diseases in hypertensive patients."

If the person with hypertension consumes alcohol, he or she should stop drinking altogether or severely limit alcohol intake. The Joint National Committee recommended that daily alcohol intake for the average person should not exceed 1 ounce (30 mL) of ethanol per day. People who are of smaller size and weight should not exceed 0.5 ounces (15 mL) of ethanol per day.

Dietary changes can also provide enhanced health benefits to the person who has hypertension. Salt should not be added to foods and high salt foods should be avoided. Some types of foods should be added while others should be cut back or eliminated. For example, it is important for the person with hypertension to ensure an adequate intake of potassium, which often may be taken care of with diet. Eating fresh vegetables may provide sufficient potassium. However, sometimes people with hypertension become hypokalemic because of medications (particularly diuretics) or for other reasons and, thus, they may need to take a potassium supplement in addition. (But people with diabetes should not self-treat, instead, potassium should be taken only by prescription, because some drugs used to treat hypertension can raise potassium levels.)

Physicians also recommend that people with hypertension cut back on their salt (sodium chloride) intake, which can help lower blood pressure levels.

Regular EXERCISE is another important lifestyle component of keeping hypertension within control. Even a brisk walk—30–45 minutes, several days a week—can be sufficient to improve health. According to the WHO-ISH 1999 report, 20 minutes per day of light-to-moderate exercise can enable a person with hypertension to reduce the risk of death from cardiovascular disease by 30 percent.

Some exercise, however, can be detrimental to the person who has hypertension; for example, heavy weight lifting or other isometric exercises can work to raise rather than lower blood pressure and, consequently, should be avoided.

Emotional stress can also raise blood pressure. People with hypertension may need to learn relaxation tactics to cope with their reactions to the problems of life. Stress cannot be altogether eliminated from life; however, it is the individual's reaction to stress that may be modified.

Treatment of Hypertension: Medication

Many people who have hypertension will also need to take medication to lower their blood pressure and many people with diabetes will need two or three different medications to optimally control their hypertension. The Joint National Committee VI stated that individuals with high-normal blood pressure and diabetes should take medication.

As of this writing, new hypertensive patients are often started off with a medication in the ACE inhibitor class. In addition to lowering blood pressure, they also help to slow the progression of renal disease in people with diabetes, independent of their overall lowering of blood pressure. ACE drugs have positive effects on the filtering units (glomeruli) in the kidney and they slow progression of neuropathy above and beyond their effects on blood pressure.

Some medications used to control diabetes also lower blood pressure, such as metformin and drugs in the thiazolidinedione class, but they should not be used solely for this purpose.

Medication may also be needed to bring DYSLIPIDEMIA under control. LDL cholesterol levels should be brought to below 100 mg/dL for patients who have both diabetes and hypertension.

Problems with Medication Adherence

Despite information that is provided to patients about the risk they face with both hypertension and diabetes as well as the emphasis upon the necessity to take their medication to decrease these risks, physicians report many problems with nonadherence to their prescribed medication regimen. There are a variety of reasons why people with hypertension and diabetes do not take their medicine.

The patient may not understand what is needed, and it's essential that doctors and patients attain clear communication. According to the WHO-ISH report, "Adequate information about BP and high BP, about risks and prognosis, about the expected benefits of treatment, and about the risks and side effects of treatment will be essential for satisfactory life-long control of hypertension, which is poor in many countries today."

Some patients don't take their medicine for hypertension regularly (or at all) for the same reason they don't take their medicine for other illnesses. For example, they may forget to take the medicine or may minimize the extent of their problem. Hypertension generally causes no symptoms and is a "silent killer."

Patients may fail to take their medication because they may not like the side effects of medication or they may not be able to afford the drugs.

Researchers have found a unique reason for why some men, especially African Americans, Mexican Americans, or Native Americans, refuse to take their medicine. The common belief among such men is that their medication will cause ERECTILE DYSFUNCTION (ED). Yet studies indicate that the incidence of sexual dysfunction with the newer medications for hypertension are low.

Bakris et al. said, "In fact, data have clearly shown that patients who achieve the lower blood pressure goals typically experience the best quality of life (including sex life)."

Followup Measurements of Hypertension

Doctors recommend follow-up measurements when patients with or without diabetes have demonstrable hypertension. The Joint National Committee VI recommended the following guidelines for rechecks of blood pressure:

Systolic	Diastolic	Follow-up Recommended
130–139	85–89	Recheck in one year
140–159	90–99	Confirm in two months (based on past BP measurements, other cardiovascular risk factors or target organ disease)
160–179	100–109	Evaluate or refer to source of care within one month

Systolic	Diastolic	Follow-up Recommended
≥180	≥110	Evaluate or refer to source of care immediately or within one week, depending on clinical situation

"White Coat" Hypertension/White Coat Effect

Some individuals have a tendency to experience an elevated blood pressure when they are in a physician's office, presumably as a reflexive act of seeing a doctor. (The white laboratory coat of the doctor is the "white coat," the sight of which may induce a temporarily elevated blood pressure in some individuals.)

Such individuals may have normal blood pressure readings when absent of this reflex. For this reason, doctors should take at least several readings that are at least two minutes apart and also take readings on different occasions before diagnosing hypertension—unless the blood pressure is so high that it would be dangerous to delay treatment. White coat hypertension is another reason why doctors advise people with diabetes and hypertension to monitor their blood pressure at home, just as they monitor their glucose. (See also ASPIRIN THERAPY, END-STAGE RENAL DISEASE (ESRD), EYE PROBLEMS, GLAUCOMA, MEDICATION NONADHERENCE, NEPHROPATHY, NEUROPATHY.)

George L. Bakris, M.D., et al., "Preserving Renal Function in Adults with Hypertension and Diabetes: A Consensus Approach," *American Journal of Kidney Diseases* 36, no. 3 (September 2000): 646–661.

John Chalmers et al., World Health Organization/International Society of Hypertension (WHO-ISH), "Practice Guidelines for Primary Care Physicians: 1999 WHO/ISH Hypertension Guidelines," Geneva, Switzerland, 1999.

Prakash C. Deedwania, M.D., "Hypertension and Diabetes: New Therapeutic Options," *Archives of Internal Medicine* 160, no. 11 (June 12, 2000): 1585–1594.

Raymond O. Estacio, M.D., et al., "Effect of Blood Pressure Control on Diabetic Microvascular Complications in Patients with Hypertension and Type 2 Diabetes," *Diabetes Care* 23, Supp. 2 (April 2000): B54–B64.

Hans-Henrik Parving, M.D., D.M.Sc., "Diabetic Hypertensive Patients: Is This a Group in Need of Particular Care and Attention?" *Diabetes Care* 22, Supp. 2 (1999).

Jennifer B. Marks, M.D., C.D.E., "Treating Hypertension in Diabetes: Data and Perspectives," *Clinical Diabetes* 17, no. 4, (1999): http://www.find articles.com/cf_0/m0682/4_17/57562552/print. jhtml.

National Academy on an Aging Society, "Hypertension: A Common Condition for Older Americans," *Challenges for the 21st Century: Chronic and Disabling Conditions* 1, no. 12 (October 2000): 1–6.

National Institutes of Health, "The Sixth Report of the Joint National Committee on Prevention, Detection, Evaluation, and Treatment of High Blood Pressure, National Heart, Lung, and Blood Institute, National Institutes of Health, NIH Publication, No. 98–4080, November 1997.

World Health Organization and the International Society of Hypertension, "1999 World Health Organization-International Society of Hypertension Guidelines for the Management of Hypertension," 1999.

hypoglycemia   Very low blood glucose (sugar) levels requiring the emergency administration of glucose. Hypoglycemia is the most common complication of diabetes, particularly Type 1 diabetes, although people with Type 2 diabetes may also experience this problem.

People who do not have diabetes at all may also become hypoglycemic, although this occurs far less frequently than was believed in the past. As many as 20 percent of all people with diabetes have at least one experience with hypoglycemia and some people have repeated incidents. Hypoglycemia may also be a problem during PREGNANCY for the woman with diabetes because most women are seeking to attain very tight levels of glycemic control. One risk that accompanies such a goal is hypoglycemia.

Symptoms of Hypoglycemia

If a person exhibits at least several of the following symptoms, he or she should be evaluated as soon as possible for possible hypoglycemia as well as for other illnesses that may be present:

- headaches/nausea
- shakiness
- rapid heartbeat
- paleness
- confusion or drowsiness
- dizziness (not vertigo)
- feeling faint
- agitation/irritability/impatience
- sweating in normal temperatures and without exerting oneself

Those Most at Risk for Developing Hypoglycemia

Any person with diabetes can develop hypoglycemia and if they exhibit symptoms, then they should be tested. Those at risk for developing hypoglycemia include:

- people with a history of hypoglycemia
- males
- people over age 65
- patients on tight glycemic control
- patients using insulin
- patients taking more than five medications
- recently hospitalized patients

The hypoglycemic newborn may have hypoglycemia that stems from the mother's diabetes or from her toxemia. The newborn may also be hypoglycemic for other reasons, such as malnutrition, a hormone deficiency, or a side effect from a medication. In very, very rare cases, the infant may have diabetes.

Adults who abuse ALCOHOL may also become hypoglycemic and alcohol abuse is the second most common reason why people with hypoglycemia present to emergency rooms. If a person with diabetes also abuses alcohol, then the risk for hypoglycemia increases further. Some people do not abuse alcohol but for a variety of reasons, they are prone to bouts of hypoglycemia. The more times that a person has a serious incident of hypoglycemia, the more likely it is that it will happen again and again.

Diagnosis/Failure to Diagnose Hypoglycemia

One key problem experienced by people with hypoglycemia is that they may appear intoxicated, drug-impaired, or even mentally ill to the physician and others. If such mistakes or misdiagnoses are made, then proper treatment is delayed or not performed at all and the person with hypoglycemia will become sicker. This could cause the individual to lapse into a coma and die.

In his article on hypoglycemia for a 2001 issue of *Emergency Medicine Report Archives,* Dr. Brady recommended that emergency room doctors consider hypoglycemia as a possible diagnosis in any patient with any apparent mental abnormality or even seizures, and that they should also perform a bedside glucose analysis to rule out hypoglycemia. He advises doctors not to listen to police officers who insist the person is intoxicated, because the police may be wrong. Instead, the doctor should make the evaluation for himself or herself.

Brady also noted that hypoglycemia may be misdiagnosed as seizure disorder, a brain tumor, psychosis, a cerebrovascular accident, a traumatic head injury, narcolepsy, multiple sclerosis, drug ingestion, depression, hysteria, and an incidence of cardiac arrhythmia.

Phases of Hypoglycemia

Hypoglycemia has two primary phases, including the sympatho-adrenal phase or "fight or flight" phase and the neuroglycopenic phase. In the first phase, most patients have symptoms that alert them to their low glucose levels. Some patients, however, do not have such symptoms, a condition called HYPOGLYCEMIC UNAWARENESS. Often they are individuals who have had repeated incidents of hypoglycemia.

In the second phase of hypoglycemia, it may be difficult or impossible for most people with hypoglycemia to recognize their own symptoms and/or to act on them. This is why it is so important for people who do recognize their symptoms in the first phase to test frequently and act right away, if they feel something is amiss. The risk is that if the problem gets worse and the person goes into a neuroglycopenic phase, he or she may no longer be able to act at that point and can become extremely ill. Hypoglycemia is usually not fatal (although it can be) but the person may sustain irreversible central nervous system damage if hypoglycemia is not treated in time. It is far better to take a little time to attend to symptoms in the first stage and avert a medical crisis.

Causes of Hypoglycemia among People with Diabetes

Individuals who have diabetes may develop hypoglycemia for the following reasons:

- imbalance of insulin/oral medications to the level of glucose
- failure to eat a meal or delayed eating
- overexertion
- excessive alcohol consumption

A combination of the above reasons or other factors beyond those listed here may also cause hypoglycemia. For example, people with diabetes who also take beta-blocker drugs for HYPERTENSION, angina, or migraine headaches may then perform strenuous exercises, leading to hypoglycemia, whose symptoms are masked by the beta-blocker. Tight glycemic control of insulin is also a very common cause of hypoglycemia.

Other causes of hypoglycemia Some foods may (rarely) cause hypoglycemia, such as the unripe ackee fruit that is found in Jamaica. Adrenal insufficiency (Addison's disease) may cause hypoglycemia. In rare cases, such as children with growth hormone deficiency, this deficiency can also cause hypoglycemia. Individuals with widely metastatic cancer to the liver or adrenal glands may develop hypoglycemia. In addition, people with severe liver or kidney disease are also more susceptible to suffering from hypoglycemia. Chronic alcohol abuse is also a frequent cause of hypoglycemia, in part because the alcoholic may be malnourished and anorexic.

Treatment of Hypoglycemia

Immediate treatment involves restoring the blood glucose level to normal by the patient taking glucose formulations or food that contains sugar, such as apple juice, fruit, or glucose tablets or gels. If the person is conscious, the glucose can be taken orally. If the person is unconscious, it is administered intravenously. In some emergencies, GLUCAGON is injected intramuscularly to treat the hypoglycemia. Solid foods such as candy should not be given unless the person has regained a completely normal mental state. Otherwise, the individual could risk choking on the candy if he or she is semiconscious, thus creating another medical emergency on top of the hypoglycemia.

People who have recurrent bouts of hypoglycemia (and even people who experience intermittent bouts of hypoglycemia) are wise to ensure that both testing equipment and a source of sugar are readily available to them at all times—including in their car, at work, and at school. They should also seek a consultation with an endocrinologist and a diabetes care team, including a registered dietitian, a registered nurse, and a certified diabetes educator, to find out how to effectively deal with this problem.

Treatment also involves identifying and working to resolve the source of the problem. The disease must be better controlled with appropriate adjustments in medication, diet, exercise, and regular physician visits.

If Hypoglycemia Is Not Treated

If the individual with diabetes or others around do not recognize that the person's blood sugar has dropped precipitously, then action may not be taken or it may be delayed. This can be very dangerous and even lead to the person suffering from seizures, coma, and/or death. For this reason, it's very important that the person with diabetes, especially one prone to hypoglycemic attacks, wear some EMERGENCY MEDICAL IDENTIFICATION in the form of an easily visible necklace, bracelet, anklet, or some other form. Emergency medical cards are good to have as well, but they may not be found in a person's purse or wallet in sufficient time to take appropriate medical action.

Complete recovery can be delayed   Another problem with hypoglycemia is that recovery is not immediate upon administration of glucose. Instead, it takes the body time to recover from hypoglycemia, even after treatment. One study of 20 people with diabetes looked at how long it took people who had a hypoglycemic attack to regain their full cognitive function as well as a stable mood. This study was reported by Strachan et al., in a 2000 issue of *Diabetes Care*.

The researchers found that although hypoglycemia did not have long-term effects when it was promptly treated, the test subjects still took about a day and a half to fully recover their cognitive function. Researchers also found that a temporary depressed and anxious state often occurred to the subject after an attack. Individuals who had many bouts with hypoglycemia had even more difficulty recovering.

The researchers said that the results "imply that acute severe hypoglycemia does not have a prolonged effect on cognitive functions, and patients with insulin-treated diabetes may be reassured that performance of activities such as work or driving is not likely to be impaired 36 h [hours] after an episode." As a result, given sufficient time, and adequate treatment, most people recover fully from a bout of hypoglycemia. But because their faculties may be somewhat impaired for a day or so afterwards, they should not engage in any difficult activities or make any important decisions during that time. (See also COMA, DEHYDRATION, GLYCEMIC CONTROL.)

William J. Brady, M.D., F.A.C.E.P., "Hypoglycemia: Current Strategies for Diagnosis and Management," *Emergency Medicine Reports Archives* (January 15, 2001).

The Diabetes Control and Complications Trial Research Group, "Hypoglycemia in the Diabetes Control and Complications Trials," *Diabetes* 46 (February 1997): 271–286.

Mark, Strachan et al., "Recovery of Cognitive Function and Mood After Severe Hypoglycemia in Adults with Insulin-Treated Diabetes," *Diabetes Care* 23, no. 3, (March 2000): 305–312.

Edith Ter Braak W.M.T., M.D., et al., "Clinical Characteristics of Type 1 Diabetic Patients with and without Severe Hypoglycemia," *Diabetes Care* 23, no. 10 (October 2000): 1467–1471.

hypoglycemic unawareness The condition when a person with diabetes has no symptoms of a low blood glucose level (HYPOGLYCEMIA). Typically, they have lost the first phase when the sympathetic nervous system induces the release of adrenaline and noradrenaline. Thus, they have no nervousness, sweating, rapid heartbeat, and other symptoms to warn them that their glucose level is declining. Patients with well-controlled diabetes will begin to experience symptoms at 55–60 mg/DL.

Hypoglycemic unawareness occurs most commonly in those who try to control their glucose levels very tightly. It is common in pregnant women for this reason. It can also be a late complication of long-standing diabetes (25 to 35 years in duration) due to AUTONOMIC NEUROPATHY.

Abnormal thinking and behavior is one of the first symptoms of hypoglycemic unawareness. At that point, the patient is unable to treat him- or herself and others must provide treatment. Some indications of such abnormal behaviors are:

- The person stops an activity and begins staring off into space
- What the person says makes no sense
- There is a sudden change in personality, facial expression, or mood

When patients have hypoglycemic unawareness, the glycemic goals are increased and the patient is asked to aim for slightly higher glucose levels to avoid hypoglycemia. The patient is also advised to monitor glucose levels more frequently, especially ensuring to check blood levels before driving. Patients are also educated about the importance of eating meals on time and avoiding missing meals or delayed meals. Patients are also advised to inform family members as well as friends and coworkers about hypoglycemic unawareness, so that they can look for subtle signs of hypoglycemia.

Hypoglycemic unawareness is reversible unless the cause is a chronic form of AUTONOMIC NEUROPATHY.

immune system   The system that protects the body from bacteria, viruses, and other substances that are considered foreign and dangerous by the body. Type 1 diabetes is considered an autoimmune disorder that results from the immune system erring by attacking the body's own pancreatic islet tissues, essential to producing and secreting insulin into the blood.

immunizations (flu/influenza, pneumococcal vaccine, and others)   Vaccines introduced into the body that cause the creation of antibodies, which are proteins made by B lymphocytes. These antibodies, in turn, protect against the disease. For those who have diabetes, it is very important to obtain flu and pneumonia immunizations, particularly among people who are over age 65. Of course, individuals with diabetes should receive periodic immunizations for tetanus and other immunizations as needed by individuals in his or her area and recommended by their physicians.

According to the Centers for Disease Control and Prevention (CDC), 10,000–30,000 people with diabetes die each year from flu and pneumonia. People with diabetes have nearly triple the risk of dying from flu or pneumonia. In addition, people with diabetes who contract flu are six times more likely to need hospitalization than are nondiabetics. Experts also recommend that family members of individuals with diabetes should be immunized as well. Not only will they be protected from the flu but they will also help their family members with diabetes by avoiding the flu and eliminating the risk of contagion.

Although a flu shot is generally a good idea for most people, individuals should be sure to check with their physicians first before receiving the immunization. Someone who is acutely ill or feverish should not take the vaccine nor should

		PERSONS WITH HIGH RISK CONDITIONS AND PERCENTAGE OBTAINING FLU AND PNEUMONIA VACCINATIONS, 1997			
	Annual Influenza and One-Time Pneumococcal Vaccination				
	Noninstitutionalized Adults Aged 65 Years and Older		Noninstitutionalized High-Risk Adults Aged 18 to 64 Years		
Select Age Groups	Influenza	Pneumococcal Disease	Influenza	Pneumococcal Disease	
	Percent				
Persons with diabetes	68	44	27	15	
Persons with heart disease	71	51	25	11	
Persons with lung disease	73	65	25	13	
Persons with kidney disease	71	46	21	13	

171

it be taken by anyone who is allergic to eggs or who has had a prior severe systemic reaction to the flu shot.

Yet despite warnings from the medical profession, many people with diabetes fail to obtain immunizations against flu or pneumonia. According to the federal data reported in *Healthy People 2010,* of those with high risk conditions, only 27 percent of diabetes patients ages 18 to 64 had obtained a flu shot and only 15 percent had received the pneumonia vaccine. Of people over age 65, they were the least likely of older people with high risk conditions of obtaining either a flu or pneumonia vaccination.

Frequency of Immunizations

Influenza is generally a problem between November and April, and pneumonia generally follows the same pattern. Most people who receive these immunizations obtain them sometime between October and mid-November. New flu shots are required each year, although pneumococcal immunizations may only need to be repeated every five to seven years, depending on the patient's physician's advice.

It may take three to four weeks for the body to develop antibodies against the flu. As a result, timing of the injection is important. For example, if a person received an injection on November 5, and then was exposed to the flu on November 11, then he or she could still develop the flu despite having received the injection. The body would not have had enough time to marshal its defenses in that time frame.

Providers and Costs of Immunizations

Flu shots and pneumococcal vaccines are covered by Part B Medicare. If the immunization must be paid for, it is generally low cost. The state health department or local clinic may provide the shot for free or at low cost, or the individual may pay to obtain the immunization from his or her doctor.

Primary Symptoms of Flu and Pneumonia

Not everyone feels the same, but most people experience common symptoms. People with the flu have at least several of these symptoms:

- fever that is greater than 101.5 degrees Fahrenheit
- sore throat (pharyngitis)
- chills
- muscle aches (myalgia)
- headache
- cough, generally dry and nonproductive

Symptoms of pneumonia are:

- fever
- coughing up sputum (generally greenish, brown or blood-tinged and *not* white or clear)
- chest pain, generally sharp

Categories of People Who Should Be Immunized

According to the CDC, an annual flu shot is particularly recommended for people who fall in one or more of the following categories. Those who:

- are over age 50
- live in a long-term care facility, such as a skilled nursing facility
- have a long-term health problem, such as diabetes, heart disease, lung disease, asthma, kidney disease, or anemia
- have a weak immune system because of HIV or medications that weaken the system, such as cancer treatments or steroids
- children ages six months to 18 years on long-term aspirin treatment (and who could develop Reye's syndrome if they caught the flu)
- doctors, nurses, and other health care providers who are likely to come in contact with people at risk of having severe flu

Minor and Major Reactions to Flu/Pneumococcal Injections

Many people have mild reactions to the injection, such as soreness at the injection site or redness. There may be some temporary achiness or slight fever for one or two days as well.

On rare occasions, individuals experience a bad reaction to the immunization. Anyone who experiences a fever of greater than 101.5 degrees F or who exhibits signs of an allergic reaction should obtain immediate medical attention. Some examples of an allergic reaction are:

- hives
- difficulty breathing/shortness of breath
- paleness/pallor
- wheezing
- rapid heartbeat
- lightheadedness

A person who experiences such a severe reaction should also ask the doctor to file a Vaccine Adverse Event Reporting System (VAERS) form with the Centers for Disease Control or, upon treatment and recovery, patients may call the VAERS later themselves at 1-800-822-7967.

Emergency treatment may be required Some individuals who have diabetes and who are ill with flu or pneumonia may need to be taken to see their medical doctor or may need to go to the emergency room or even be hospitalized in order to avoid severe consequences. Circumstances when the sick person with diabetes should see his doctor or, if this is not possible, go to the hospital emergency room are:

- if the individual is too ill to monitor his or her blood glucose levels and has no one to help with monitoring
- if he or she has high ketone levels in his urine
- if the person has severe nausea and vomiting and is unable to keep up with the needed intake of fluids (and there is no one else available to provide assistance). This could lead to DEHYDRATION

Other Immunizations That Are Needed

Individuals who have diabetes should also obtain diphtheria-tetanus (dT) shots every 10 years. Children should obtain hepatitis B injections, as should adults who are at risk of contracting the disease. Children should also have the hemophilus vaccine.

Steven A. Smith, M.D., and Gregory A. Poland, M.D., "Use of Influenza and Pneumococcal Vaccines in People with Diabetes," *Diabetes Care* 23, no. 1 (January 2000): 95–108.

impaired glucose tolerance (IGT)   A condition in which the blood glucose levels are higher than normal but they are not high enough that the person could be diagnosed with diabetes. Former names of IGT, no longer in use (because they are inaccurate), are "borderline diabetes," "subclinical diabetes," "chemical diabetes," and "latent diabetes."

People with IGT may go on to develop diabetes as well as the MICROVASCULAR complications that accompany this disease. Studies of the PIMA INDIANS of Arizona, a tribe with an extremely high rate of Type 2 diabetes, have revealed that there is about a three-year period from the development of impaired glucose tolerance to the onset of Type 2 diabetes.

These same studies from the Pima Indians reveal that patients with IGT appear to more likely have HYPERINSULINISM, i.e., they are more insulin resistant and thus need to attempt to overproduce insulin to compensate than those with impaired fasting glucose (IFG). The Pima Indians in these studies who developed IFG appeared to have more beta cell dysfunction, which means that they are less able to secrete enough insulin to normalize the blood glucose. (It is necessary for patients to have both insulin resistance and impaired insulin secretion to develop Type 2 diabetes mellitus.)

IGT seems to be a better predictor of the future development of Type 2 diabetes as well as the development of cardiovascular disease.

The DIABETES PREVENTION PROGRAM is a study that is ongoing in the United States, as of this writing, and seeks to determine if changes made by a person who has impaired glucose tolerance (in lifestyle and medication) can delay or altogether slow down the progression to diabetes. We know from the UNITED KINGDOM PROSPECTIVE DIABETES STUDY (UKPDS) that patients who eventually develop Type 2 diabetes have metabolic abnormalities that can precede the diagnosis by as much as 10 years. As a result, most experts feel that any efforts to slow down the progression to diabetes will have a positive effect in terms of preventing and delaying complications.

In 2001, researchers who studied 522 middle-aged adults with impaired glucose tolerance sought to determine if lifestyle changes could prevent or delay the onset of diabetes. Their findings were reported in the *New England Journal of Medicine*. (See PREVENTION OF DIABETES.) The researchers definitively proved that lifestyle changes such as weight loss, increased exercise, and dietary changes such as decreased sugar consumption and increased vegetable and fiber consumption, dramatically reduced the risk of diabetes for subjects, even when followed up four years after the study. The "intervention group" that made lifestyle changes had an incidence of diabetes of 11 percent while the control group had an incidence of diabetes of 23 percent. (See also SYNDROME X.)

M. J. Davies, N. T. Raymond, and J. L. Day, et al. "Impaired Glucose Tolerance and Fasting Hyperglycemia Have Different Characteristics," *Diabetes Medicine* 17 (2000): 433–440.

impotence   See ERECTILE DYSFUNCTION (ED).

India   An Asian country with an increasing problem with Type 2 diabetes. Experts estimate that by 2005, there will be 30 to 35 million people with diabetes in India, about 20 percent of the world population with diabetes. It will be extremely difficult for hospitals in India to meet this growing need.

Complications of diabetes will be difficult to cope with. An analysis of complications among approximately 3,000 people with diabetes in India revealed that about 28 percent had DIABETIC NEUROPATHY, about 24 percent of the patients had DIABETIC RETINOPATHY, and about 6 percent had DIABETIC NEPHROPATHY. In addition, 38 percent had HYPERTENSION and 11 percent had heart disease.

Experts urge that awareness of the problem is one step toward taking action to cope with the escalating problem of diabetes in India.

infants and preschool children with diabetes
The presence of Type 1 diabetes in babies and preschool children, an uncommon condition. According to authors Denis Daneman, Marcia Frank, and Kusiel Perlman in their book, *When a Child Has Diabetes,* less than 1 percent of the cases of diabetes are diagnosed in a child's first year and less than 10 percent are diagnosed before the child is age five. When a small child does have diabetes, the illness is often not diagnosed until the child becomes severely ill with DIABETIC KETOACIDOSIS (DKA).

Children can also develop Type 2 diabetes but when it occurs among children, it nearly always develops during or after puberty. Type 2 diabetes is unknown in babies and preschool children.

An infant or toddler with diabetes suffers from the same symptoms as older children or adults with Type 1 diabetes, exhibiting thirst, weight loss, and fatigue. The AMERICAN DIABETES ASSOCIATION advises against tight glycemic control for children under the age of two.

According to Daneman et al., a healthy baby or toddler with controlled diabetes will grow normally and have a normal weight gain. The child will also meet normal developmental milestones for sitting up, crawling, standing, and so forth. There will be no KETONES in the child's urine when diabetes is under control and the child will have good energy levels.

Because babies and small children cannot check their own blood levels or inject insulin, this task must be performed by adult caregivers. Whenever possible, it should be shifted among adults, so that one person does not always have to be the "bad guy." The child's feelings about finger pricks should be acknowledged but they should also not be delayed, because the child's health is at stake.

Alternate site glucose monitoring, by testing the blood in other parts of the body such as the arm, may be preferable in infants and preschool children. Obviously, noninvasive monitoring will be very helpful when it becomes available.

A helpful educational game, "Wizdom Kids," is offered at www.diabetes.org/wizdom.

Some helpful books for parents include the following:

The Ten Keys to Helping Your Child Grow Up with Diabetes by Tim Wysocki (NTC Publications Group, 1997).

Sweet Kids: How to Balance Diabetes Control and Good Nutrition with Family Peace by Betty Page Brackenridge, M.S., R.D., C.D.E. and Richard R. Rubin, Ph.D., C.D.E. (NTC Publications Group, 1996).

American Diabetes Association Guide to Raising a Child with Diabetes by Linda M. Siminerio, R.N., M.S., C.D.E. and Jean Betschart, R.N., M.N., C.D.E. (NTC Publications Group, 2000).

Denis Daneman, M.B., B.Ch., F.R.C.P.C., Marcia Frank, R.N., M.H.Sc., C.D.E., and Kusiel Perlman, M.D., F.R.C.P.C., *When a Child Has Diabetes* (New York, N.Y.: Firefly Books, 1999).

infections Bacterial, fungal, or viral invasions of the body. People with diabetes are more prone to contracting a variety of infections than are nondiabetics. They are also at graver risk for contracting and becoming very ill from influenza or pneumonia. The greatest risk is seen in patients with poor glycemic control. High glucose levels prevent the immune system from working well, particularly impairing the abilities of the white blood cells to work at an optimal level to fight off infection. Yet only an estimated 50 percent of those who know they have diabetes obtain an annual flu or pneumonia IMMUNIZATION.

When individuals with diabetes suffer from DIABETIC NEUROPATHY, they are also at a greater risk for developing infections of the foot which, if not treated, may progress to GANGRENE and the necessity for an AMPUTATION of a limb.

Rates of kidney infections (pyelonephritis) are similar in people with and without diabetes; however, patients with diabetes are twice as likely to need hospitalization when they do have a kidney infection. Diabetic neuropathy that leads to a NEUROGENIC BLADDER tends to significantly increase the number of bladder infections. This problem may also occur after surgery, especially in cases of surgery for cardiac, chest, or abdominal areas. People with good glycemic control and with fewer complications are likely to be discharged from the hospital sooner.

Women with diabetes are susceptible to Candida vaginitis (yeast) and men to Candida balanitis. Candida grows well in warm, moist environments where glucose is plentiful. (See also BALANITIS, FLU, FOOT CARE, GINGIVITIS, IMMUNIZATIONS, URINARY TRACT INFECTION, VAGINITIS.)

Douglas S. Paauw, M.D., F.A.C.P., "Infectious Emergencies in Patients with Diabetes," *Clinical Diabetes* 18, no. 3 (Summer 2000): 102–106.

inhaled insulin Insulin that is delivered as a dry powder or fine solution through an inhaler rather than through injections. As of this writing, inhaled insulin is being tested and appears to be a viable alternative for at least part of the insulin needed by all people with Type 1 diabetes and some people who have Type 2 diabetes. This method of delivery may be more acceptable to people with diabetes than the three to four injections per day that some people require.

Inhaled insulin as a therapy is under clinical study, as of this writing. It appears to be an effective method of delivery, but further study is necessary to ensure that it is safe for the lungs over the long term.

injection devices Devices used to introduce medications into the body. The majority of people with diabetes in the United States and Canada who self-inject insulin use traditional insulin syringes with 29- and 30-gauge needles. There are now "short" needles available for thin patients to avoid inadvertent intramuscular injections. (Insulin should be injected into the subcutaneous fat.) In Europe, most insulin is injected with pen devices with 30- and 31-gauge needles.

All syringes in the United States and Canada are calibrated to U-100 (100 units of insulin/1 cc or mL). Syringes are available in $^1/3$ cc (30 units), $^1/2$ cc (50 units) and 1-cc (100 unit) sizes.

There are also insertion aids available that will inject the needles when triggered. Some will also automatically release insulin, while others need to be manually activated after the needle is in place.

Jet injectors that force insulin through the skin via air pressure are available but they are expensive. Since standard needles have become very small and also very sharp, there has been much less demand for these devices. They can also cause some bruising and need to be cleaned regularly.

Multiple devices are also available for the visually impaired. These devices help patients measure the insulin dose and guide and stabilize the needle, while also magnifying the syringe so that they can read the dose correctly.

injections Method to deliver medications directly into the body. In most cases, individuals with TYPE 1 DIABETES must inject themselves with insulin at least twice daily and usually on a more frequent basis. As they age, individuals with TYPE 2 DIABETES may have an increasingly impaired insulin secretory system and may also need to self-inject insulin. Insulin is injected into subcutaneous fat, where it is absorbed into small blood vessels.

Because many people dislike not only testing their blood but also injecting insulin, and because this dislike often leads to failure to self-test or to self-inject, scientists have sought other solutions. One such solution is the implantable pump, which provides insulin on a regular basis to the patient. Inhaled insulin is an alternative

that is being tested in 2001 and which appears to be a viable alternative to injected insulin for many patients with diabetes.

Some patients actually inject their medicine through their clothes, although there is considerable controversy among physicians as to whether this is an acceptable or safe procedure.

Glucagon, which is administered for severe hypoglycemia, is generally injected into a large muscle, such as the muscle in the shoulder or the thigh. (See also SELF-MONITORING.)

injection site rotation The practice of giving oneself an injection in different sites of the body so that one particular part of the body doesn't become overly inflamed or harmed. Repeated injections in the same site could result in lumps that are called "lipodystrophies" or "lipohypertrophies." For people with Type 1 diabetes, this is a key reason for rotating the location of the insulin injection.

Most people inject insulin in areas of the body that are easy to reach, such as the outer arm, close to the waist, the upper buttock, and the thigh. Sometimes people give themselves their morning injection in one part of the body and then administer their evening injection in another part. In the future, medical experts hope that many people with diabetes will be able to use BLOODLESS TESTING, so that they may easily and painlessly monitor their glucose levels.

With the newer pure insulin available today, patients can use one site to inject as long as they move 1-2 finger widths away with each injection. They should follow a pattern of moving from left to right or up and down to rotate within one area.

Absorption of insulin varies from site to site and it is absorbed most quickly and consistently in the abdomen and slowest in the buttocks. Absorption and injection in the arms and thighs provide medium absorption. If the person exercises a leg or arm after an injection, it will increase the speed of absorption. (See also FINGER PRICK, LANCET.)

insulin A medication used to treat people with diabetes and the single most important factor enabling many people with diabetes to survive and thrive, particularly those with Type 1 diabetes.

Insulin was first discovered as a treatment for diabetes in 1921 at the University of Toronto in Canada by Dr. Frederick Banting, a Canadian physician and Charles Best, his medical student assistant. Prior to that time, people with Type 1 diabetes died at young ages or suffered greatly until death in young adulthood.

Insulin is produced by the beta cells of the islets of Langerhans, found in the pancreas. The pancreas then secretes it in order to regulate the levels of glucose in the bloodstream. Insulin is a polypeptide (protein) hormone made of two chains and derived from proinsulin. The C-PEPTIDE (connecting peptide) is removed before use. It is this C-peptide fragment that can be measured in the body to determine if a patient is still producing insulin.

Individuals with Type 1 diabetes have very low (for the first few years after diagnosis) or no insulin (thereafter) because their illness has destroyed the beta cells. As a result, they need insulin that is injected or pumped into the body on a daily basis.

People with Type 2 diabetes have a different problem. Although their bodies produce insulin, they suffer from insulin resistance, which means that the body is unable to use the insulin effectively. As a result, they generally need oral medication to control their diabetes as well as careful blood glucose monitoring and dietary control. Because people with Type 2 diabetes are often obese, they are frequently advised to lose weight by eating less and increasing their activity levels. Patients with Type 2 diabetes may need to take

---

INSULIN FORMS AND SPEED AND LENGTH OF ACTION

	When Insulin Begins to Work	PEAK Effect	Typical Length of Effect
Rapid			
Lispro* (Humalog)	15 minutes	1 hour	3–5 hours
Aspart (Novolog)	15 minutes	1 hour	3–5 hours
Short			
Regular* (Humulin and Novolin)	45 minutes	2–3 hours	5–8 hours
Intermediate			
NPH* (Humulin and Novolin)	2–4 hours	4–10 hours	10–16 hours
Lente* (Novolin and Humolin)	3–4 hours	4–12 hours	12–18 hours
Long			
Ultralente (Humulin)	6–8 hours	10–18 hours	16–24 hours
Glargine† (Lantus)	2–4 hours	No peak	20–26 hours

* Also available in pen devices.
† Glargine is an acidic insulin that cannot be combined with other insulins.

Premixed Forms of Insulin

70/30 Insulin* (Humulin and Novolin)	70% NPH/30% Regular
75/25 Insulin* (Humulin)	75% Neutral protamine lispro/25% lispro
50/50 Insulin (Humulin)	50% NPH/50% Regular

*Available in pen devices.

Note: Onset, peak, and length of effects are significantly affected by injection site, activity, smoking, kidney function, and a variety of other factors.

insulin, especially during pregnancy or after many years of the illness.

Types of Insulin

When insulin was first discovered, there was only one form. Today, there are five primary types of insulin and people who use insulin generally take two of these types. Most insulin is now U-100, which means it comes in 100 units/cc. U-500 (500 units/cc) can be special ordered for patients who require very large doses of insulin. Currently, Eli Lilly & Company, Novo Nordisk, and Aventis Pharmaceuticals supply insulin in the United States.

Extra insulin should be stored in the refrigerator and discarded after its expiration date, if not used. Once opened, insulin can be stored in the refrigerator for three months and then discarded. INSULIN GLARGINE should be discarded 28 days after the vial has been opened.

If kept at room temperature (55 to 75 degrees F), insulin should be discarded after one month.

Insulin in cartridges in pen devices are generally used for seven days after opening at room temperature. Patients should throw away any insulin in cartridges that seem "frosted" or that have clumps in them.

HUMALOG and novolog are fast-acting forms of insulin that start to work within five to 15 minutes from an injection. They work best at lowering blood sugar about 45 to 90 minutes after injection.

Short-acting or regular insulin starts to work in 45 minutes. It peaks at two to three hours from the injection and will last up to 8 hours.

Intermediate-acting NPH (N) or Lente (L) insulin starts working from two to four hours from injection and has a peak action for four to 12 hours after injection.

Long-acting, ULTRALENTE insulin starts to work from four to six hours after the injection and has a peak action that occurs from eight to 20 hours after the injection.

Peakless insulin or glargine lasts 20 to 24 hours and cannot be combined in the same syringes of other insulin.

Another type of insulin is a combination of two forms in the same bottle, such as NPH and Regular or NPH and Humalog/Novolog insulin mixture. Being premixed, it is easier to use and more convenient for patients.

(See also GLYCEMIC CONTROL.)

insulin allergy   An allergic reaction to insulin. If the allergy is localized, the skin becomes red, irritated, and itchy at the site of the injection. If the allergy becomes systemic, this means the whole body is affected and the person may develop hives, wheezing, or low blood pressure.

Insulin allergy was more common with beef and pork insulins but still can occur with human recombinant insulins. Patients can also be allergic to the preservatives in insulin or to the protamine in NPH. A local reaction can be treated with ice, antihistamines, and steroid creams. Systemic reactions will require emergency room evaluation, antihistamines, and steroids, as well as a follow-up evaluation by an allergist.

Both types of allergies are very uncommon to rare.

insulin-dependent diabetes mellitus (IDDM)
The former name for Type 1 diabetes. The disease was also called "juvenile onset diabetes" in past years, until researchers realized that not only children but also adolescents and even adults may be diagnosed with this form of diabetes. In addition, sometimes people with what was formerly called "non-insulin dependent diabetes" develop the need to take insulin after many years or during pregnancy or at other times. As a result, for clarity, the illness was renamed Type 1 diabetes.

Note: the Arabic number "1" is used rather than the Roman numeral I for the purposes of clarity. The Arabic number "2" is used for what was formerly called non-insulin dependent diabetes or adult onset diabetes. The reason for this numbering choice was that experts feared that if, for example, they used "Type II," some people would misread it as "Type Eleven." However, there still is some confusion and some people continue to mistakenly use the Roman numerals rather than the correct Arabic numbers.

insulin glargine   A very long-acting form of INSULIN that may enable some people with diabetes to function well on only one injection per day. It is an acidic insulin that cannot be mixed with other insulins. Insulin glargine is "peakless," which means that it provides a continuous level of insulin (basal insulin) over a 20- to 26-hour period.

The amino acid sequence in the two chains in insulin were manipulated to create this basal insulin. It is manufactured by Aventis Pharmaceuticals.

insulin pen   A special device that resembles a ballpoint pen but which contains specific amounts of insulin and a needle that the person with diabetes may self-administer by the press of a button. Insulin pens are used as substitutes for syringes. Typically, pens have 300 units of insulin. The person uses the pen by turning the top to dial up or click up on the dosage.

There are many different brands of insulin pens. Some use removable cartridges of insulin that can be refilled while others are prefilled and disposable after the insulin is gone. Eli Lilly and Novo Nordisk pharmaceutical companies make insulin pen devices containing Humalog, Novolog, regular insulin, NPH, Lente, and premixed combinations of 70/30 insulin and 75/25 insulin. (See also PEN DEVICES.)

insulin pump   Typically an external device (although experimental implantable pumps are also available) that metes out continuous dosages of insulin to the person with diabetes. This battery-driven device is used instead of regular injections of insulin. The individual using the insulin pump needs to give extra bolus doses to cover meals and snacks.

Individuals who have fluctuating blood levels of glucose and/or people who have a great deal of trouble controlling their diabetes may be good candidates for pump therapy, although this is a decision that should be discussed between the patient and his or her physician. Sometimes women who are pregnant have difficulty maintaining good glycemic control and a pump may be a good temporary solution for them.

External pumps connect to flexible tubing that ends with a needle which is inserted in the skin in the abdominal area. This pump is about the size of a package of cards and it can be worn on a belt or in a pocket. The pump is set by users to provide a continuous "basal" amount of insulin all day. Bolus units are released at meal time or at other times when the extra insulin is needed. Blood glucose monitoring is required to verify that the insulin was received and in the correct dosages.

The internal or implantable insulin pump is surgically inserted in the abdomen on the left side. It weighs about six ounces and delivers a continuous basal dose of insulin, controlled through a remote control unit. The key advantage of the implantable pump is that the insulin goes directly into the liver, as it would with insulin that was produced naturally by the pancreas. As of this writing, the implantable pump is not FDA-approved in the United States for clinical use.

Candidates for pump therapy must be motivated enough to monitor their glucose levels six to 10 times per day, learn how to do CARBOHYDRATE counting and be fastidious in pump preparation. They should also not be individuals with severe end-stage complications. Patients with GASTROPARESIS may be candidates for the insulin pump, as may individuals desiring tight control but who have been unable to achieve it via multiple daily doses of insulin.

Wayne Clark, "Pumped Up: But Is It for Everyone?," *JDF International Countdown* 18, no. 2 (1997): 20–21, 24, 26–28.

Marina Scavini, M.D., and David S. Schade, M.D., "Implantable Insulin Pumps," *Clinical Diabetes* 14, no. 2 (1996): 30–35.

insulin reaction   Another name for HYPOGLYCEMIA. Also called "insulin shock." Refers to a precipitous drop in blood glucose, which may occur because the individual has not eaten enough, has injected too much insulin, or had excessive activity.

insulin resistance The impaired ability of the body to efficiently utilize the insulin that is produced by the pancreas. Insulin resistance is a necessary requisite to develop Type 2 diabetes. It is also an intrinsic part of SYNDROME X, also known as INSULIN RESISTANCE SYNDROME.

Insulin resistance may be a problem for years before the insulin resistance and/or diabetes is actually diagnosed. Most insulin resistance occurs in muscle cells. The problem in diabetes is not due to a lack of insulin receptors but rather due to a problem within the cell. It does not allow the insulin "message" to be appropriately transmitted.

Using the analogy of locks and keys, the key is insulin. The locks are the insulin receptors in the muscle cells. These locks must be opened to allow insulin inside the cell to be used for fuel, stored for future use, or converted to another compound. The locks are plentiful in a person with diabetes but, in this analogy, can be considered "rusty." Therefore, they must be forced open. Clinically, one can force these locks open by using more insulin, exercising, eating less and losing weight, or taking oral medications such as THIAZOLIDINEDIONES (TZDS) or METFORMIN.

insulin resistance syndrome A metabolic syndrome which involves several conditions, including IMPAIRED GLUCOSE TOLERANCE/diabetes/ dyslipidemia/HYPERLIPIDEMIA, HYPERTENSION, polycystic ovarian syndrome, OBESITY, CORONARY HEART DISEASE, and ATHEROSCLEROSIS. People with this syndrome are at high risk for developing abnormal clotting in blood vessels as well as any of the aforementioned medical problems. (See also HYPERINSULINISM, SYNDROME X.)

insulin sensitivity Ability to effectively use the insulin that the pancreas produces. A key feature of Type 2 diabetes is that although the body produces some insulin, it is not able to use it because of insulin resistance. Insulin sensitivity is the opposite of insulin resistance.

Ken C. Chiu, M.D., F.A.C.E., "Insulin Sensitivity Differs among Ethnic Groups with Compensatory Response in Beta Cell Function," *Diabetes Care* 23, no. 9 (September 2000): 1353–1358.

insurance Medical or life coverage that is provided by private, state, or federal organizations. Such coverage is important to individuals with diabetes, who may otherwise be unable to afford medication and physician visits. Studies indicate that people with health insurance are more likely to have dilated eye examinations, foot examinations, and annual dental examinations, all methods to screen for and prevent COMPLICATIONS of diabetes.

Health Insurance

What is covered by insurance varies; for example, some insurance, such as Medicaid and some private insurance carriers, provide for the coverage of medications, while other insurance, such as Medicare, does not cover medications as of this writing. (There may be a predetermined copayment amount for Medicare patients through some carriers that offer prescription drug coverage.)

In 1998, the federal government began offering Medicare recipients payment of insulin, syringes, and related material that are needed by individuals with diabetes. Prior to that time, they were responsible for this expense on their own unless they qualified for a low income program such as Medicaid. Another relatively new offering for Medicare recipients was coverage for therapeutic shoes. (See SHOES, THERAPEUTIC, and ORTHOTICS.)

Racial/ethnic differences in health insurance coverage Researchers considering data from the Third National Health and Nutrition Examination Survey (NHANES III) looked at the health insurance coverage of people with diabetes among a group of approximately 1,500 adults.

According to author Maureen Harris, there were marked differences in insurance coverage between races. In looking at all patients with diabetes, the researchers found that 93 percent had some form of insurance, and 73 percent were covered by private health insurance, 48 percent were on Medicare, 15 percent were on Medicaid, and 5 percent were on Champus/VA (military-related insurance). About half the people with diabetes had dual coverage.

Of those with no insurance, 4.7 percent were non-Hispanic white, 7 percent were non-Hispanic black and a much higher percentage, 23.2 percent of Mexican Americans, had no health insurance at all.

Non-Hispanic whites were most likely to have private insurance only (40.8 percent), followed by non-Hispanic blacks (35.9 percent). Mexican Americans were *least* likely to have private insurance only (29.9 percent). Non-Hispanic blacks were *most* likely to have government-sponsored insurance only (Medicare or Medicaid), and 37.3 percent of this group had only government insurance. They were followed by Mexican Americans at 32.2 percent.

Non-Hispanic whites, in sharp contrast, had only 14 percent receiving government-sponsored insurance only.

These racial groupings were found to be similar for nondiabetics, with the exception that people with diabetes are more likely to be receiving government health insurance than nondiabetics.

Life and Accident Insurance

Accident and/or life insurance is another form of insurance purchased by individuals with diabetes, and premiums are generally higher for those with Type 1 diabetes. Several researchers studied the mortality and accident rates of people with Type 1 diabetes over three years, including approximately 7,600 members of the Danish Diabetes Association who had purchased group accident insurance. About 6,200 were using insulin and the other individuals were being treated with oral medications or by diet only. The researchers looked at accidents such as falls (the most common injury), as well as sports injuries, and traffic accident injuries.

Although the researchers found that the death rate among diabetics was higher than the nondiabetic population, they did not find a higher rate of accidents. They also looked at permanent injuries and found no difference from what would be expected from the nondiabetic population. In some cases, the numbers of accidents were lower for people with diabetes. For example, the average number of accidents in the two nondiabetic groups were 4.5 and 5.5 per 1,000. The average for the people with diabetes was 0.7 per 1,000 person-years. "Based on the data from control group 1, a total of 102 accidents were expected, while 16 were observed," said the authors.

They further commented on their findings,

This suggests that insurance premiums and conditions have been based on assumptions rather than scientific evidence from actuarial studies. The fact that diabetic patients have an increased mortality and a risk of developing late diabetic complications (neuropathy, retinopathy, macroangiopathy, etc.) has led to the assumption that the diabetic individual has an increased risk of experiencing an accident and that the degree of permanent injury after an accident may be higher in a diabetic than in a nondiabetic individual.

The authors suggest that insurance companies look at facts rather than relying on perceptions only. (See also HMOs, MANAGED CARE, MEDICAID, MEDICARE, SSI.)

Maureen I. Harris, Ph.D., M.P.H., "Racial and Ethnic Differences in Health Insurance Coverage for Adults with Diabetes," *Diabetes Care* 22, no. 10 (October 1999): 1679–1682.

Brent Mathiesen, M.D., and Knut Borch-Johnsen, M.D., "Diabetes and Accident Insurance," *Diabetes Care* 20, no. 11 (November 1997): 1781–1784.

International Diabetes Federation (IDF)

Global organization for practitioners who care for people with diabetes as well as for those who have diabetes.

Founded in June 1949 in Brussels, Belgium, and also known as the Fédération Internationale du Diabète (FID), the International Diabetes Federation has 132 national organizations in 108 countries, including the United States. The organization promotes World Diabetes Day, which is November 14th of each year. It works to promote global awareness of diabetes. Publications include *IDF Newsletter, IDF Bulletin, IDF Triennial Report,* and others.

International Diabetes Federation
IDF Secretariat
1 rue Defacqz
B-1050 Brussels, Belgium

www.idf.org

islet cell transplantation   The removal of pancreatic islets of Langerhans from a donor (a cadaver) and transplantation into individuals with diabetes. In 2000, the procedure was greatly improved by Dr. James Shapiro and his colleagues at the University of Alberta in Edmonton, Canada, who used specialized enzymes when they removed the islets from the pancreases of the cadavers. Dr. Shapiro and his team treated eight patients with Type 1 diabetes in 1999, and as of 2001, these patients continue to be completely free of diabetes. The successful procedure was subsequently named the "Edmonton Protocol."

In 2000, the National Institutes of Health (NIH), with the Juvenile Diabetes Research Foundation International, announced funding of a clinical trial to test the Edmonton Protocol in 40 people at locations around the world. The trial would last for seven years and include patients who fit the following criteria:

- had Type 1 diabetes for five years or more
- between the ages of 18 and 65 years
- unable to control glucose levels, even with intensive therapy

- unable to sense the onset of hypoglycemia (HYPOGLYCEMIC UNAWARENESS)
- at least one hypoglycemic episode within the past 1.6 years that required medical care but that could not be explained
- diabetes complications, such as DIABETIC RETINOPATHY, or problems with kidneys (nephropathy), nerves (neuropathy), or blood vessels

The Islet Cell Transplant Procedure

The procedure takes about an hour or less for the surgeon to perform. A special catheter is placed in a blood vessel and threaded into the liver. The islets are injected into the catheter. The cells then attach to blood vessels within the liver and start releasing insulin. Insulin will continue to be needed until tests reveal that the cells are supplying a sufficient amount of insulin.

Pros and Cons of Islet Cell Transplants

The biggest risk/problem with this transplant, as with other forms of transplanted organs, is rejection by the body. The immune system may react to the new organ or cells as invaders and create antibodies to destroy them, as if they were diseases. For this reason, transplant patients need antirejection (immunosuppressive) drugs, which they must take for the rest of their life.

Another problem is that the procedure, as of this writing, requires two pancreases for each transplantation in order to obtain adequate numbers of islet cells, and pancreases are in scarce supply. There are about 3,000 pancreases available each year for transplant, but there are nearly 1 million people with Type 1 diabetes.

For more information on islet transplantation, contact the:

Immune Tolerance Network (ITN)
Patient Information
5743 South Drexel Avenue
Suite 200
Chicago, IL 60637

(773) 834-4535 (in the United States)
(780) 407-1501 (in Canada)
www.immunetolerance.org

J. Kovarik and T. E. Mandel, "Islet Transplantation," *Transplantation Proceedings* 31, Supp. 1/2A (1999): 45S–48S.

R. Paul Robertson, M.D., et al., "Pancreas and Islet Transplantation for Patients with Diabetes," *Diabetes Care* 23, no. 1 (January 2000): 112–116.

Islets Neogenesis Associate Protein (INGAP)
One of a family of recently discovered naturally occurring proteins that has been synthesized in the laboratory. It can stimulate the growth of the insulin-producing beta cells in the pancreas. In initial animal studies, INGAP has increased insulin levels and has apparently cured the diabetes in these animals, at least for the short term.

As of this writing, INGAP is being tested in 62 human patients. Theoretically, INGAP has the potential to cure Type 1 diabetes because it stimulates the individual's own pancreas to produce new beta cells that make insulin.

The only cure for Type 1 diabetes available as of this writing is the transplantation of an entire pancreas or the transplantation of beta cells from organ donors. Two pancreases are required for each beta cell transplantation in order to obtain an adequate number of cells, and insufficient numbers of pancreases are available. In addition, the transplantation recipients will need to take antirejection drugs for their lifetime. Hopefully, this problem will not occur if INGAP is successful as a treatment.

islets of Langerhans   A structure within the pancreas that contains alpha, beta and delta cells. Together these cells produce and secrete hormones that aid in the digestion of food and the maintenance of normal glucose levels. In a person with Type 1 diabetes, the beta cells cease to function. Supplemental doses of insulin, either through injection or pump, are needed as a substitute.

In 1999, physicians using the "Edmonton Protocol" successfully transplanted islet cells from the pancreases of recently deceased individuals into eight patients with Type 1 diabetes. In 2001, the patients continued to do well and did not need any insulin or other medications for diabetes. (See also ISLET CELL TRANSPLANTATION.)

itching skin   Dry and itchy skin, a condition that is also known as PRURITIS is one possible symptom of diabetes. Combined with other common symptoms, such as constant thirst, increased appetite, etc., severe itching (in the absence of other obvious causes) may mean that an undiagnosed individual does have diabetes. In such a case, the person should obtain a medical diagnosis. Severe hyperglycemia may lead to itchy skin, although the most common cause is dryness. (See also SKIN PROBLEMS, XEROSIS.)

Joslin Diabetes Center Nonprofit diabetes treatment, research, and educational institution that is affiliated with the prestigious Harvard Medical School. The Joslin Diabetes Center specializes in treating patients with diabetes and performing cutting edge research on diabetes treatment and prevention. It is the largest organization in the United States that devotes its energies and efforts solely to diabetes research and care, providing clinic services including endocrinology, ophthalmology, nephrology, pediatric endocrinology, obstetrics, mental health, nutrition, and exercise physiology.

The Joslin Diabetes Center was originally formed in 1898 by Elliott P. Joslin, M.D., a noted Boston physician and author who was extremely active in the field of diabetes both prior to the discovery of insulin as well as afterwards. Today the Joslin Diabetes Center has affiliates at 23 locations in 12 states and serves more than 40,000 patients with diabetes.

A Research Organization

Researching both Type 1 and Type 2 diabetes as well as diabetic complications, the Joslin Diabetes Center is actively involved with cutting edge research on such issues as possible cures for diabetes and genetic causes. For example, Joslin researchers are studying the linkage between diabetes and OBESITY and possible causes for both conditions. One cause may be a substance called leptin.

Other researchers at the Joslin Diabetes Center are working on methods to cause non-insulin producing cells to produce insulin, thus alleviating the disease altogether. Even if current islet cell transplantation procedures are perfected, a limiting problem is that each transplantation still requires two pancreases and there are not enough cadaver pancreases to accommodate all individuals with Type 1 diabetes. (Live donors cannot be used, as with kidney donations, since no one can live without a pancreas.)

The Joslin protocol to stimulate non-insulin producing cells may be one of the many breakthroughs needed by people with diabetes.

An Educational Organization

The Joslin Diabetes Center provides professional education to over 30,000 physicians and health care professionals in courses nationwide and globally. The Joslin website also provides a wealth of information to patients and medical professionals.

Support and outreach Recognizing that many minorities are at high risk for developing Type 2 diabetes, the Joslin Diabetes Center has spearheaded a variety of successful programs to encourage blacks and Hispanics to obtain testing and treatment.

Another group helped by Joslin has been parents of teenagers with diabetes. Joslin provides education as well as meetings and support groups so individuals can share information as well as learn from professionals.

For more information, contact:

Joslin Diabetes Center
One Joslin Place
Boston, MA 02215
(617) 732-2415
www.joslin.harvard.edu

(See Appendix for names and addresses of Joslin Affiliates.)

juvenile-onset diabetes   Former name for Type 1 diabetes, also formerly known as insulin-dependent diabetes (IDDM). An estimated 5–10 percent of people with diabetes suffer from Type 1 diabetes. The illness is often diagnosed in children and adolescents although it may not develop until early adulthood or later. (See also ADOLESCENTS, CHILDREN, INFANTS, TYPE 1 DIABETES.)

Juvenile Diabetes Research Foundation (JDRF) International   An organization that concentrates on fundraising for research on Type 1 diabetes.

Founded in 1970, the Juvenile Diabetes Research Foundation (formerly known as the Juvenile Diabetes Foundation International), is an organization that primarily supports research and promotes advocacy for individuals with Type 1 diabetes. Its primary goal is finding a cure for Type 1 diabetes. According to the organization, they are the leading nonprofit and non-governmental funding source for diabetes research, and spend 84 cents of each dollar on research and education. They anticipated spending $120 million on research and education in 2001.

The organization offers two publications: *Countdown* magazine and *Countdown for Kids* magazine. They also offer books and other helpful information on Type 1 diabetes.

As of this writing, actress Mary Tyler Moore is the organization's international chairman. She has Type 1 diabetes.

Juvenile Diabetes Research Foundation (JDRF)
    International
120 Wall Street
19th Floor
New York, NY 10005
(800) 223-1138 or (212) 889-7575
www.jdrf.org

(See also TYPE 1 DIABETES.)

ketones   Chemicals that the liver derives from fat and that may accumulate rapidly in the blood when the body has insufficient insulin and thus, it must consequently break down body fat rather than use carbohydrates for energy.

There are two types of ketones: ACETOACETATE and B-HYDROXYBUTYRATE. Standard REAGENT STRIPS for the urine only measure acetoacetate. There is now a reagent strip that will measure B-hydroxybutyrate in the blood. It is probably best used in physician offices.

"Ketosis" is the state in which fat is being broken down and accumulates in excessive amounts in the bloodstream. This may become a problem for people with diabetes when they become ill with an intercurrent illness such as flu, thus increasing both stress on the body and resistance to insulin and consequently, throwing the body out of balance. It can also become a problem if they undergo a rigorous or special diet or fasting. Anyone may develop mild fasting ketosis after an overnight fast. This is not considered a pathological condition.

People with diabetes may become extremely ill when they enter DIABETIC KETOACIDOSIS (DKA), a life-threatening condition that requires immediate emergency medical treatment.

Contrary to popular belief, if a person with diabetes is unable to eat because of nausea or vomiting, this does *not* mean that it is all right to ignore glucose levels. Quite the contrary: the person who takes insulin may need even more insulin. An imbalance of ketones is also the reason why people with diabetes need to learn SICK DAY RULES, so that they will know what to do when they become ill.

ketosis   A process in which the body begins to break down stored fat in order to supply sufficient energy to the body. A person who has Type 1 diabetes and is not monitoring their glucose levels and insulin intake because of illness or another reason may develop ketosis. Ketosis may further advance to DIABETIC KETOACIDOSIS (DKA), a risky condition which, if untreated, may lead to organ damage, coma, or even death.

The key symptoms of ketosis are abdominal stomach pain, nausea, and vomiting. (See also DIABETIC KETOACIDOSIS (DKA), KETONES.)

kidney disease   See DIABETIC NEPHROPATHY.

Kimmelstiel-Wilson lesions   A distinctive lesion that was first noted in pathology specimens of the kidney by Drs. Paul Kimmelstiel and C. Wilson in 1936, which they then called "intercapillary glomerulosclerosis," i.e., scarring in the filtering units of the kidneys. The lesion was later named after these two physicians. The doctors observed that certain illnesses occurred together in some patients, including diabetes, ALBUMINURIA, HYPERTENSION, retinal deterioration, and kidney failure.

In 1950, ophthalmologist Jonas Friedenwald of the University of Maryland wrote about the relationship between lesions caused by Kimmelstiel-Wilson disease to retinal lesions found in diabetes.

Kumamoto Study   A small controlled study that was performed at the Kumamoto University

School of Medicine on 110 Japanese men with Type 2 diabetes and was reported in 1995. The subjects were leaner than their American counterparts who have diabetes; however, this study definitively proved that improved GLYCEMIC CONTROL of multiple injections of insulin significantly decreased the risk of the complications of diabetes. For example, a 2 percent decrease in the HbA1C of the subjects resulted in the dramatic reduction of 68 percent fewer incidences of DIABETIC RETINOPATHY and 70 percent fewer incidences of DIABETIC NEPHROPATHY.

Intensive therapy also reduced the deterioration to microalbuminuria by 57 percent. (See also CLINICAL STUDIES.)

Kussmaul's respiration Rapid and heavy panting type of breathing which is exhibited by those who have DIABETIC KETOACIDOSIS (DKA). It is the body's attempt to decrease carbon dioxide levels and thus, help improve the body's acid base balance. The condition was named after Adolph Kussmaul, a physician from the 19th century who first discovered it.

lancet The sharp needle-like device used by people with diabetes (or physicians, or laboratory workers) to prick the finger in order to obtain a droplet of blood that will be tested for glucose levels. Pricking the side of the finger is much less painful than pricking the finger tip as there are far fewer pain receptors present at that location. Newer devices enable the user to obtain a blood drop from alternate sites of the body with even fewer pain receptors than the fingertip or side of the finger.

There are a number of lancing devices with accompanying meters that allow for lancing alternate sites such as the forearm. There are also devices that will allow the patient to individualize the force of the automatic lancing action as well as the depth of penetration, thus making the process much more comfortable. (See also BLOODLESS TESTING, FINGER PRICK.)

lawsuits Litigation filed by individuals who believe they have been wronged in some way. Because of problems with perceived discrimination against individuals with diabetes in the workplace, school, and other environments, individuals with diabetes have filed many lawsuits. Many people hoped that the AMERICANS WITH DISABILITIES ACT would correct many of the problems faced by individuals with disabilities; however, apparent inequities continue.

Organizations such as the AMERICAN DIABETES ASSOCIATION (ADA) have found it necessary to assist individuals in cases where their rights were violated. For example, in some cases, schools have refused to provide testing for children with diabetes or to allow school-age children to test their own blood. In some cases, schools or even laws have required that a physician perform the testing, and thus a conflict occurs between clashing federal laws and the needs of children.

The ADA prevailed in a lawsuit in which a daycare center denied admission to a child solely because of her Type 1 diabetes and need for testing and medication. (See also DISCRIMINATION, DISABILITY, SCHOOL, WORK.)

LDL Refers to low density lipoprotein cholesterol, which, in contrast to high density cholesterol (HDL), is often called "bad" cholesterol. People with diabetes have a greater than normal risk for heart attacks and strokes. Because high levels of LDL can increase the probability of either a heart attack or stroke, it's important for people with diabetes to work at lowering their LDL levels through diet, EXERCISE, and other lifestyle changes, such as losing weight and quitting smoking.

LDL levels should be lower than 100 mg/dL. Studies are ongoing to determine if even lower levels will be advantageous to people with diabetes. LDL should be measured in the fasting state and can be calculated if total cholesterol, trigylceride level, and HDL are also measured. It can also be measured directly, which is preferable in patients with diabetes. (See also CHOLESTEROL, HDL.)

leprechaunism A very rare disease caused by a genetic mutation that also causes HYPERGLYCEMIA and INSULIN RESISTANCE. It is characterized by severe mental and physical retardation and causes the progressive wasting away and death of the afflicted infants. These children are very small but leprechaunism should not be confused with dwarfism, which is a general term for all people of short stature.

According to the *Encyclopedia of Genetic Disorders and Birth Defects,*

The nasal bridge is flat, nostrils flared, the ears low-set. Infants may have excessive facial hair (hirsutism). The features are quite coarse, not cute as the leprechaun label might suggest. Excessive skin folds, lack of subcutaneous tissue and low birth weight give infants an emaciated appearance. Breast enlargement is common in males and females, as are penile and clitoral enlargement. The hands and feet are also large. The striking physical appearance is usually sufficient for diagnosis.

James Wynbrandt and Mark D. Ludman, M.D., F.R.C.P.C., *The Encyclopedia of Genetic Disorders and Birth Defects,* Second Edition (New York, N.Y.: Facts On File, Inc., 2000).

leptin   A hormone that is secreted by fat cells and that acts on cells in the brain and tissues to regulate food consumption and overall energy levels.

Some researchers have found, as of this writing, a genetic link between obesity and diabetes, based on testing with rats. Further research may indicate that manipulation among human subjects can control the serious problem of OBESITY.

Researchers have also found a link between DIABETIC RETINOPATHY and high levels of leptin in the eye.

Circulating leptin levels may be related to INSULIN RESISTANCE. In patients with HYPERTENSION, leptin may also be increased.

J. Agata et al., "High Plasma Immunoreactive Leptin Level in Essential Hypertension," *American Journal of Hypertension* 10, no. 10, part 1 (1997): 1171–1174.

K. L. Segal et al., "Relationship between Insulin Sensitivity and Plasma Leptin Concentrations in Lean and Obese Men," *Diabetes* 45, no. 7 (1996): 988–991.

life expectancy   The number of years the average person can expect to live. Experts report that diabetes decreases life expectancy by five to 10 years, primarily due to the COMPLICATIONS that diabetes can cause in many individuals. Thus, much research is aimed at primary prevention, especially among patients with Type 2 diabetes. (See also DEATH.)

lipids   Fatty substances stored and circulating as lipoproteins in the body for the purpose of energy reserve. Cholesterol and triglycerides are both forms of lipids. High levels of lipids are seen in individuals suffering from such diseases as ATHEROSCLEROSIS, which is often a problem that people with diabetes face. (See also HDL, LDL.)

lipoatrophy   Refers to indentations in the skin where a person with Type 1 diabetes has repeatedly injected insulin into the same spot. It is preferable to rotate the body sites that receive the medication to avoid this problem, though it is now unusual to see lipoatrophy with the very pure human insulin that is available. It was a common problem in the past with pure animal insulin. (See also INJECTION SITE ROTATION.)

macrovascular/microvascular disease   A general term that refers to damage to the large (macrovascular) or smaller (microvascular) blood vessels. This damage results from a build up of fat, blood clots, and oxidation to the endothelium (the lining of the blood vessels). Macrovascular disease is the most common cause of death among individuals with Type 1 and Type 2 diabetes.

Macrovascular Diseases

Macrovascular diseases include coronary artery disease, cerebrovascular disease, and peripheral vascular disease. Some complications of macrovascular disease are ischemic heart disease, heart attack (myocardial infarction), intermittent claudication, lower extremity ulcer, and STROKE.

Microvascular Diseases

Some complications of microvascular diseases are DIABETIC NEPHROPATHY, DIABETIC NEUROPATHY, and DIABETIC RETINOPATHY.

Microvascular diseases harm the small blood vessels and can occur in people who have had diabetes for many years.

The Diabetes Control and Complications Trial Research Group, "Effect of Intensive Diabetes Management on Macrovascular Events and Risk Factors in the Diabetes Control and Complications Trial," *The American Journal of Cardiology* 75 (May 1, 1995): 36–51.

macular edema   A swelling in part of the retina known as the "macula," and also a frequently seen complication of DIABETIC RETINOPATHY. This generally occurs due to formation of many microaneurysms that lead to leaking of retinal capillaries. It is diagnosed by an examination with a device called a slit lamp and by fluorescing angiography (a procedure in which a colored dye is injected into an arm vein and special photos of the retina are taken). The macula provides fine central vision or reading vision. There are about 75,000 new cases of diabetic macular edema each year. (See also BLINDNESS, EYE DISEASE.)

malignant otitis externa   An outer ear infection (in the external auditory canal) that is found in a person with diabetes, usually someone over age 65. It is usually caused by bacteria in the *Pseudomonas* genus. This problem needs to be considered in all external ear infections diagnosed among patients who have diabetes so that appropriate antibiotics may be started. The standard antibiotics that are used for ear infections typically will not kill *Pseudomonas*. Malignant otitis externa can affect facial nerves and cause a facial droop. In the worst case, surgery may be needed. (See also ELDERLY.)

malnutrition   Severe lack of basic nutrition, leading to starvation. In developing-world countries, malnutrition is a risk factor for developing diabetes. In the United States and other developed countries, patients with diabetes who develop malnutrition suffer slow healing of wounds and an increased risk of DIABETIC NEPHROPATHY.

managed care   See HMOS/MANAGED CARE.

Maturity Onset Diabetes of the Young (MODY)

An uncommon to rare subset of Type 2 diabetes in which the diagnosis is typically made prior to the age of 25. MODY is generally found in slender African-American adolescents, and is rarely found in white adolescents. This type of diabetes runs in families, and more than 50 percent of these patients have an abnormal glucokinase enzyme (a protein in the beta cells of the pancreatic islets that senses the glucose level in the blood). Other genetic abnormalities have also been found. Inheritance is often autosomal dominant.

Typically the patients are not insulin dependent and do not develop ketosis, although they may require insulin for the glucose control.

Carla R. Scott, M.D., et al. "Characteristics of Youth-onset Noninsulin-Dependent Diabetes Mellitus and Insulin-dependent Diabetes Mellitus at Diagnosis," *Pediatrics* 100, no. 1 (July 1997): 84–90.

meals, timing of   Planning for when and what to eat, based on factors affecting a person with diabetes.

People with diabetes need to be careful about not only *what* they eat but also *when* they eat. For example, if an extended period occurs between meals, the person's blood sugar levels may drop to a dangerous level. Timing of meals also affects the choice of the type of insulin one uses, and whether the person uses a rapid, short-acting, intermediate, or long-acting insulin—or some combination of these various types of insulin preparations.

Blood testing results are also affected by the timing of meals. Studies indicate that postprandial (after a meal) testing provides a far better indicator of the individual's health than does a blood test that is administered before a meal. (See also CARBOHYDRATE COUNTING, DIET, GLYCEMIC CONTROL, NUTRITION.)

Medicaid   Refers to the medical insurance program under Title IX of the Social Security Act, which was first enacted in 1965. This program is both federally and state funded in its mission to provide medical benefits to indigent individuals who are disabled and who are also often ineligible for other federal or private programs. At the federal level, Medicaid (and also MEDICARE) is overseen by the Centers for Medicare and Medicaid Services (CMS), formerly known as the Health Care Financing Administration (HCFA). Medicaid affects many people with diabetes who are elderly, disabled, and who earn a low income.

To qualify for Medicaid, people must be "categorically eligible" for Medicaid, which means that being poor is not sufficient by itself to guarantee eligibility. Instead, the person must also receive Temporary Aid to Needy Families (TANF) payments or receive Supplemental Security payment benefits (SSI) due to a disability or qualify in some other category of public assistance. Some other categories of individuals who are also eligible for Medicaid, include the following groups:

- children under age six whose family income is at or below 133 percent of the federal poverty level
- pregnant women whose family income is at or below 133 percent of the federal poverty level
- recipients of foster care assistance or adoption assistance under Title IV of the Social Security Act
- some Medicare beneficiaries who are indigent

Some states extend Medicaid coverage to more groups, depending on their state plan.

Types of services   Medicaid provides coverage for the following forms of medical services:

- inpatient hospital care
- outpatient physician care
- prenatal care
- medications
- vaccines for children

- laboratory and x-ray services
- family planning services
- skilled nursing facility services

Some states also provide dental and optometric care in their Medicaid plans, as well as other services. Another option chosen by many states is a form of managed care or HMO coverage for Medicaid enrollees, in which a particular physician or group will be the one(s) to provide care. This service has proven to be cost-effective for states and the federal government because it diverts individuals on Medicaid from seeking their routine medical care at hospital emergency rooms. (See also DISABILITY.)

Deborah Shatin, Ph.D., et al., "Health Care Utilization by Children with Chronic Illnesses: A Comparison of Medicaid and Employer Insured Managed Care," *Pediatrics* 102, no. 4 (October 1998): 102–106.
Social Security Administration, Office of Policy, Office of Research, Evaluation and Statistics, *Annual Statistical Supplement 2000 to the Social Security Bulletin*, Baltimore, Md., Social Security Administration, 2000.

Medicare A massive federal medical program for individuals who are eligible for monthly checks in relation to their retirement or disability benefits, not including Supplemental Security Insurance (SSI). Medicare provides medical coverage for 95 percent of the aged population in the United States and also provides medical coverage for many disabled adults. As of 1999, Medicare payments totaled $213 billion for the year. Contrary to the SSI program, individuals receiving Medicare benefits need not be indigent as a requirement of eligibility. Instead, they must meet age or disability requirements, among other conditions of eligibility.

The Centers for Medicare and Medicaid Services (CMS), formerly known as the Health Care Financing Administration (HCFA), is the federal organization that oversees the Medicare program, including the care of an estimated 40 percent of all Americans with diabetes (more than 4 million individuals). CMS also administers the End-Stage Renal Disease Program to pay for dialysis and kidney transplants in Medicare patients whose kidneys fail them.

At the outset of the program, Medicare was part of the Social Security Amendments of 1965, under Title XVIII of the Social Security Act. The program originally covered only eligible people who were ages 65 and older. In 1973, the program was amended to include people under age 65 who were entitled to either Social Security disability benefits or Railroad Retirement disability benefits. At that time, most people with END-STAGE RENAL DISEASE (ESRD) were also added to the program, which is still a feature of the program today. This is important for many people with diabetes whose DIABETIC NEPHROPATHY devolves into renal failure.

Parts of Medicare

There are two parts to Medicare, Part A and Part B. Medicare Part A covers inpatient hospital care and very limited periods of SKILLED NURSING FACILITY care. Part B benefits primarily cover outpatient (office) physician visits. There is also a third part of Medicare known as the "Medicare+ Choice" program, established by the Balanced Budget Act of 1997, which allows members to participate in private health care plans. There are about 40 million people in the United States who are enrolled in Medicare and most have both Part A and B benefits. Of these, about 6 million participate in a Medicare+Choice plan.

Supplies and Equipment Covered and Not Covered by Medicare

Medicare also pays for some HOME HEALTH CARE, as well as some approved medical equipment, such as wheelchairs, prosthetic devices, and oxygen equipment. As of this writing, prescription medications are not covered by Medicare, with the exception of IMMUNIZATIONS for pneumonia, flu, and hepatitis B, as well as some anticancer drugs.

Coverage for devices such as syringes, needles, supplies, and meters that are needed by some individuals with diabetes, particularly those with Type 1 diabetes who must self-inject insulin, are partly covered under Medicare. To receive coverage, the patient's doctor must fill out a form every six months. Medicare may cover special shoes as well, if needed. In general, the individual must pay for 20 percent of the Medicare-approved amount.

As of this writing, insulin itself is not covered under Medicare. Medicare also does *not* cover dental services, eyeglasses, or hearing aids.

Paying for Noncovered Items

Because Medicare does not cover all medical needs as of this writing, most seniors purchase what is called "Medigap" insurance, to pay for such items as medications and chiropractic care. Some Medigap insurers provide prescription coverage. Medigap insurance also covers the copay for Medicare recipients. If a retired person has health insurance from a private company, usually that insurance company pays for medical costs first and then, if there are still costs remaining, Medicare will consider paying some of the balance.

For more information on Medicare, contact the local Social Security Administration office or contact CMS at:

Centers for Medicare and Medicaid Services
7500 Security Boulevard, C2-26-112
Baltimore, MD 21244
(800) 444-4606
www.medicare.gov

National Diabetes Information Clearinghouse
National Institute of Diabetes and Digestive and
   Kidney Diseases (NIDDK)
1 Information Way
Bethesda, MD 20892-3560
(800) 860-8747 or (301) 654-3327
www.niddk.nih.gov/health/diabetes/ndic.htm

(See also DISABILITY, ELDERLY, MEDICARE THERA-
PEUTIC SHOE ACT.)

Claresa Levetan, M.D., "Mastering Diabetes at Medicare," *Clinical Diabetes* 18, no. 2 (Spring 2000): 74–79.

Social Security Administration, Office of Policy, Office of Research, Evaluation and Statistics, *Annual Statistical Supplement 2000 to the Social Security Bulletin,* Baltimore, Md., Social Security Administration, 2000.

Medicare Therapeutic Shoe Act   Passed in 1993, this act allows for the coverage of special protective shoes and/or inserts or shoe modifications for people who have diabetes along with certain other medical problems, such as PERIPHERAL NEUROPATHY, a history of foot ulcers, a severe foot deformity, impaired circulation or prior amputation of part or all of a foot.

Medicare recipients must obtain a prescription for such shoes from the physician who is treating them for diabetes, and an approved podiatrist or other approved foot expert must fit the shoes. As of this writing, Medicare will pay for 80 percent of the reasonable charge for the shoes or shoe modifications.

Experts say that many patients with diabetes are not taking advantage of this benefit. According to Michael S. Pinzur, M.D., a study of about 400 long-term patients with diabetes, who were an average of 62 years old, revealed that only a minority (about 12 percent) of patients wore special shoes. (See also FOOT CARE, MEDICARE, ORTHOTICS.)

"Letters: American Orthopaedic Foot Ankle Society Diabetic Shoe Survey," *Diabetes Care* 22, no. 12 (December 1999): 2099.

medication adherence/compliance   Refers to a patient following a physician's orders for the timing and amount of medication. Medication nonadherence is a very serious problem for people who have diabetes for a variety of reasons; for example, it results in worse control of glucose and blood pressure. Over the long-term, failure to take medications prescribed by physicians can lead to eye, kidney, cardiac, and other diseases, as well as an earlier death that would not have occurred if the medication were taken as ordered by the physician.

Reasons for Nonadherence

Some reasons why people with and without diabetes do not follow their doctor's orders for taking their medication are:

- not understanding the physician's instructions

- deciding after a few doses that they are not "really sick" and thus, no longer need medicine

- confusing one medication with another and consequently taking the wrong one

- becoming confused because the patient takes many medications. The patient may skip a medicine if she isn't sure she took it. Or she may take it anyway, possibly administering an unwitting second dose

- forgetting to take the medicine

- losing the medicine

- other individuals administering the medicine fail to provide it on time, because they forget or lose the medicine or don't think the person needs it

- not taking medication because of side effects it causes

- being unable to afford medications

Nonadherence among People With Diabetes

Several recent studies indicate that noncompliance is a very serious problem among those with diabetes, particularly with individuals diagnosed with Type 2 diabetes, who may not take the illness as seriously as they should.

A study reported at the American Diabetes Association's 60th Annual Scientific Sessions provided data on individuals with diabetes in Scotland and gave insight on medication adherence problems. Medical records were studied on 400,000 residents over three years, including 3,000 individuals who were diagnosed with diabetes.

Only about one third of the individuals taking sulfonylureas or metformin refilled their prescriptions sufficiently to maintain acceptable blood glucose levels. When individuals were prescribed both drugs, only 13 percent complied.

Adherence to the medication plan varied with the number of pills that were prescribed. Patients who only had to take one pill per day had a higher compliance rate than those who had to take two or more pills daily. Researchers found a 22 percent decrease in compliance with each additional drug that was added to the medication regimen.

In another study reported in Belgium in 1999 for the period 1991–97, researchers found very poor rates of compliance among people with Type 2 diabetes. About half the patients taking acarbose did not refill their prescription within a one-year period. In addition, about one third of those taking metformin apparently discontinued the drug altogether.

Failure to take their medications did have a serious impact on the subjects with diabetes. Researchers in the Belgium study found that the patients who stopped taking their oral antidiabetic medications were nearly twice as likely to require emergency hospital treatment.

Nonadherence among adolescents   According to researchers in Scotland who reported their findings in a 1997 issue of *The Lancet*, it is likely that adolescents and young adults with Type 1 diabetes who suffer from complications are not taking their insulin as directed. They found that among 89 patients, 16 patients (18 percent) had been hospitalized 37 times over the period 1993–1994. Of these, 36 of the 37 hospital admissions were for acute complications stemming from their diabetes, including 15 with DIABETIC KETOACIDOSIS (DKA) and 21 with HYPOGLYCEMIA. Some of the patients had failed to take any insulin at all. The authors said,

> The reasons for failing to take insulin are complex, but may include deliberate failure as part of a weight-loss strategy, manipulation, recklessness, error, or simple fatigue in the day-to-day effort of managing diabetes. Overall adherence were excellent before puberty and improved again in the adult years; we maintain this is related to behavioural factors. Parents

will supervise the treatment regimen for their children, and this may explain the positive adherence index.

Improving Medication Adherence

Because medication compliance is so critically important for individuals with diabetes and other illnesses, doctors try to make compliance as easy as possible. Some ways that doctors simplify the drug regimen, whenever possible, are the following:

- They order time-release medications that can be used once a day.
- Medication is ordered to be taken at meals or upon arising or before bed.
- When possible, combination medications are ordered.
- Doctors review the medication regimen, each time they see the patient.
- Medications given in calendar blister packs may be easier for patients to comply with.
- Medication containers (with one section for "Monday," "Tuesday," and so forth) that are set up in advance by the patient or visiting nurse or family members.

Medication Packaging Can Help

In a study reported in a 2000 issue of *Diabetes Care,* researchers sought to find if individuals with diabetes were more likely to take their medication at the proper time and in the designated dose if a calendar blister pack were provided.

The researchers ran the test for eight months on 68 patients with diabetes in New Zealand. About half the patients took three or more medications per day. Their patients using the calendar blister pack were given both their oral antidiabetic medication and antihypertensive medicine. The results: researchers found that both the glucose levels and the hypertension levels of those who were using the calendar blister pack dropped significantly versus the levels for the control group subjects who did not receive the blister pack.

Probably the key problem with blister packing multiple medications is that many individuals take medications produced by different pharmaceutical companies and would require some means of cooperation between sometimes heavily competitive companies. For example, to illustrate just one problem, would the packaging be done at Pharmaceutical Company A's plant or Pharmaceutical Company B's plant? Of course, if one pharmaceutical company produced both the antidiabetic medicine and the antihypertensive, this would not present the same problem.

All patients with diabetes should carry a list of their medications, both prescribed and nonprescribed medications. The list should also include all vitamins, herbs, and other supplements the person may take, as well as dosages of each drug. This information should be provided to all healthcare providers that they see.

Patients with diabetes should also attempt to obtain all their medications and supplements from one pharmacy only, in order to minimize errors and drug to drug interactions that may occur. The patients should be sure to tell the pharmacist about supplements they plan to use, so that he or she can enter the information into the computer. (See also ADOLESCENTS, GLYCEMIC CONTROL.)

Jayant Dey, M.D., et al., "Factors Influencing Patient Acceptability of Diabetes Treatment Regimens," *Clinical Diabetes* 18, no. 2, (Spring 2000): 61–67.

Andrew Morris et al., "Adherence to Insulin Treatment, Glycaemic Control, and Ketoacidosis in Insulin-Dependent Diabetes Mellitus," *The Lancet* 350, no. 9090 (November 22, 1997): 1505–1510.

D. Simmons, F.R.A.C.P., M.D., et al., "Can Medication Packing Improve Glycemic Control and Blood Pressure in Type 2 Diabetes?," *Diabetes Care* 23, no. 2 (2000): 153–156.

medications and diabetes   Drugs prescribed for people with diabetes. Insulin formulations and oral medications are very important for individuals with diabetes. In most cases, the individual with Type 2 diabetes needs medications to keep their glucose at an acceptable level. However, all individuals with Type 1 diabetes, and some with Type 2 diabetes, must use insulin.

Many physicians use three or more drugs to control Type 2 diabetes and sometimes this causes a problem with MEDICATION ADHERENCE. According to a 1999 study performed by the American Association of Clinical Endocrinologists, 90 percent of the 348 physician respondents said they prescribed three or more medications for their patients with Type 2 diabetes.

Some commonly prescribed medications for Type 2 diabetes, as of this writing, are: tolbutamide, chlorpropamide, tolazamide, metformin, glyburide, glipizide, ACARBOSE, miglitol, micronized glyburide, nateglinide, and repaglinide. Some commonly prescribed medications for patients with Type 1 diabetes are various forms of insulin (regular, lispro, NPH, Aspart, lente, ultra-lente, semi-lente, and glargine).

Although not a common cause of diabetes, it is true that some drugs may interfere with the secretion of insulin and can thus precipitate Type 2 diabetes in people who have a genetic predisposition to INSULIN RESISTANCE and beta cell dysfunction. Most physicians are aware of the potential risks of these medications and are also alert to symptoms that may indicate the development of diabetes.

If an individual taking such a medication exhibits symptoms of diabetes, and if laboratory tests then confirm the presence of diabetes, the doctor may decide to take the person off the medication altogether. Or, if the medication is deemed necessary to the patient's health, the physician may instead opt to decrease the dosage or continue it at the same level. Of course, the doctor should treat the patient for diabetes as well and perform regular follow-up checks, whether the medication that induced diabetes is discontinued, decreased, or is kept at the same level.

Some examples of medications that sometimes induce diabetes are:

- glucocorticoids (steroids prescribed to reduce severe inflammation)
- nicotinic acid/niacin (prescribed for hyperlipidemia). Generally has a small effect
- alpha-adrenergic agonists, prescribed to increase blood pressure in patients with low blood pressure
- thiazides that cause low potassium levels (Some diuretics prescribed for edema [water retention])
- dilantin (anti-epileptic drug, prescribed for seizures). This rarely induces diabetes
- pentamidine, used to treat infections in HIV positive individuals
- interferon-alpha therapy (prescribed for hepatitis B and C and some cancers)
- diazoxide (used to treat insulin-producing tumors)

(See also MEDICATION ADHERENCE/COMPLIANCE, MEDICATION INTERACTIONS.)

medication interactions The effect that medications may have on each other when taken by a person at about the same time or together. Some medications may boost ("potentiate") the impact of other drugs. They may also lower the efficacy of other medications. Some medications, when taken together, can result in medical problems that would not occur if they were not combined.

Medication interactions are a potential problem for any person who takes any medicines, including over-the-counter drugs. Even alternative remedies can cause a problem, for example, ginkgo biloba can cause blood thinning and boost the impact of other blood thinners such as warfarin (Coumadin). If a physician did not know a patient was taking an herbal remedy, then he could not provide a warning. Many individuals, particularly older people who have diabetes, are likely to be on more than two or three medications for chronic conditions such as hypertension, cardiac problems, and other ailments. It's a good idea for patients to use just one pharmacy, if possible, so that the pharmacist can help track possible drug interactions. It's also a good idea for patients to keep a complete list of all medications and supplements, so that this information can be provided to new physicians or to pharmacists. (See also MEDICATION ADHERENCE/ COMPLIANCE, MEDICATION.)

meglitinides   A class of medication prescribed for people with Type 2 diabetes in order to maintain glycemic control. As of this writing, Prandin (repaglinide) is the only FDA-approved drug in this class. A meglitinide drug is a "secretagogue" medication, which means that it induces a greater secretion of insulin. Sulfonylurea drugs also are secretatogues but they act differently.

Prandin helps restore "first phase insulin" secretion, which is important to control glucose levels after meals. The rates of HYPOGLYCEMIA and weight gain are lower with Prandin than is seen with sulfonylurea medications. Thus, it appears safer although slightly less effective. Prandin is usually prescribed to be taken three to four times a day in dosages ranging from 0.5 mg to 4.0 mg (0.5 mg three to four times a day up to 4.0 mg for three to four times per day.)

The drug is taken with the first bite of a meal. It can be used in patients with renal insufficiency and mild liver disease.

men and diabetes   The effect and overall impact of diabetes on males. Both men and women are at risk for diabetes; however, men have a higher risk for DEATH from diabetes. In the United States, about 7.5 million men have diabetes, although it's estimated that about one third have not yet been diagnosed with the disease. Most males with diabetes have Type 2 diabetes. Some studies indicate that men feel much more confident about handling their diabetes than women do, or at least, they report that is how they feel.

Attitudes and Emotions Toward Their Illness

In studies performed or analyzed by Richard R. Rubin and Mark Peyrot, reported in a 1998 issue of *Diabetes Spectrum,* the authors found that men felt more in control of their illness than women did and more confident that they could affect the outcome of their diabetes. Their spouses mirrored their views, as did the spouses of the less-confident women.

These beliefs were carried through in behaviors; for example, men were less likely to delay meals or insulin injections than women and they were less likely to engage in binge eating than females. The men also had fewer complications related to diabetes, with the exception of erectile dysfunction.

The men were half as likely or less than women to exhibit symptoms of depression or anxiety nor did the men worry as much about their weight gain as the women. In addition, about 26 percent of the men with diabetes in one study worried about their appearance, compared to 52 percent of the women with diabetes.

It is also possible that some of the male patients may be denying real medical problems. Rubin and Peyrot say,

> We often see patients who are clearly struggling both physically and emotionally, yet actively resist acknowledging the seriousness of their problems and our efforts to help them deal with these problems. Such patients may present with clear signs of depression, persistent chronic hyperglycemia, and even with diabetes-related complications, yet say something like, "I'm doing just fine. I'm still walking around, right?"

Gender-related Complications of Diabetes

Although both men and women suffer from the symptoms or complications of diabetes, some symptoms that men experience from diabetes are uniquely gender-related, such as IMPOTENCE, also known as ERECTILE DYSFUNCTION. This problem may be caused by DIABETIC NEUROPATHY or by peripheral vascular disease. Men with diabetes typically develop erectile dysfunction about 10 to 15 years before their nondiabetic peers.

Men with diabetes may also suffer from retrograde ejaculation. This means that with intercourse and orgasm, the semen is secreted backwards into the bladder. This can affect fertility. If a man has such a problem, he should be evaluated by a urologist.

Men who developed diabetes before the age of 30 are more likely than women with diabetes to develop DIABETIC RETINOPATHY, which can then lead to BLINDNESS. Men with diabetes also face a risk of AMPUTATION that is at least double the risk suffered by women who have diabetes.

Work-Related Problems

Some men with diabetes have experienced difficulty with DISCRIMINATION at work, especially if they have Type 1 diabetes and must take insulin injections. The AMERICAN DIABETES ASSOCIATION provided a "friend of the court" brief on a case in which a police officer who had been previously employed in police work was denied a job solely because he had Type 1 diabetes. His individual situation was disregarded because of a blanket policy against any person who needed insulin. The court ruled for the man with diabetes, but a higher court ruled against him. The U.S. Supreme Court reversed the lower court, thus the man prevailed.

Richard R. Rubin, Ph.D., C.D.E., and Mark Peyrot, Ph.D., "Men and Diabetes: Psychosocial and Behavioral Issues," *Diabetes Spectrum* 11, no. 2 (1998): 81–87.

Rebecca K. Stellato, S.M., "Testosterone, Sex Hormone-Binding Globulin, and the Development of Type 2 Diabetes in Middle-Aged Men," *Diabetes Care* 23, no. 4 (April 2000): 490–494.

menopause Refers to the process of the cessation of ovulation and the end of menstruation in middle-aged or older women. It begins with a lowering of production of estrogen and progesterone and occurs over five to 16 years. If the woman has not menstruated for over a year and is over age 45, the probability is high that she has experienced menopause, although she should consult with a physician and request confirming laboratory tests to verify if this is true. Women with diabetes may have more difficulty with menopause than nondiabetics.

The average age for menopause is 51 years. In addition, if women have had both their ovaries surgically removed, an artificial menopause will occur at whatever age the surgery is performed.

Menopause may upset glycemic control and a perimenopausal woman (woman in early menopause) may need to consult with her diabetes care team to review her program. As progesterone levels fall, women become less insulin resistant. However, many perimenopausal women exercise less and consequently will gain weight. As a result, this is an important time for women with diabetes to review their exercise program.

Hormone replacement therapy Many physicians prescribe HORMONE REPLACEMENT THERAPY (HRT) to women who are menopausal. There are many pros and cons to this choice and each woman should discuss this decision with her gynecologist. In addition, the woman with diabetes should remind her gynecologist about her diabetes, in the event that a medication might affect her glucose levels.

The number of incidents of urinary tract infections, vaginitis, and yeast infections may also increase during menopause, as the lack of estrogen leads to vaginal lining atrophy. Eating low fat yogurt with active cultures (acidophilus) may help.

For more information, contact:

American College of Obstetricians and Gynecologists (ACOG)
409 12th Street, SW
P.O. Box 96920
Washington, DC 20090
(202) 484-8748
www.acog.org

North American Menopause Society
P.O. Box 94527
Cleveland, OH 44101

(216) 844-8748
www.menopause.org

Planned Parenthood Federation of America, Inc.
810 Seventh Avenue
New York, NY 10019
(800) 230-PLAN
www.plannedparenthood.org

(See also HORMONE REPLACEMENT THERAPY, WOMEN AND DIABETES.)

Rhoda H. Cobin, M.D., F.A.C.E., Chairman, "AACE Medical Guidelines for Clinical Practice for Management of Menopause," *Endocrine Practice* 5 no. 6 (November/December 1999): 354–366.

menstruation   Refers to the monthly flow of menstrual blood that occurs after puberty and continues regularly until interrupted by pregnancy, menopause, or the removal of the uterus in a hysterectomy. Diabetic control may become more difficult for a female during menstruation, because hormonal changes can drastically affect the hormonal balance and make tight control even more difficult than at other times. Typically, glucose levels tend to rise just prior to menstruation and then drop when bleeding starts, although this is not always the case.

Good GLYCEMIC CONTROL is associated with more normal menstrual cycles in adolescent girls, based on a study reported in a 2000 issue of *The Journal of Reproductive Medicine*.

Researchers reported on their retrospective review of the medical records of 46 adolescent females with Type 1 diabetes, including 37 girls (81 percent) with normal cycles and nine girls (19 percent) with menstrual problems. The girls were seen every three to six months, at which time their menstrual function, glycemic level, and any problem areas were evaluated. The girls were similar in BODY MASS INDEX and the age when they began menstruating. The average blood glucose levels were significantly higher for the girls with menstrual difficulties. The researchers also noted that as glucose levels of the girls increased, problems with menstruation also increased. In addition, the girls with menstrual problems had a higher rate of hospital admissions for DIABETIC KETOACIDOSIS (DKA).

The researchers noted that menstrual problems may be greater among females with diabetes than among the general population.

In a study of females with Type 1 diabetes, researchers found that 61 percent had an increase in their blood glucose prior to menstruation, causing 36 percent of them to change their insulin dosing.

Women who do not have diabetes have also been found to have an increase in insulin resistance prior to menstruation. Some clinicians hypothesize that some women may increase their intake of carbohydrates prior to menstruation.

To date, there is no evidence that women with diabetes suffer more from premenstrual syndrome (PMS) or from premenstrual dysphoric disorder (PMDD) than nondiabetic women. When such a problem does occur, antidepressants such as Prozac (fluoxetine) or Zoloft (sertraline) have been found to work effectively to combat these symptoms. (See also WOMEN WITH DIABETES.)

Janine Roumain, M.D., M.P.H., et al., "The Relationship of Menstrual Irregularity to Type 2 Diabetes in Pima Indian Women," *Diabetes Care* 21, no. 3 (1998): 346–349.
Betsy Schroeder et al., "Correlation between Glycemic Control and Menstruation in Diabetic Adolescents," *Journal of Reproductive Medicine* 45, no. 1 (January 2000): 1–5.

metabolic syndrome   See SYNDROME X.

metabolism   The series of chemical and physical processes that all cells use to maintain life. One part of metabolism is catabolism, which refers to the breakdown of chemicals (including foods) to release energy. The other part of metabolism is anabolism, which refers to the process during which the body uses food to either build up or to mend damaged cells. Insulin is an essential part of the anabolic process.

When patients with Type 1 diabetes have inadequate insulin, they are in a catabolic state, i.e., they are unable to store amino acids in protein, fatty acids in triglycerides, or convert glucose into glycogen and thus, their bodies begin breaking down the muscle protein and fat.

Anabolism is the process in which the body integrates simple molecules into larger ones. This is a healthy build-up state. This is also the reason why a person with poorly controlled diabetes and who then becomes well-controlled will gain weight. He or she goes from a catabolic state to an anabolic state and is able to store energy.

metformin One of the medications in the BIGUANIDE class that is used to treat people with Type 2 diabetes. Metformin has been available worldwide for 35–40 years but became available as Glucophage (produced by Bristol-Myers Squibb) in the United States in about 1995. The drug is only effective if a person's body still makes some insulin, thus it is not helpful for patients with Type 1 diabetes.

Metformin works by decreasing the amount of glucose that the liver produces and thus, it has a good effect on fasting glucose levels. Sophisticated studies have shown that this effect is most likely due to the suppression of the synthesis of new glucose (gluconeogenesis). By improving glucose levels, the drug will diminish glucose toxicity and indirectly will also decrease resistance to insulin. Because it does not cause an increase in insulin secretion when used alone (as monotherapy), it will not cause HYPOGLYCEMIA (low blood glucose).

If metformin is added to insulin or to an insulin secretagogue (a compound that stimulates the pancreas to make more insulin), this addition can contribute to hypoglycemia. In such a case, the physician will usually decrease the dose of either the insulin or the secretagogue.

Because it does not cause weight gain, metformin is favored as the first line therapy for overweight patients with Type 2 diabetes. (Most Type 2 diabetes patients are either overweight or obese.) Some patients with diabetes who are taking metformin lose a few pounds. In nondiabetic patients, the drug has not been effective in aiding with weight loss.

The primary adverse effect of metformin is gastrointestinal upset and it may cause diarrhea and a change in bowel habits. These effects can be minimized by starting the patient on a low dose and slowly titrating upwards to the maximally tolerated and effective dose.

Formulations of Metformin

Glucophage is available in the United States in dosages of 500-, 850-, and 1,000-mg tablets. The maximum allowed dose is 2,550 mg/day, generally given in two doses, although clinical studies have shown that most people achieve a maximal effect at a dose of 2,000 mg per day. The drug is also available as a sustained release preparation, known as Glucophage XR, which comes in 500-mg tablets that can be taken in one dose. This preparation seems to be as effective as Glucophage and causes fewer side effects.

Metformin is also available in a combination medication called Glucovance, which contains both metformin and the sulfonylurea drug, glyburide. It is formulated in a glyburide/metformin combination in tablets of 1.25/250 mg, 2.5/500 mg, and 5/500 mg. Many patients who were on the two medications are pleased to take one pill instead of two and to have one insurance co-payment (if they have copayments). Studies have also revealed that MEDICATION ADHERENCE/COMPLIANCE is also better with this regimen.

In the UNITED KINGDOM PROSPECTIVE DIABETES STUDY (UKPDS), patients treated with metformin had the lowest cardiac mortality of all treatment groups.

Patients Who Should Avoid Metformin

Metformin should not be used in patients with active congestive heart failure, significant liver disease, or in patients with renal insufficiency. It should also be used cautiously in patients over the age of 80 years. If a patient has had surgery or a radiological procedure that used contrast dye, the metformin should be withheld for 48 hours to ensure adequate urine flow. It is customary to recheck the patients' blood creatinine level 48 hours after the procedure.

One rare and very serious adverse effect of metformin is lactic acidosis. This is fatal in up to half of the patients who develop it. It is almost always seen in patients who have liver or kidney disease and in those who should not have been taking metformin.

microalbuminuria   Minute amounts of albumin found in the urine and which may be early indicators of DIABETIC NEPHROPATHY (kidney disease) or even atherosclerosis. If a standard urine dipstick is negative, the patient with diabetes should be tested for microalbuminuria. This can be done in the office with a color-coded dipstick or it can be sent to a lab for a more precise radioimmunoassay measurement.

Microalbuminuria is defined as 30–300 mg of albumin per g of creatinine, as measured in a spot urine sample. Less than 30 is normal and greater than 300 is overt albuminuria/proteinuria.

Poor glycemic control, fever, and exercise can cause transient increases in albumin excretion. Generally, the level is determined two to three times before committing a patient to therapy. Generally an ACE inhibitor drug is prescribed, even if the patient has normal blood pressure.

In patients with Type 1 diabetes, microalbuminuria is an indication of early kidney damage, even within the first five years of diagnosis. In patients with Type 2 diabetes, microalbuminuria is also predictive of progression to overt proteinuria. In addition, for Type 2 patients, microalbuminuria is also a risk for the development of early cardiovascular disease.

The microalbuminuria syndrome has been associated with hypertension, abnormal lipid profiles, insulin resistance, an increased prevalence of "silent killer" heart disease, diabetic neuropathy, and peripheral vascular disease, as well as a variety of clotting and cellular abnormalities.

M. B. Mattock et al., "Prospective Study of Microalbuminuria as a Predictor of Mortality in NIDDM," *Diabetes* 41 (1992): 736.

J. Messent et al., "Prognostic Significance of Microalbuminuria in Insulin-Dependent Diabetes: A Twenty-three Year Followup Study," *Kidney International* 41 (1992): 836.

myocardial infarction   Refers to the death of the myocardial cells (the muscle cells) of the heart and usually associated with ATHEROSCLEROSIS; also known as a heart attack. Myocardial infarction, along with angina (chest pain) is a problem experienced by people with CORONARY HEART DISEASE (CHD). Patients with long-term diabetes are more prone to myocardial infarctions and other manifestations of cardiac diseases. A heart attack is a life and death emergency and an ambulance should be called immediately for a person exhibiting symptoms of a heart attack.

According to the American Heart Association (AHA), the following symptoms are the most common warning signs of a heart attack:

- an uncomfortable pressure, fullness, squeezing, or pain in the center of the chest that lasts longer than a few minutes
- Pain that spreads to the shoulders, neck, or arms
- Chest discomfort that is accompanied by lightheadedness, fainting, sweating, nausea, or shortness of breath

The AHA says that there are also some less common indicators of a heart attack, such as:

- unusual pain in the chest, stomach, or abdomen
- nausea or dizziness
- difficulty with breathing or shortness of breath
- heart palpitations

- a cold sweat or paleness
- unexplained anxiety, fatigue, or weakness

(See also COMPLICATIONS, CARDIOVASCULAR DIS-EASE.)

nateglinide   See PHENYLALINE DERIVATIVES.

National Diabetes Eye Examination Program

A program launched in 2001 in the United States by the Foundation of the American Academy of Ophthalmology (FAAO) and the American Optometric Association (AOA), in conjunction with the Centers for Medicare and Medicaid Services (CMS), formerly the Health Care Financing Administration (HCFA). The CMS is an organization that administers the payment aspect of the MEDICARE program.

Many people with diabetes and especially older Americans with diabetes fail to obtain dilated-eye examinations. This failure to be examined on at least a yearly basis to detect the many eye problems that may lead to visual loss and BLINDNESS (such as DIABETIC RETINOPATHY, CATARACTS, MACULAR EDEMA/DEGENERATION and GLAUCOMA) is a tragedy and quite costly to society. Earlier diagnosis will lead to earlier treatment and preservation of vision.

To increase the number of people over age 65 with diabetes who receive dilated-eye examinations and treatment based on those exams, the National Diabetes Eye Examination Program was created. It helps patients find participating eye professionals who will perform the needed eye exam coverage at no cost to MEDICARE patients over age 65 who have diabetes and have not had a dilated eye examination for three or more years. If eye illnesses are discovered during the examination, the patient may receive up to one year of treatment from a participating OPHTHALMOLOGIST, at no cost to the patient.

According to the Foundation of the American Academy of Ophthalmologists, 7,400 doctors have signed up for the program and over 16,000 seniors were referred to receive free eye examinations by March 2001. For further information and to locate a participating ophthalmologist, call the 24-hour toll-free number: (800) 222-3937. To locate a participating optometrist, call the American Optometric Association's Diabetes Hot Line between 7 A.M. and 7 P.M. central time, at (800) 262-3947.

National Diabetes Information Clearinghouse (NDIC)

Under the direction of the National Institute of Diabetes and Digestive and Kidney Diseases (NIDDK), the National Institutes of Health, the National Diabetes Information Clearinghouse provides information and education for professionals and the general public. Information is either free or at low cost.

NDIC
1 Information Way
Bethesda, MD 20892-3560
(301) 654-3327
www.niddk.nih.gov/health/diabetes/ndic.htm

National Institute of Diabetes and Digestive and Kidney Diseases (NIDDK)

Established in 1950 by Congress as an adjunct to one of the National Institutes of Health (NIH). The NIDDK performs research and provides information on diabetes and digestive and kidney ailments. It is the lead agency for diabetes research at the NIH.

The NIDDK also supports 12 Diabetes Research Centers, including six Diabetes and

Endocrinology Research Centers (DERCs) and six Diabetes Research and Training Centers (DRTCs) and funds extremely important clinical trials. For example, the Diabetes Control and Complications Trial (DCCT), a massive 10-year study of over 1,400 patients in 27 research centers, was an NIDDK project. This study definitively proved the importance and efficacy of tight GLYCEMIC CONTROL in preventing or delaying complications from diabetes.

For further information, contact the NIDDK at:

National Institute of Diabetes and Digestive and
  Kidney Diseases
National Institutes of Health
Building 31, Room 9A04
31 Center Drive, MSC 2560
Bethesda, MD 20892-2560
(301) 496-3583
www.niddk.nih.gov

National Institutes of Health (NIH) Based in Bethesda, Maryland, the National Institutes of Health is a major federal government agency in the United States, and one of eight health agencies within the U.S. Department of Health and Human Services. It is this agency that contracts for (or itself performs) major health studies. The NIH was the agency that administered the DIABETES CONTROL AND COMPLICATIONS TRIAL (DCCT), a very important 10-year study of subjects with Type 1 diabetes that definitively proved that tight GLYCEMIC CONTROL can limit complications stemming from diabetes.

Within the NIH are other agencies that are important to people with diabetes and others interested in the disease, for example, the NATIONAL INSTITUTE OF DIABETES AND DIGESTIVE AND KIDNEY DISEASES (NIDDK).

nephrologist Medical doctor who specializes in treating diseases of the kidneys, such as DIABETIC NEPHROPATHY and END-STAGE RENAL DISEASE (ESRD). Nephrologists generally train for three years in internal medicine and then an additional two to three years in a nephrology fellowship.

When patients with diabetes have a creatinine level of 1.8 mg/dL or greater, then a nephrology consultation should be considered. Nephrologists also evaluate structural problems of the kidneys and bladder. (Patients with kidney and bladder problems may also see a urologist.)

The nephrologist also treats patients with a PROTEINURIA level that is greater than 1,000 mg or 1 g per day, or one that has changed rapidly. In addition, they treat patients with hard to control blood pressure and other unexplained abnormalities seen on urinalysis (red blood cells, casts, and other findings).

nephropathy See DIABETIC NEPHROPATHY.

nephrotic syndrome A kidney disorder that is often caused by DIABETIC NEPHROPATHY. It is marked by damage to the glomeruli of the kidneys. These are blood vessels that filter waste and extra water from the blood and transport them to the kidney in the form of urine.

Key characteristics of nephrotic syndrome are:

- high levels of protein in the urine (PROTEINURIA) that exceed 3.5 grams
- swelling of the body, especially around the feet, hands, and eyes
- high levels of cholesterol

The treatment for nephrotic syndrome depends on the cause. If the main problem is high blood pressure, then the physician will work with the patient to control HYPERTENSION. If there is a possibility of glomerulonephritis, then a kidney biopsy is usually needed and the patient may also require immunosuppressive therapy. All patients with this syndrome should be referred to a NEPHROLOGIST.

For more information, contact the following organizations:

American Kidney Fund
6110 Executive Boulevard
Rockville, MD 20852
(800) 638-8299

National Heart, Lung, and Blood Institute
Information Center
P.O. Box 30105
Bethesda, MD 20824-0105
(301) 592-8573

National Kidney Foundation
30 East 33rd Street
New York, NY 10016
(800) 622-9010

nerve conduction velocity   A clinical study of the speed of a nerve function. This test may determine if a person is in the early stages of the nerve damage of DIABETIC NEUROPATHY. Unfortunately, it is better at measuring large nerve fibers that conduct motor impulses and thus, nerve conduction velocities may be normal in the early phases of sensory neuropathy.

neurogenic bladder   Refers to a bladder that does not empty properly and is prone to infections and to CYSTITIS. Such problems are most common among people with diabetes and often stem from DIABETIC NEUROPATHY. (See also BLADDER PROBLEMS.)

neurologist   Physician who treats disorders of the nervous system. A person with diabetes may need to see a neurologist because of problems with DIABETIC NEUROPATHY, as well as other problems of the nervous system, such as STROKE, seizures, DEMENTIA, or headache.

Neurontin (gabapentin)   An antiseizure medication that is also used to treat people with DIABETIC NEUROPATHY because it can alleviate neuropathic pain symptoms. The exact mechanism of the medicine is unknown. If the medication is started at lower doses, it is generally well tolerated. The patient may eventually need 3,000 to 7,000 mg a day to relieve pain symptoms. Neurontin can cause some side effects, such as sleepiness, fatigue, dizziness, and irritability. It has been studied for its use in treating seizures.

M. Backonja et al. "Gabapentin for the Symptomatic Treatment of Painful Diabetic Neuropathy in Patients with Diabetes Mellitus: A Random Controlled Trial," *JAMA* 280 (1998): 1831–1836.

neuropathy   See DIABETIC NEUROPATHY.

nocturnal hypoglycemia   Low blood glucose experienced at night, especially while an individual with diabetes is asleep. Nearly 50 percent of severe hypoglycemia occurs when patients are asleep and thus, their response to it is much slower. Testing blood glucose levels at bedtime is critically important.

People with Type 1 diabetes need to be vigilant about their food intake and blood glucose levels and to be especially watchful that they work to avoid a lapse into hypoglycemia while asleep. To avert such a problem, most people with Type 1 diabetes are advised to eat a small snack before bedtime, especially if the glucose level is less than 140 mg/dL. Milk and crackers is one commonly recommended snack.

Working with their physicians and registered dietitians, people with nocturnal hypoglycemia may adjust the timing and dosage of their insulins to avoid HYPOGLYCEMIA. If the nocturnal hypoglycemia is recurrent, the use of the continuous glucose monitor may be helpful.

non-insulin-dependent diabetes mellitus (NIDDM)   The former name for what is now called Type 2 diabetes. This name was changed because it was misleading. Many people with Type 2 diabetes do not require insulin injections and may manage their diabetes with medication, diet, and exercise. However, as most people with Type 2 diabetes age, and their pancreas secretes less insulin, most will eventually require insulin therapy.

non-invasive monitor/testing   A device that can measure blood glucose levels without pricking the skin and drawing blood. Because most people don't like to prick their fingers with a sharp instrument (LANCET), they may fail to test their blood glucose level as frequently as their doctor recommends (or they may fail to test their blood at all). For this reason, researchers have been working on noninvasive and non-painful methods to attain the same information about glucose levels. For example, some devices can extract blood from the forearm or other body parts where nerve endings are less sensitive than the finger. The Glucowatch, developed by Cygnus Therapeutics, can actually test blood through the skin using special sensors. It was on the market in 2002 in the United States. Other researchers are working with infrared technologies to measure glucose levels. (See also BLOODLESS TESTING.)

nursing homes   See SKILLED NURSING FACILITIES.

nutrition   Intake of food. People with both Type 1 and Type 2 diabetes need to pay attention to eating a healthy and balanced diet, while at the same time maintaining good GLYCEMIC CON-TROL through regular blood testing and acting on the results of the test. One problem is that the average American, including people with and without diabetes, does not eat the recommended five or more servings of fruits and vegetables per day. According to the Centers for Disease Control and Prevention (CDC), poor nutrition and also lack of regular exercise is responsible for an estimated 300,000 deaths in the United States per year, second only to smoking as a cause of death.

Rates of good nutrition vary from state to state. Of those adults not eating recommended amounts of fruits and vegetables, Arizona is the worst, at 91 percent of all adults. Although still not eating sufficient levels of fruits and vegetables, Minnesota scores the best, at 68 percent of adults who fail to maintain good nutritional habits.

Portion control is a critical aspect of nutrition for patients with diabetes. Many patients initially need to weigh and measure foods in order to learn how to accurately estimate their portions. (See also CARBOHYDRATE COUNTING, DIETITIAN.)

American Diabetes Association, Position Statement: Nutrition Recommendations and Principles for People with Diabetes Mellitus," *Diabetes Care* 24, Supp. 1 (2001): 544–547.

Marie Karlsen et al., "Efficacy of Medical Nutrition Therapy: Are Your Patients Getting What They Need?," *Clinical Diabetes* 14, no. 4 (May–June 1996): 54–61.

obesity Excessive body fat for an individual's height and build. An estimated 20 percent of all adult Americans are obese according to the guidelines of the National Heart, Lung, and Blood Institute of the National Institutes of Health. About 80 percent of individuals with Type 2 diabetes are obese.

Usually a chronic disease, obesity can become very dangerous because it may lead to Type 2 diabetes as well as to a variety of other medical problems, such as heart disease, gallbladder disease, and even cancer. Obesity causes INSULIN RESISTANCE which can progress to diabetes. Weight loss can reduce the risk for developing Type 2 diabetes.

Obesity is rarely found among people with Type 1 diabetes, although insulin may cause some people to become overweight. Some medications for people with Type 2 diabetes may also cause an increase in weight.

Obesity is linked to many other serious illnesses, such as HYPERTENSION, DYSLIPIDEMIA, CORONARY HEART DISEASE, and STROKE. When an individual loses weight, often other medical problems improve, such as hypertension or dyslipidemia. In some cases, a person with an early case of Type 2 diabetes may revert to normal if sufficient weight is lost.

An Epidemic in the United States and Other Developed Countries

The NATIONAL INSTITUTES OF HEALTH and many experts are concerned that obesity is at an epidemic level in the United States and other developed countries such as the United Kingdom and Australia. Obesity has also been found to be a sig-nificant factor in congenital defects among infants when their mothers were both obese and had diabetes. Women who are both diabetic and obese have a greatly increased risk of bearing a child with a serious birth defect. (See PREGNANCY.)

In the United States the CENTERS FOR DISEASE CONTROL AND PREVENTION (CDC) said that in 1998, 55 percent of all Americans were overweight with a BODY MASS INDEX or BMI equal or greater than 30. The prevalence of overweight individuals varied from state to state; for example, from a low of 48 percent of overweight people in Hawaii to a high of 60 percent in both Alabama and Minnesota.

It is possible for people who are not overweight in terms of their total pounds to be obese because of a high percentage of body fat. This condition, however, is not the norm. Instead, most people who are obese have excessive weight as well as excessive amounts of fat deposits.

Most experts believe that obesity is a function of both genetic influences and environmental impacts. Much of the dramatic increase in obesity in the latter part of the 20th century has been attributed to overeating combined with a sedentary lifestyle.

In children and adolescents, obesity commonly leads to psychosocial effects, hyperlipidema, abnormal glucose metabolism, early puberty, asthma, and POLYCYSTIC OVARIAN SYNDROME (PCOS). One indicator of the problem is that for adolescents, daily participation in physical education in high school has declined. According to information presented at the 61st American Diabetes Association annual conference in 2001 by Dr. William Dietz and Dr. Jack Yanovski, their research revealed that for boys, participation in physical education declined by 13 percent over an eight-year period: from 45 percent in 1991 to 32 percent in 1999. The rate of participation declined 12 percent for girls, from 37 percent in 1991 to 25 percent in 1999.

At the same meeting, Dr. Giammattei presented data on the relationship of BMI with hours of television viewing. His study of boys and girls in the sixth and seventh grades in Santa Barbara County, California revealed a direct correlation: the more TV the children watched, the more body fat they had. Among the children who watched television fewer than two hours per week, 28 percent were overweight and 12 percent were obese. Among children who watched television more than two hours a week, 52 percent were overweight and 28 percent were obese.

Rise in Incidence of Obesity

Obesity is a worsening problem in the United States and other developed countries. Researchers performing a nationwide telephone survey found that the incidence of Type 2 diabetes had increased by 33 percent in 43 states in the United States from 1990 to 1998. They reported these findings in a 2000 issue of *Diabetes Care.* Increases were particularly high among younger individuals; for example, among respondents ages 30–39, the rate of diabetes increased by 76 percent.

The rise in obesity was found in all races; for example, the obesity rate among Hispanics increased by 38 percent, the rate among whites rose by 29 percent, and the rate for African Americans increased by 26 percent.

The authors said,

When an increase of 33% in diabetes in just 8 years is considered with the disturbing reality that the effects of the obesity epidemic have not fully unfolded, an alarming scenario indeed unfolds. Regardless of whether this increase relates partly to an increased awareness of diabetes, it is clear that the need for diabetes care will rise dramatically in the future.

Scandinavians and obesity Americans are not the only people with an obesity problem that often leads to diabetes: a study of Norwegian adults, reported in a 1999 issue of *Diabetes Care,* revealed that Norwegians and residents of other Scandinavian countries have become increasingly overweight and also prone to developing Type 2 diabetes.

Norwegian researchers compared the results of two studies, one encompassing subjects studied during the period 1984 to 1986 and another study that ran from 1995 to 1997. They found that the prevalence of obesity among men doubled by the time of the second study, among both diabetic and nondiabetic populations. The researchers were particularly concerned about a rise in obesity and the increased incidence of diabetes among younger subjects, ages 40–42 years.

Adipose fat Researchers have also found that excessive fat sited around the waistline is more predictive of diabetes, coronary artery disease, and other ailments than is fat located in the hips or lower body. Stated very simply, individuals with an "apple" body shape are at greater risk for diabetes than are those with a "pear" body shape. This issue was also discussed in a 2000 issue of *Diabetes,* entitled "The Perils of Portliness."

Defining Obesity: The Body Mass Index

The federal government in the United States uses a term called Body Mass Index (BMI) to denote both overweight and obesity, which is a more extreme problem than "overweight." BMI is a gender-neutral term, which takes into account weight and height.

Causes of Obesity

It would seem obvious that the cause of obesity is that an individual takes in more calories than he expends, thereby increasing stored food. However, it is not a simple problem for people who are obese. Some obese people insist that they eat no more than others, and in some cases, this is verifiable. Many people may have the "thrifty gene," wherein their body works to keep them at a stable weight. As they eat less, their bodies adjust to use the food more efficiently and maintain their weight. Thus, some people need to severely limit their calories in order to lose weight.

In some rare cases, the obese individual may have an underlying medical problem such as a THYROID DISEASE. Hypothyroidism is a common problem but it rarely causes obesity.

Scientists in 2000 discovered that some types of obesity appear to be caused by factors other than mere overeating and under-exercising. Apparently there are brain pathways that control the appetite "thermostat," and which can go awry, possibly because of a malfunction that triggers a genetic predisposition. Scientists have also linked the substance LEPTIN to predispositions to obesity and overweight. If leptin is adjusted in rats, the rats become thinner or fatter.

Scientists in 2001 also found a hormone called Resistin that may be linked to both obesity and the development of Type 2 diabetes. Further study is ongoing.

Genetic factors   In April 2000, a British firm, Gemini Genomics, reported that, in collaboration with Kyowa Hakko Kogyo Co., Ltd., a Japanese pharmaceutical company, they discovered a unique gene linked to both obesity and diabetes. This discovery, as well as other ongoing research, may lead to treatments or GENETIC MANIPULATION that could eventually result in curing obesity and/or diabetes.

Treating Obesity

Thousands of books and magazine articles have been written for people who need to lose weight, but for most people, the basic answer still appears to be to increase activity levels and decrease the total amount of calories that are consumed. Others require more in-depth solutions. Some people who are 100 pounds or more overweight have bariatric surgery, which is surgery that limits the amount of food their stomachs can process. It is considered for people with a BMI of over 40 or people with a BMI that is over 35 who also have concurrent medical problems.

Some individuals have had success with medications for weight loss, although some past weight loss medications such as Redux were found to be dangerous and were ordered by the Food and Drug Administration (FDA) to be removed from the market. Newer medications are Xenical (orlistat) and Meridia (sibutramine), both approved by the FDA.

Exercise is an important remedy for weight loss; however, people with diabetes need to test their glucose levels before and after very active physical activity in order to avoid a problem with HYPOGLYCEMIA. Experts say that exercise need not be difficult or even especially strenuous; for example, walking for 20 minutes a day can make a difference in weight as well as in the health of the individual.

For further information, contact:

Weight-control Information Network (WIN)
1 WIN Way
Bethesda, MD 20892
(800) WIN-8098 or (301) 984-7378
www.niddk.nih.gov/health/nutrit/win.htm

(See also EXERCISE, LEPTIN, MEDICATION.)

George A. Bray, M.D., "Physiology and Consequences of Obesity," Medscape Continuing Medical Education (CME), December 2000.

Kathryn S. Bryden, R.N., "Eating Habits, Body Weight, and Insulin Misuse," *Diabetes Care* 22, no. 12 (December 1999): 1956–1960.

Dana K. Cassell and David H. Gleaves, Ph.D., *The Encyclopedia of Obesity and Eating Disorders* (New York: Facts On File, Inc., 2000).

David N. Leff, "Many Are Fat But Few Are Diabetic: Analyzed by DNA Chips, Genes in Adipose Cells Aim to Predict Diabetes Onset Well in Advance," *BIOWORLD Today* (October 18, 2000).

Ali H. Mokdad, Ph.D., et al., "Diabetes Trends in the U.S.: 1990–1998," *Diabetes Care* 23, no. 9 (September 2000): 1278–1283.

Carl T. Montague, "The Perils of Portliness: Causes and Consequences of Visceral Adiposity," *Diabetes* 49, no. 6 (2000): 883–888.

Ardre J. Scheen, M.D., Ph.D., and Pierre J. Lefebvre, M.D., Ph.D., F.R.C.P., M.A.E., "Management of the Obese Diabetic Patient," from *Diabetes Reviews* 7, no. 2, 1999, in *Annual Review of Diabetes 2000* (Alexandria, Va.: American Diabetes Association, 2000).

onset of diabetes   Some individuals may be diagnosed with diabetes as children (as with Type 1 diabetes, although the illness may not be diagnosed until adolescence or adulthood), while others are not diagnosed until they are adults or even elderly individuals. In general, when the individual has Type 1 diabetes, the onset is usually sudden and severe, and it is clear that the person is very ill. Often there has been considerable weight loss and other apparent symptoms.

In contrast, when adults (and some children and adolescents) are diagnosed with Type 2 diabetes, they may have no symptoms for years until they exhibit such symptoms as extreme thirst, excessive urination, and other classic symptoms of diabetes.

Unfortunately, damage may have already occurred prior to the time of diagnosis.

ophthalmologist   A surgical doctor who specializes in diagnosing and treating diseases of the eye both medically and surgically, such as CATARACTS, GLAUCOMA, MACULAR EDEMA, or DIABETIC RETINOPATHY.

Many experts believe that eye exams should begin within five years for patients with Type 1 diabetes. Patients with Type 2 diabetes should be examined shortly after diagnosis. It's best to have a dilated eye examination, in which the doctor inserts special eye drops that enlarge the pupils of the eyes so that the doctor can see the entire retina. Patients often will need to wear sunglasses home after such an exam because their dilated eye will be extremely sensitive to light. They may prefer to have someone drive them home.

Children who have been diagnosed with Type 1 diabetes should receive regular eye exams within five years after diagnosis. Children with Type 2 diabetes may need screening exams sooner because they may have metabolic abnormalities that precede the diagnosis of their diabetes.

Interestingly, it is quite rare for children with Type 1 diabetes to develop any complications prior to puberty even with poor glycemic control (other than a possible delayed growth and/or feeling ill).

For further information, contact the following organizations:

American Academy of Ophthalmology
655 Beach Street
San Francisco, CA 94109-7424
(415) 561-8500
www.eyenet.org

National Eye Institute
P.O. Box 20/20
Bethesda, MD 20892-3655
(301) 496-5248
www.nei.nih.gov

(See also BLINDNESS, BLURRED VISION, CATARACT, DIABETIC RETINOPATHY, EYE DISEASE, GLAUCOMA.)

optometrist   An eye professional who is specially trained to determine whether or not people need glasses or contact lenses, and to detect eye diseases such as GLAUCOMA or DIABETIC RETINOPATHY. The optometrist is not a medical doctor but is aware of the risks and problems that diabetes can bring. Anyone who has diabetes should be sure to alert the optometrist to this condition at the time of an eye examination.

For more information, contact:

American Optometric Association
243 North Lindbergh Boulevard
St. Louis, MO 63141
(314) 991-4100
www.aoanet.org

oral glucose tolerance test (OGTT)   A test to determine if a person has diabetes. After fasting for eight to 14 hours, plasma glucose levels are measured and levels are taken again about one or two hours later and after the individual ingests 75 g of glucose provided by the person administering the test. An alternative test is the FASTING PLASMA GLUCOSE (FPG) test.

Extending the test to three, four, or five hours is not necessary. In fact, a large number of people with normal glucose metabolism will become hypoglycemic between the third and fifth hour. Thus, the OGTT should *never* be used to diagnose hypoglycemia.

Generally, urine measurement of the level of glucose provides no significant extra information.

	Fasting Glucose	2-Hour Glucose
Normal	Less than 110 mg/dL	Less than 140 mg/dL
Impaired Fasting Glucose	110–125 mg/dL	140–199 mg/dL
Diabetes	≥126 mg/dL	>200 mg/dL

oral hypoglycemic agent (OHA) A category of oral medications used to decrease blood glucose levels by causing the pancreas to release more insulin. Also known as insulin secretagogues. Drugs in the following classes are secretagogues: sulfonylureas, meglitinides, and phenylalanine derivatives. (See appendix for medication data.) (See also MEDICATIONS, MEGLITINIDES, PHENYLALA-NINE DERIVATIVES, SULFONYLUREAS.)

oral medications Drugs that need not be injected but can be consumed by mouth. Often people who are diagnosed with Type 2 diabetes do not need insulin but may instead use oral agents to lower their glucose levels. It is also true, however, that sometimes people who have had Type 2 diabetes for many years may need supplemental insulin. Regular testing and periodic physical examinations and laboratory tests will enable the physician and patient to make decisions about medications to help control diabetes.

There are currently four general classes of oral medications: the insulin secretagogues (sulfonylureas, meglitinides, and phenylalanine derivatives), biguanides (metformin), alpha glucosidase inhibitors (miglitol, acarbose) and thiazolidinediones (TZDs, such as rosiglitazone and pioglitazone).

(See also MEDICATIONS, MEDICATION ADHERENCE/COMPLIANCE, MEDICATION INTERACTIONS.)

orthostatic hypotension Refers to a decrease in blood pressure that may occur when the afflicted person changes position, for example from lying down to sitting, from sitting to standing or from lying down to standing. The result may be fainting (syncope).

Individuals with diabetes are at greater risk for orthostatic hypotension than are nondiabetics, primarily because they are more likely to have autonomic DIABETIC NEUROPATHY and are also more susceptible to DEHYDRATION. Other risk factors for experiencing orthostatic hypotension are:

- Medications
- Atherosclerosis
- Prolonged bed rest

Symptoms of orthostatic hypotension are dizziness or lightheadedness, as well as blurred vision. The person may also feel off-balance or experience vertigo.

Treatment depends on the cause of the orthostatic hypotension; for example, if the physician believes a medication is the cause, he may change the dosage or prescribe another medicine. If the problem is dehydration, the patients receives fluids and salts intravenously and, when discharged from the hospital or emergency room, will be encouraged to consume copious quantities of fluids.

Sometimes medications are used, such as flurinef, a synthetic steroid that helps the body retain both salt and water and also helps to constrict the blood vessels. Alpha agonists such as midodrine (Proamatine) may also be used to constrict the blood vessels. In addition, patients are counseled to move slowly from a lying down position to a sitting position, and then to a standing position.

orthotics   Custom-made inserts for shoes, often for a person with diabetes who suffers from DIABETIC NEUROPATHY and has little or no feeling in the feet. The MEDICARE THERAPEUTIC SHOE ACT (1993) provided for Medicare coverage (at the 80 percent rate) for people with diabetes and other serious and related problems, and who need specially made protective footwear. Many people who are eligible for such therapeutic shoes have not taken advantage of this option.

Made-to-order shoes are created by a pedorthist, who should be familiar with the U.S. Medicare requirements for payment. (See also SHOES, THERAPEUTIC.)

osteoporosis   A medical condition in which not only is total bone mass decreased but there are also microarchitectural abnormalities in the bones that lead to an increased risk for fractures. People with diabetes have a slightly increased risk for developing osteoporosis compared to nondiabetics.

About 80 percent of those with osteoporosis are female. The hip fractures that osteoporosis can cause are especially dangerous and about 20 percent of these patients die within a year and 50 percent lose their independence.

Anyone can have osteoporosis although people with Type 1 diabetes have a slightly greater risk for developing this problem. Often still thought of as a disease of the elderly, the reality is that osteoporosis can occur in middle-aged or younger people. Some experts have expressed concern, however, that osteoporosis among men has been virtually ignored as an issue.

According to the National Institute of Arthritis and Musculoskeletal and Skin Diseases, 10 million people in the United States have osteoporosis. Eighteen million more experience decreased bone mass and they are at risk for osteoporosis. The disease causes 1.5 million fractures per year in the United States, including about 300,000 hip fractures, 700,000 spinal fractures, 250,000 wrist fractures, and 300,000 fractures found elsewhere in the body.

Causes of Osteoporosis

Aging is clearly one factor in the development of osteoporosis, although middle-aged and younger people can develop osteoporosis. The disease may also be due to a genetic predisposition. For example, according to the National Institutes of Health, one study showed that women age 65 and older who had the apolipoprotein E gene on chromosome 19 had twice the risk of those without the gene to experience fractures of the hip and wrist. The loss of naturally occurring sex steroid hormones, such as estrogen in women and testosterone in men, play a pivotal role in the development of osteoporosis.

Lifestyle factors clearly play a role and less active people are more likely to develop osteoporosis.

Secondary causes of osteoporosis   A study of 56 patients with Type 1 diabetes, 68 patients with Type 2 diabetes and 498 nondiabetic control subjects, reported in a 1999 issue of *Diabetes Care*, revealed that those with Type 1 diabetes faced a significantly greater risk for osteoporosis, unexplained by insulin treatment or other factors. Other secondary causes of osteoporosis include anorexia nervosa, ACROMEGALY, alcoholism, steroid use, malnutrition, primary hyperparathyroidism, and hypogonadism.

Risk Factors

According to the National Resource Center for Osteoporosis and Related Bone Diseases, a subsection of the National Institutes of Health, the key risk factors for developing osteoporosis are:

- gender (females are at greater risk)
- thin or small-boned stature
- age (risk increases with age)
- a family history of osteoporosis

- postmenopausal status
- eating disorders such as anorexia nervosa or bulimia
- diets low in calcium
- medications such as corticosteroids and anti-convulsants
- inactive life
- smoking cigarettes
- race (greatest risks are for Caucasians or Asians)

Diagnosis and Treatment

The doctor may strongly suspect a patient has osteoporosis because of a fracture from a minor fall or because he or she has risk factors for the disease. The only way to know for sure if the patient has osteoporosis is to run tests and most doctors order bone mass density tests. In most cases, the dual-energy X-ray absorptiometry (DXA) is used to measure bone density, although other tests are available.

Medications are usually the treatment for osteoporosis. Many doctors prescribe estrogen for postmenopausal women, although studies indicate estrogen may serve better as a prevention from osteoporosis rather than a treatment for the disease after it is known to occur. All patients should be on adequate calcium and vitamin D, 1000–1500 mg/day and 400–800 IU respectively. Other drugs that are prescribed are:

- Fosamax (alendronate) if the osteoporosis was drug-induced by taking glucocorticoid medications
- Actonel (risedronate)

- Evista (raloxifene)
- Miacalcin (calcitonin)

Other treatments under investigation are vitamin D metabolites, sodium fluoride, and injectable parathyroid hormone, which may become available in 2002.

For more information, contact:

National Institutes of Health
Osteoporosis and Related Bone
  Diseases—National Resource Center
1232 22nd Street, NW
Suite 500
Washington, DC 20037-1292
(202) 223-0344 or (800) 624-BONE
www.osteo.org

National Osteoporosis Foundation
1150 17th Street, NW
Suite 500
Washington, DC 20036-4603
(202) 223-2226
www.nof.org

(See also ELDERLY, HORMONE REPLACEMENT THERAPY, MENOPAUSE.)

Cheryl L. Lambing, M.D., "Osteoporosis Prevention, Detection, and Treatment: A Mandate for Primary Care Physicians," *Postgraduate Medicine* 107, no. 7 (June 2000): 37–41, 47–48.

Kelly A. McGarry, M.D., et al., "Postmenopausal Osteoporosis: Strategy for Preventive Bone Loss, Avoiding Fracture," *Postgraduate Medicine* 108, no. 3 (Sept 2000): 79–82, 85–88, 91.

Jussi T. Tumoninen et al., "Bone Mineral Density in Patients with Type 1 and Type 2 Diabetes," *Diabetes Care* 22, no. 7 (July 1999): 1196–1200.

Pacific Islanders   See ASIANS/PACIFIC ISLANDERS. See also RACE/ETHNICITY.

pain   Moderate or severe discomfort. When patients have diabetes, their pain from the disease most commonly stems from DIABETIC NEUROPATHY. This pain is usually treated with analgesics such as aspirin or acetaminophen and more serious pain may be treated with prescribed analgesic medications or even narcotics.

Sometimes physicians prescribe tricyclic antidepressants (TCAs) for the pain of neuropathy and other chronic pain. In the book *Pain: What Psychiatrists Need to Know*, physician Augusto Caraceni and colleagues describe studies in which patients who were depressed and in pain were compared to nondepressed patients who had pain. Both groups were given tricyclic antidepressants. The results revealed that TCAs were successful at decreasing pain for both groups, although it is not entirely clear how the medications worked. Imipramine is one form of TCA that has been shown to be successful at reducing the pain of diabetic neuropathy. Currently, Elavil (amitriptyline) and Pamelor (nortriptyline) are most commonly used.

In addition, drugs in the adrenergic agonist class, such as Catapres (clonidine) and tizanidine have also proven effective at decreasing pain from diabetic neuropathy and other forms of chronic pain.

An antiseizure drug, NEURONTIN, is also frequently used for pain. Tegretol (carbamazepine) is another antiseizure medication that is often tried when a person has lightning-like pain.

Sometimes it is the absence of pain rather than its presence that presents a problem to the person with diabetes; for example, if neuropathy is advanced, then when part of the body is injured, there is no pain. The person with diabetes is particularly at risk for harming the foot and should be vigilant about FOOT CARE. If an unnoticed infection continues, the person may suffer from GANGRENE and may require an AMPUTATION of a limb.

Augusto Caraceni, M.D., et al., "Pain Management: Pharmacological and Nonpharmacological Treatments," in *Pain: What Psychiatrists Need to Know* (Washington, D.C.: American Psychiatric Press, 2000).

pancreas   A vital digestive organ that is located in the mid-posterior abdomen, behind the stomach. Malfunction of the beta cells in the pancreas leads to diabetes.

The pancreas is an endocrine (it secretes hormones) gland as well an exocrine (secretes digestive enzymes) organ. It secretes insulin, glucagon, somatostatin, and a variety of other hormones. The enzymes it makes include lipase and amylase.

Individuals cannot survive without a pancreas, although it is possible to have a TRANSPLANT of a donor pancreas. In the case of people with Type 1 diabetes, their pancreas fails to produce insulin. As a result, they must self-inject insulin in order to live. However, people with Type 1 diabetes have some normal endocrine function.

It is the pancreas that contains the BETA CELLS, and those cells produce the much-needed

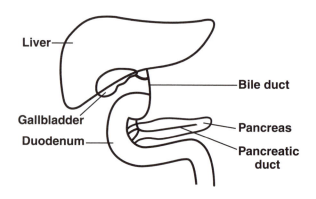

insulin. The alpha cells in the pancreas control the release of GLUCAGON into the blood. The delta cells make a substance called somatostatin. There are also other pancreatic functions about which little is known, although research continues.

As can be seen from the drawing, the pancreas is in close proximity to the liver and the gall bladder. Pancreatitis is an inflammation of the pancreas that can be caused by gallstones, alcohol, or very high triglyceride levels.

pediatric endocrinologist   A pediatric medical doctor who specializes in treating endocrine disorders (diabetes, thyroid diseases, growth problems, abnormal puberty, and others) that are suffered by children and adolescents. Pediatric endocrinologists usually train for three years in pediatrics and then an additional two to three years in endocrinology. They will generally treat children until the children are in their late teen years and sometimes into their early 20s, at which time most then switch to an adult endocrinologist who has had training in internal medicine.

There are very few pediatric endocrinologists nationwide and many of them have full-time academic appointments at medical schools. When treating children with diabetes, the pediatric endocrinologist usually works with a diabetes team (registered nurse, registered dietitian, social worker, etc.) to care for children with dia-

betes. (See also ADOLESCENTS, CHILDREN, INFANTS, ENDOCRINOLOGIST.)

pen devices   See INSULIN PEN.

periodontal disease   Bacterial infections that cause inflammation and, if untreated, result in destruction of the soft tissues and bone that surround the teeth and gums. As a result of this damage, the teeth are not held as firmly and the disease can lead to the loss of teeth. People with diabetes are at greater risk for developing periodontal disease than nondiabetics.

According to the National Institutes of Health, about 22 percent of adults who are ages 35–44 have periodontitis, an advanced gum disease. GINGIVITIS, an inflammation and infection of the gums, is an early stage of periodontal disease that always comes before periodontitis. If treated, gingivitis usually will not get any worse. Some very controversial research indicates that the bacterium that is linked to periodontal disease may be associated with a greater risk for HEART DISEASE and STROKE.

Symptoms of Periodontitis

There are often no symptoms at all until the periodontal disease is advanced. (Periodontal disease can be detected in a dental examination, which is a key reason why people with diabetes should have dental checkups twice a year or more frequently, if the dentist recommends it.) At that point, the individual will feel pain and loosening of at least some of the teeth. The patient will need the services of a periodontist and may also need surgery as well. Regular brushing of the teeth and flossing will no longer be sufficient, as it would have been when the disease was gingivitis.

Diabetes and Periodontitis

Periodontal disease is a frequent problem among people with diabetes, many of whom fail to see a dentist even annually, although they are at greater risk for gum and tooth disease than nondiabetics. Unfortunately, research has revealed that many individuals with diabetes are apparently unaware of the importance of regular dental visits. Dentists can detect cavities and gum diseases and are also educated to detect oral cancers.

Diagnosis and Treatment

The severity of destructive periodontal disease is measured by the loss of the surrounding tissue attachment to the teeth and by the depth of gum pockets. Special treatments can minimize tissue damage if they are done in time. For example, in the early stages of periodontitis, the dentist or a technician can perform deep cleaning of the gum surfaces and can also smooth the damaged root surfaces of the teeth.

When the disease is advanced, the person will usually need gum surgery to save the teeth. The surgery will be performed by a periodontist, a dentist who has special training in this area. An antibiotic may also be ordered to stem any further bacterial growth. Before receiving treatment for periodontitis, the person with diabetes should ask his or her medical doctor to contact the dentist and provide information on the medical status before any complicated procedures are started. Tight glycemic control will aid in the healing of tissue and infection.

Prevention of Periodontal Disease

The best prevention is an annual dental examination, or more frequent examinations, if the dentist recommends them. An annual examination often can enable the dentist to detect and treat problems before they become severe. Yet, only about 58 percent of those over age two who have diabetes have an annual dental examination. The federal government in the United States hopes to increase the annual dental examination rate for people with diabetes to 75 percent by 2010.

As can be seen from the following table, there are also significant racial, age, educational, and disability status differences among those who receive annual dental examinations and those who do not. For example, Blacks have the best percentage (63 percent) of annual exams, followed by Whites at 58 percent. However, only about 32 percent of Hispanics or Latinos receive an annual dental examination. This is likely to translate into a greater risk of periodontal disease and loss of teeth for larger numbers of Hispanics and Latinos who have diabetes.

Persons Aged 2 Years and Older with Diabetes, 1997	Annual Dental Examination
	Percent
TOTAL	58
Race and ethnicity	
Asian or Pacific Islander	56
Black or African American	63
White	58
Hispanic or Latino	32
Gender	
Female	59
Male	57
Education level (aged 25 years and older)	
Less than high school	40
High school graduate	52
At least some college	65
Disability status	
Persons with disabilities	42
Persons without disabilities	66

Source: *Healthy People 2010: Objectives for Improving Health.* Chapter 5, Diabetes.

Education clearly plays a role in those who have an annual dental examination. Only 40 percent of those with less than a high school education have their teeth checked once a year. That percentage rises to 52 percent for the high school graduate and still further to 65 percent for the person with diabetes who has at least some college education.

Only 42 percent of persons with diabetes who have disabilities get an annual exam, compared to 66 percent without disabilities. Apparently healthier people with diabetes are more likely to see their dentists; however, it is important for all to have annual checkups. Also, sicker people probably are in even greater need of a checkup.

As for age discrepancies, the probability of having an annual dental examination decreases with age. Sixty percent of people with diabetes who are 18–44 years old see their dentist annually. The percentage falls to only 50 percent for people ages 45 to 64 and continues to fall. (See also GUM DISEASE.)

peripheral neuropathy Refers to nerve damage that is directly caused by diabetes and that usually involves sensory nerves or sometimes motor nerves. DIABETIC NEUROPATHY is a form of peripheral neuropathy. Peripheral neuropathy can also be caused by other diseases, such as AIDS, alcoholism, or nutritional deficiencies, such as an insufficiency of vitamin B_{12}. People with diabetes are at greater risk of experiencing peripheral neuropathy than nondiabetics.

People experiencing peripheral neuropathy have varied complaints ranging from numbness and tingling to pain and burning, and the loss of sensation. Patients may also have abnormal sensations, such as feeling like they are walking on balls or that there is an extra sock in their shoe, even though the patient knows that nothing is there. The cause is believed to be an excess of glucose in the nerve, which results in changes in the cell that make it unable to nourish itself. In essence, the nerve cell's "battery" runs down.

The most common complaint voiced by those suffering from a peripheral neuropathy is that their bedding bothers their feet at night, and they feel compelled to get up and walk around or at least remove their feet from under the sheets. This type of neuropathy can cause a great deal of suffering. It is treated by pain medications, based on its severity. They range from aspirin and acetaminophen to antidepressant medications, antiseizure drugs, or narcotics.

Peripheral neuropathy may also cause weakness, particularly occurring in the legs and feet, although it may also occur in the hands or arms.

In its most extreme case, peripheral neuropathy may lead to ulceration, which, if due to a lack of feeling, can then lead to GANGRENE. At that point, amputation of the affected limb is the only treatment.

Another form of peripheral neuropathy involves the lateral femoral cutaneous nerves in the upper thigh. It can cause numbness, tingling or pain in the legs. It generally disappears on its own, but can be very annoying while the person experiences the problem. Often this form of peripheral neuropathy occurs in both legs.

Early symptoms of peripheral sensory neuropathy are aches and pains in the feet and hands that tend to be worse when the patient is inactive, especially when they go to bed. Patients should avoid SMOKING, maintain tight GLYCEMIC control, and also keep their blood pressure down to as close as normal as possible.

Both the DIABETES CONTROL AND COMPLICATIONS TRIAL (DCCT) and the UNITED KINGDOM PROSPECTIVE DIABETES STUDY (UKPDS) revealed that tight glycemic control can help prevent the development and progression of peripheral sensory neuropathy.

For further information contact the following organizations:

American Chronic Pain Association (ACPA)
P.O. Box 850
Rocklin, CA 95677
(916) 632-0922
www.theacpa.org

Neuropathy Association
60 East 42nd Street
Suite 942
New York, NY 10165
(212) 692-0662
www.neuropathy.org

(See also DIABETIC NEUROPATHY, PAIN.)

S. J. Benbow et al., "Diabetic Peripheral Neuropathy and Quality of Life," *QJM: Monthly Journal of the Association of Physicians* 91, no. 11 (1998): 733–737.

peripheral vascular disease (PVD)   Disease of the large blood vessels found in the arms, legs, and feet. This is also known as a "macrovascular" disease. People with long-term diabetes are most prone to developing PVD. Symptoms include pain and aching in the arms, legs and feet, especially during walking (intermittent claudication) and may also lead to foot ULCERS that are slow to heal.

PVD is best prevented by preventive FOOT CARE as well as by avoiding or quitting SMOKING, keeping HYPERTENSION under control, and maintaining good GLYECMIC CONTROL.

Physicians evaluate a patient's blood flow by palpating the pulses in the feet, groin and arms. They also inspect for the presence or absence of hair as well as the health of fingernails and the general skin condition. This inspection helps the doctor make a clinical assessment for PVD because people with PVD lose hair and their fingernails are less healthy and grow less well. A noninvasive evaluation can also be done with blood pressure cuffs and Doppler ultrasound to measure pressure and wave forms.

Patients who appear to have PVD are typically referred to a vascular surgeon, who will often request a standard angiography or magnetic resonance imaging (MRI) to delineate the extent of the disease. Some diseases can be improved with balloon angioplasty while others require bypass surgery. Medication therapy includes aspirin and clopidogrel (both antiplatelet agents), pentoxiphyllin, and cilostazol.

Patients are encouraged to walk until pain occurs, then rest and walk again. This process will encourage new arterial blood growth around the blocked area.

phenylalanine derivatives   A medication for people with Type 2 diabetes. Starlix (nateglinide) is the only drug in this class, as of this writing. It works in a manner analogous to Prandin (repaglinide) and has a similar efficacy and side effect profile. It is dosed 60–120 mg. each, three times a day and is taken with the first bite of a meal.

Pima Indians   A tribe of Native Americans. In Arizona, they have been studied by researchers from the National Institutes of Health since 1965. The Pima Indians suffer from the highest known rate of diabetes in the world. About half of all U.S. Pima Indians develop Type 2 diabetes after the age of 35 years. The children of Pima parents who have DIABETIC NEPHROPATHY appear to inherit their parents' risk for the disease.

Experts believe that the high rate of Type 2 diabetes among the Pima Indians is partly a function of genetics but also stems from such environmental factors as obesity and a sedentary lifestyle. They point to the Pima Indians living in Mexico (who still apparently have an agrarian, active lifestyle, a low fat diet and overall, much lower BMIs) whose prevalence of diabetes is very low.

Pima Indians in the United States are also at much greater risk of suffering from diabetic complications such as END-STAGE RENAL DISEASE, BLINDNESS, AMPUTATIONS, and other complications related to diabetes.

With Pima Indians, an elevation in blood pressure before the onset of diabetes predicts abnormal PROTEINURIA. (See also AMERICAN INDIANS/NATIVE AMERICANS, COMPLICATIONS, RACE/ETHNICITY.)

pneumonia   See IMMUNIZATIONS.

podiatrist   A specialist in diseases of the foot. Some people with diabetes, particularly those who have had long-term diabetes, experience problems with their feet stemming from DIABETIC NEUROPATHY, such as pain, lack of feeling, or tingling. They may need to see a podiatrist for regular foot examinations. Individuals with diabetes should also regularly check their feet for cuts or infections.

It should be noted that some podiatrists concentrate on routine care while others are more likely to specialize in surgery or other aspects of foot care.

Many insurance plans, including MEDICARE, will cover regular podiatric visits for patients with diabetes who have problems such as ulcer, pre-ulcerative callus, use of anticoagulant medications, or the presence of neuropathy or PERIPHERAL VASCULAR DISEASE. (See also FOOT CARE, ORTHOTICS.)

polycystic ovarian syndrome (PCOS)   A condition that, if untreated, causes enlarged cystic ovaries. It is frequently accompanied by irregular MENSTRUATION and infertility. Women who have INSULIN RESISTANCE SYNDROME or Type 2 diabetes are at greater risk for this medical problem.

Previously known as Stein-Leventhal syndrome, PCOS is more common among women who are obese. Other co-occurring syndromes are ACANTHOSIS NIGRICANS and HYPERTENSION. Many also have HYPERLIPIDEMIA. The women with this condition also have a problem with excessive body hair (hirsutism). Treatment is aimed at lowering insulin resistance with medications such as METFORMIN, rosiglitazone, or pioglitazone, although these drugs are not FDA-approved for this indication. An overweight woman who has not menstruated or who menstruated erratically and who is then placed on one of these drugs is advised to use BIRTH CONTROL unless pregnancy is her intention. The drugs may alleviate years of infertility.

Treatment will decrease the levels of male hormones and thus the hirsutism will decrease.

polydipsia/polyphagia/polyuria (the three "Ps" or the "polys")   Polydipsia refers to extreme and continuous thirst and is one of the three primary symptoms of diabetes. Polyphagia refers to excessive hunger, and it is yet another sign of diabetes. Lastly, polyuria alludes to frequent urination, a third very common symptom exhibited by those who have diabetes but have not yet been diagnosed. Individuals who exhibit all three of these symptoms should advise their physician, who will in most cases order diagnostic laboratory tests for diabetes. (See also SYMPTOMS OF DIABETES.)

positronic emission tomography (PET)   A radiologic test that can reveal the metabolism of glucose within the body, particularly in the brain. As of this writing, the PET test is very expensive and is rarely used in the diagnosis or treatment of diabetes. Instead, it is used experimentally to see how the brain, heart, and kidneys utilize glucose in a variety of conditions. Currently PET is typically used in the evaluation of diseases involving cancer, and neurological and heart disorders.

postprandial blood glucose levels   Blood glucose levels that are tested from one to two hours after eating and that may give a better picture of the person's glycemic control than only pre-meal testing could provide. In a person with normal digestive and stomach emptying functions (and who does not have GASTROPARESIS), the peak glucose level generally occurs one hour after the start of a meal.

The advent of bioengineered and very rapidly acting human insulin, such as insulin lispro (HUMALOG) and insulin Aspart (Novolog) has been a great help to improve GLYCEMIC CONTROL. This is primarily because the level of these insulins peaks one hour after injection and thus, coincide with the peak of the blood glucose rise. As a result, the increased insulin levels can meet the increased levels of glucose after meals.

Postprandial glycemia is better correlated with macrovascular complications (versus microvascular complications), such as heart attack (MYOCARDIAL INFARCTION) and STROKE, as well as death. In 1987, the Honolulu heart study showed that there was a significantly increased risk of fatal coronary heart disease in those patients who had the highest blood glucose levels after having an oral glucose tolerance test.

If premeal glucose levels seem well controlled and the hemoglobin A_{1C} level is elevated (i.e., it is not consistent with the glucose levels), then the physician will request that the patient measure postprandial glucose levels.

Prandin   See MEGLITINIDES.

Precose See ACARBOSE.

pregnancy Gestation of a fetus. Pregnancy may bring many fears and joys to women. When pregnancy is complicated by the presence of diabetes, the woman's concerns are usually magnified. The realization that the health of her baby is heavily dependent on the woman's ability to maintain good glucose levels can be a frightening burden. The additional medical treatment, more frequent testing, and other requirements of managing diabetes may also seem daunting to the woman.

To face these special challenges, experts emphasize a TEAM MANAGEMENT approach to help the pregnant woman with diabetes. It is best if she consults with an obstetrician, a DIABETOLOGIST, a registered DIETITIAN, and any other experts that her physicians deem necessary, such as a neonatologist, a NEPHROLOGIST, and an OPHTHALMOLOGIST.

Excellent GLYCEMIC CONTROL is critical in the first weeks of pregnancy, and most experts prefer that women seek medical advice before conception even occurs. According to the authors of a 2000 article in *Early Human Development,* poor glycemic control in very early pregnancy is predictive of the baby's longer stay in a neonatal unit after the birth. Inadequate glycemic control is also predictive of infant malformations and even death.

Gestational Diabetes

Women who have never had diabetes may develop GESTATIONAL DIABETES, which may abate after delivery. Sometimes women who are diagnosed with gestational diabetes actually had Type 2 diabetes before their pregnancies, but it had not been diagnosed.

Demographic Data on Pregnant Women with Diabetes

According to statistics provided by the National Center for Health Statistics in 2000, there were about 27 women per 1,000 in the United States in 1998 with diabetes and who had babies born to them. The incidence varied greatly by race,

with white and black new mothers experiencing about the same rates of diabetes. In contrast, American Indian and Asian/Pacific Islanders had much higher rates (nearly double), as follows:

TABLE 1 RATE PER 1,000 OF WOMEN WITH DIABETES WHO HAD BABIES IN 1998	
All Women	26.7
White	25.9
Black	25.1
American Indian	48.5
Asian or Pacific Islander	42.2

Source: National Center for Health Statistics, National Vital Statistics Report 48, no. 3 (March 28, 2000).

Other research bears out these differences in age and ethnicities among women with diabetes who are pregnant. Researchers who reported their findings in a 1998 issue of *Morbidity and Mortality Weekly Report (MMWR)* found an overall rate of maternal diabetes of 25.3 per 1,000 women of all races and they also discovered broad differences between ethnic groups. For example, the highest incidence of 56.1 of 1,000 was found among Asian Indian women and the lowest incidence of maternal diabetes (19.3) was found among Korean women. (See Table 2.)

According to this study, the risk for maternal diabetes increases steadily with age and continues to vary greatly by ethnicity. In all groups, younger women are less likely to have diabetes than older women. Researchers found that maternal diabetes was lowest (8.3 per 1,000 women) for women under age 20. (See Table 2.)

In considering racial background, American Indians/Alaskan Natives under age 20 had the highest risk of 12.9 per 1,000 births, followed by Hawaiians at 11.4. The racial groups with the lowest rates of maternal diabetes for women under age 20 were found among Central or South Americans, at 5.6 per 1,000 and Mexicans, at 6.4 per 1,000.

The risk for all racial groups was highest for women who were between the ages of 40–49 years, at 65.6 per 1,000 of all women. The risk was highest for American Indians/Alaska Natives,

TABLE 2   NUMBER AND RATE* OF DIABETES DURING PREGNANCY,
BY RACE/ETHNICITY AND AGE OF MOTHER—UNITED STATES, 1993–1995

Race/Ethnicity	No.†	Age (yrs) of mother						Total	
		<20	20–24	25–29	30–34	35–39	40–49	Unadjusted	Age-adjusted§
Non-Hispanic									
White	6,996,046	10.0	17.8	24.5	30.3	41.3	56.1	**25.3**	**24.3**
Black	1,770,102	6.5	14.0	26.1	40.3	57.4	81.1	**22. 6**	**27.5**
Hispanic									
Mexican	1,331,361	6.4	12.5	23.7	41.9	63.8	88.8	**22.8**	**27.5**
Puerto Rican	161,065	8.8	21.4	36.3	56.9	79.7	107.7	**31.6**	**38.7**
Cuban	35,148	¶	14.7	23.6	30.2	40.4	53.4	**24.9**	**22.7**
Central or									
South American	271,639	5.6	11.4	21.7	35.8	56.4	79.9	**25.4**	**24. 3**
American Indian/									
Alaskan Native	108,982	12.9	26.8	49.5	77.3	110.2	150.6	**43.9**	**52.4**
Asian/									
Pacific Islander									
Chinese	77,359	¶	11.5	26.7	40.4	60.8	75.1	**39.1**	**27.3**
Japanese	25,885	¶	20.3	16.9	26.3	37.4	67.4	**26.8**	**21.6**
Hawaiian	16,982	11.4	16.8	33.3	47.5	67.1	¶	**28.9**	**32.6**
Filipino	88,487	8.0	16.2	28.8	47.5	69.5	100.0	**39.8**	**32.0**
Asian Indian**	31,574	¶	26.0	45.2	70.5	109.9	108.0	**56.1**	**48.3**
Korean>**	24,918	¶	9.0	13.3	22.9	31. 0	48.6	**19.3**	**16.1**
Samoan**	4,855	¶	¶	27.4	42.4	69.8	¶	**25.7**	**28.7**
Vietnamese**	34,140	¶	6.5	16.6	34.6	41.4	70.8	**24.3**	**19.5**
Total††	**11,384,926**	**8.3**	**16.3**	**25.1**	**33.8**	**47.4**	**65.6**	**25.3**	–

* Per 1000 singleton live-born infants in specified population.
† Women for whom diabetes status was reported.
§ Directly standardized to the aggregate population of all race/ethnicities.
¶ Numbers were too small for meaningful analysis.
** Data available for seven states (California, Hawaii, Illinois, New Jersey, New York, Texas, and Washington).
†† Includes races other than those listed.

at 150.6 per 1,000 births. They were followed by Puerto Ricans, at a risk of 107.7 per 1,000 births. The lowest risks for older mothers were among Korean mothers, at 48.6 per 1,000 births, followed by Central or South American mothers, at 54.4 per 1,000 births.

One major positive indicator that the researchers found was that women with diabetes are more likely to begin prenatal care in the first trimester than are nondiabetic pregnant women. (Although many doctors believe that the number of diabetic women seeking prenatal care is still not high enough. (See Table 3.)

As can be seen from Table 3, 84.3 percent of all women with diabetes in the United States received prenatal care during the first one to three months of their pregnancies. This compared favorably to the 79.9 percent of women without diabetes who had obtained prenatal care in the first trimester. However, again, broad racial variations were found; for example, Cuban woman (90.4 percent) and Japanese women with diabetes (90.2 percent) were the most likely to obtain medical care in the first trimester. Those least likely to obtain early prenatal care were Samoans (59 percent), followed by American Indians/Alaskan Natives (71.1 percent).

Experts warn that it can be extremely dangerous for both mother and baby if prenatal care is not obtained, and this failure increases the risk

TABLE 3   PERCENTAGE DISTRIBUTION OF MONTH PRENATAL CARE BEGAN AND ANNUAL AVERAGE NUMBER OF WOMEN WITH LATE, INADEQUATE, OR NO PRENATAL CARE, BY RACE/ETHNICITY AND DIABETES STATUS OF MOTHER—UNITED STATES, 1993–1995

Race/Ethnicity	No.*	1–3 Months		4–7 Months		8–9 Months or No Care		Average Number of Mothers per Year with Late or No Care†	Average Number of Mothers per Year with Inadequate or No Care§
		With Diabetes	Without Diabetes	With Diabetes	Without Diabetes	With Diabetes	Without Diabetes		
Non-Hispanic									
White	6,987,365	89.2	86.2	10.1	12.3	0.8	1.5	35,2 33	319,333
Black	173,029	77.3	67.9	20.5	26.6	2.2	5.5	31,539	183,867
Hispanic									
Mexican	1,313,659	72.0	66.9	25.6	27.6	2.4	5.6	24,047	144,495
Puerto Rican	155,355	77.1	71.6	20.6	24.5	2.3	4.0	2,023	14,627
Cuban	34,927	90.4	89.3	8.7	9.6	¶	1.1	132	1,241
Central or South American	263,138	71.8	71.0	25.3	25.0	2.9	4.0	3,482	25,452
American Indian/ Alaskan Native	108,831	71.1	64.7	25.6	29.1	3.3	6.2	2,111	12,705
Asian/ Pacific Islander									
Chinese	76,028	88.4	85.4	10.5	13.0	1.1	1.7	415	3,681
Japanese	25,429	90.2	88.6	9.1	10.0	¶	1.4	1 15	961
Hawaiian	16,373	79.8	74.3	19.6	22.4	¶	3.3	175	1,392
Filipino	87,176	85.6	80.3	13.3	17.5	1.0	2.3	641	5,671
Asian Indian**	30,675	82.6	81.5	14.6	16.0	2.8	2.5	261	1,888
Korean**	24,111	80.8	79.8	17.7	17.7	¶	2.6	203	1,623
Samoan**	4,673	59.0	56.1	36.1	35.2	¶	8.7	134	682
Vietnamese**	33,344	85.1	81.4	13.1	16.2	¶	2.5	272	2,061
Total††	11,286,002	84.3	79.9	14.4	17.3	1.3	2.8	105,122	751,673

* Women for whom month prenatal care began and diabetes status were reported.
† Care beginning in the eighth or ninth month of pregnancy or no care.
§ Care beginning after the third month of pregnancy or no care.
¶ Numbers were too small for meaningful analysis.
** Data available for seven states (California, Hawaii, Illinois, New Jersey, New York, Texas, and Washington).
†† Includes races other than those listed.

of miscarriage, fetal harm, and/or delivering a very large baby (macrosomia).

Preconception Planning

When women with diabetes receive medical advice about pregnancy before conception occurs, major advantages accrue; for example, their babies have a rate of congenital malformations that is about equal to women who do not have diabetes, or about 2 percent or less. However, when women with diabetes do not receive preconception care, the rate of small to severe birth defects among their infants can be high as 11 percent. Also, studies have found lower death rates among the newborns of mothers with diabetes when the mothers had received preconception care. Clearly, preconception care is very important for the children of women with diabetes.

Although physicians strongly recommend that women with diabetes plan ahead before becoming pregnant, many women do not. In a study performed by Holing et al., on 85 women with diabetes in Washington State who gave birth (reported in a 1998 issue of *Diabetes Care*), researchers compared women who planned their pregnancies to women who did not. Only 41 percent of the women had planned their pregnancies.

The researchers found that women who had planned their pregnancies were more educated and had a higher socioeconomic status. The preplanners were also more likely to have private health insurance. Also, they were more likely to have consulted with an endocrinologist before becoming pregnant.

Another difference: the women in the preplanned pregnancy group reported more frequently (80 percent of the preplanned pregnancy group) that the baby's biological father was aware of issues related to diabetes and pregnancy. Only 16 percent of the women with unplanned pregnancies said their male partners were well informed.

The perception of their physicians was also reported as very different between the preplanners and the nonplanners. The women with

planned pregnancies reported receiving positive feedback from their doctors before their pregnancies. Seventy-five percent said they had received positive and encouraging advice.

In sharp contrast (and almost a complete reversal), 70 percent of the women with unplanned pregnancies reported negative feedback from their physicians. They said that they had either been discouraged from pregnancy by their physicians before the pregnancy or they had received mixed messages from the doctor. (Perhaps because the physician believed the woman was not yet able to manage her diabetes.)

When asked about their relationship with their doctor, 71 percent of the women with planned pregnancies reported positive relationships versus 28 percent of the women with unplanned pregnancies.

The researchers said,

> In spite of innumerable reports documenting outstanding pregnancy success for women with well-controlled diabetes, many women still perceive the message that pregnancy should not occur. In addition to the content and consistency of care, the nature of the interaction [with the health care system] may be crucial. It is vital that couples be supported and reassured that with pre-conception glucose control, almost all women with diabetes can have healthy babies; the essential step is planning the pregnancy.

Some researchers have studied the cost effectiveness of preconception care and have found a financial savings of thousands of dollars. Healthier mothers and babies incur fewer medical expenses.

Women with Type 1 Diabetes

In a study reported by Baha M. Sibai in a 2000 issue of the *Journal of Maternal-Fetal Medicine*, researchers looked at pregnancy complications among women with Type 1 diabetes. They found that some women were more at risk for developing preeclampsia, a dangerous condition related to the combination of HYPERTENSION, PROTEINURIA, and EDEMA. The women who were most at risk were those with their first pregnancies (nulliparous), and also women with the following factors:

- pre-existing DIABETIC NEPHROPATHY (kidney disease), including proteinuria of 190–499 mg/d before 20 weeks of pregnancy and microalbuminuria before pregnancy
- elevated HbA1C level in early pregnancy
- chronic hypertension
- Duration of maternal diabetes (the longer the woman had diabetes, the worse the risk)

The author said, "At the present time, it appears that aggressive control of maternal hypertension and blood sugars before pregnancy and throughout gestation may be the most effective ways to reduce the rate of preeclampsia in such women."

Women with Type 2 Diabetes

Although many people consider Type 1 diabetes to be far more serious than Type 2 diabetes, both conditions can be dangerous to a developing fetus. Some studies indicate a high risk of death for the babies of women with Type 2 diabetes, particularly if the women are obese.

In a study performed in New Zealand and reported in *Diabetic Medicine* in 2000, the researchers reviewed the records of 434 women with Type 2 pregnancies, 160 with Type 1 diabetes and 932 who had gestational diabetes, over the period 1985–1997. They found the newborn death rate for the children of women with Type 2 diabetes was 46.1 per 1,000 pregnancies. The rate for the general population was 12.5. The researchers found that the mortality rate for women with Type 1 diabetes was also 12.5 and the rate for women with gestational diabetes was even lower (8.9). The researchers said,

> There was a seven-fold increase in the rate of late fetal death and 2.5-fold increase in the rates of intermediate fetal and late neonatal death. Subjects with Type 2 DM were significantly older and more obese than subjects with Type 1 DM, and presented later to the diabetes services.

Obesity among pregnant women with diabetes was also a critical factor in another study reported in a 2000 issue of *Epidemiology.* Researchers Lynn Moore and colleagues studied data from nearly 23,000 pregnant women. They found that pregnant women who were both obese and diabetic had about triple (3.1 times) the risk of having a child with a major birth defect. Women who had diabetes but were not obese had a much diminished risk of having a child with a medical problem other than having a higher prevalence of babies with musculoskeletal defects. The authors said, "Approximately 65% total major defects among [the children of] women who were obese and had some form of diabetes was attributable to the interaction of the two factors."

Risks of miscarriage   Women with pre-existing diabetes have a 3–5 percent rate of miscarriage, which is higher than the rate of 1.5 percent for women without diabetes. But very tight blood glucose control has been demonstrated to reduce the risk of miscarriage to near the rates seen among pregnant women without diabetes. (See DIABETES CONTROL AND COMPLICATIONS TRIAL (DCCT).) However, with tight control also comes the risk for HYPOGLYCEMIA, requiring even further vigilance on the part of the pregnant woman, her life partner, and her health care providers.

Researchers studying pregnant women with Type 1 diabetes found that the risk of developing hypoglycemia was highest in the first half of pregnancy, peaking between the 10th and 15th week of pregnancy. They were uncertain as to the cause. (This information was reported in "Medical Complications of Diabetes Mellitus in Pregnancy" in *Clinical Obstetrics and Gynecology.* See citations at the end of this essay.)

Risks to the Child

The children born to women with diabetes have a higher rate of birth defects when blood glucose levels are not optimal. The types of birth defects may vary from cleft palate or cleft lip to heart, lung, or intestinal problems as well as developmental or motor delays. These malformations are found more frequently among the babies of women who have not had good prenatal care and who did not work to attain close to normal glucose levels.

According to Reece and Homko in their article on infant malformations born to women with diabetes in a 2000 issue of *Clinical Obstetrics and Gynecology*, most congenital defects happen before the eighth week of gestation. Researchers have also found a direct relationship between hemoglobin A1C levels in early pregnancies and subsequent birth defects or spontaneous abortions (miscarriages).

Treatment: Medications

All women with Type 1 diabetes as well as many women with Type 2 diabetes will require insulin during their pregnancy. (After the pregnancy, many women with Type 2 diabetes may return to taking their oral medications.) Women who need insulin during their pregnancies will also usually require insulin intravenously during labor and delivery, to protect both the mother and her baby. Some women with diabetes may require other medications as well, and doctors will work to balance any possible dangers that medication may present to both mother and child during the pregnancy.

In countries other than the United States, physicians have added glyburide to treat gestational diabetes and METFORMIN to treat Type 2 diabetes during pregnancy. These drugs are not FDA-approved for this usage in the United States and it is not a standardized treatment.

The insulin pump   Some pregnant women have found that the insulin pump has made the management of their diabetes much easier. In a study reported in a 2000 issue of the *American Journal of Obstetrics and Gynecology*, the researchers evaluated women who used an insulin pump before pregnancy and also women who initiated therapy of the pump during pregnancy. They found high satisfaction among both groups, although there were some problems that were mostly self-managed, such as an infection at the site of the infusion.

Of the women who started using the pump during pregnancy, 95 percent continued to use it after the birth of their babies. The authors noted that many women with diabetes who do not use insulin pumps are still able to attain excellent glycemic control during pregnancy. However, this high level of control nearly always rapidly falls off after the birth of the baby. The pump is one way to maintain good control.

Treatment: Tests

Many doctors rely on ULTRASOUND imaging tests to determine the size and health of the fetus. According to Dr. David Hadden in a supplementary article to *Diabetes Care* in 1999, women with Type 1 diabetes should have at least three ultrasounds during pregnancy. The first should be performed in early pregnancy to determine growth problems and any congenital defects. The second ultrasound should be performed at about the 28th-week point to determine the size of the fetus, possible congenital defects, and any excessive amount of amniotic fluid (polyhydramnios). Then, at around the 36-week point, an ultrasound should be done to determine if the baby is overly large.

The fetal Biophysical Profile (BPP) is one form of ultrasound test that has been used successfully with pregnant women who have diabetes. It can ascertain the volume of amniotic fluid and also identify malformations. This test looks at fetal breathing, gross body motions, fetal tone, and amniotic fluid, and awards scores of "2," for normal, down to zero, for an absence of the characteristic being evaluated. (No amniotic fluid, no fetal breathing, and so forth.)

A normal fetus scores eight out of 10. A fetus that may be in trouble scores six or lower. One study of 98 women with Type 1 diabetes revealed that the BPP was predictive of normal Apgar scores (scores given to newborns at birth) in 99 percent of the cases. This means that if the BPP said the baby was normal, in almost every case the infant is normal at delivery. The reverse is also true.

Another testing option is Doppler velocimetry, which measures uterine waveform data and can help determine if there is a problem with the pregnancy.

Some physicians rely upon the nonstress test to determine the fetal heart rate and possible problems. The test may be given at 32 weeks or may be administered earlier if the woman also has hypertension or other medical problems in addition to diabetes. If the woman is using insulin, the test may be performed twice a week after the 32-week point.

Self-Care Is Important

HOME BLOOD GLUCOSE MONITORING is important for all people with diabetes, but it becomes even more important for the pregnant woman. Depending on the individual, the doctor may ask that the woman screen her blood as many as eight times per day, as well as adjust her diet and exercise plans. This frequent screening also has the advantage that it will help the woman to know if she may have a problem with hypoglycemia.

Medical Risks to the Mother and Child

The pregnant woman with diabetes incurs risk to her own body as well as to her fetus or newborn child. For example, the risks for developing DIABETIC RETINOPATHY are increased, as is the risk for already existing retinopathy to worsen with pregnancy.

Tight glycemic control can prevent such worsening. In a study reported in Sweden in 2000, 112 pregnant women with Type 1 diabetes and with problems with retinopathy were studied over the period 1993–1997. The goal was normal glucose levels and this was attempted through outpatient clinic visits made by the women as well as by having the women increase the number of blood testings per day and also increasing their insulin administration to four to six times per day.

Researchers found that the women's levels of HbA1C (blood glucose) significantly decreased from their pre-pregnancy rates. Retinopathy among the women did not worsen sufficiently to require treatment. Of the few women who did have retinopathy that worsened, they had experienced an earlier onset of Type 1 diabetes than did the women whose retinopathy stayed the same or for those whose condition improved.

Hypoglycemia is a risk with tight glucose control and four of the women did experience severe hypoglycemic episodes, although it did not affect their babies.

The researchers also reported that the tight control maintained during pregnancy did not last after the delivery, stating,

> During pregnancy motivation is high for maintaining a tight metabolic control, not only because of the beneficial effect on retinopathy, but also because this may improve the prognosis of the perinatal outcome. However, after delivery the obstetric counseling is less and irregularities in the day rhythm unavoidably result from nursing the newborn child.

Clearly, the implication from this statement is not that women with diabetes should avoid breastfeeding, but rather that their lives are even busier after their babies are born than before and thus, it is more difficult to maintain tight glycemic control.

Pregnancy can also exacerbate any pre-existing medical problems of the pregnant woman with diabetes. For example, if the pregnant woman has kidney disease stemming from diabetes, then her pregnancy outcome is affected as well. According to Rosenn and Miodovnik in their 2000 article in *Clinical Obstetrics and Gynecology,*

> The presence of diabetic nephropathy significantly affects the outcome of pregnancy, primarily for three reasons: (1) the increased risk of maternal hypertensive complications, (2) the increased risk of fetal prematurity caused by worsening maternal hypertension and preeclampsia, and (3) the increased risk of fetal growth restriction and fetal distress. In general, the worst prenatal outcomes occur in women

who have measurable impaired renal function, with decreased creatinine clearance and increased serum creatinine concentrations.

The experts report that nearly all of the infants will survive but may have problems with developmental delays (retardation) or motor delays.

Some physicians worry that glycemic control could become overly strict Although a consensus of physicians agrees that tight glycemic control during pregnancy is critically important, there are some physicians who worry that the overall definition of good glycemic control is too vague. They are also concerned that pregnant women who rigidly adhere to glucose control guidelines run a greater risk of developing hypoglycemia. In addition, these physicians say that not enough attention is paid to the fact that women with diabetes may have babies who are small for their gestational age (SGA), and such babies are at risk for developing diabetes as adults.

According to Barak M. Rosenn and Menachem Miodovnik, in their 2000 article for the *Journal of Maternal-Fetal Medicine,* the biggest risk of tight glycemic control is hypoglycemia. The authors say,

> The risks of hypoglycemia are far from trivial; indeed, it can be a life-threatening complication of intensive insulin therapy in patients with Type 1 diabetes. Hypoglycemia is the most common side effect in patients with diabetes receiving intensive insulin therapy, and it is also their greatest fear. Approximately 25 percent of these patients experience at least one episode of severe hypoglycemia in a given year. Such episodes include need for glucagon or intravenous glucose administration, emergency room treatment, seizures, loss of consciousness, coma, or even death. In fact, current estimates attribute 4% of all deaths in patients with Type 1 diabetes to hypoglycemia.

Cesarean deliveries Some studies have shown that women with diabetes have a four times greater risk of having a cesarean section (C-section) over nondiabetic women. The rea-son for this may be that the fetus is overly large and it is determined safer to perform a C-section. Some doctors are also more likely to perform cesarean sections on women with diabetes because of health concerns and risks, even the infant is normal-sized.

Induction of labor Even if a vaginal delivery is planned, sometimes doctors will induce labor, particularly if they are concerned that the child is large or will become too large by the time of delivery. Prior to induction, an amniocentesis test on the fetus is usually performed to determine the maturity of the lungs.

The authors also reported several studies on pregnant women with Type 1 diabetes who had hypoglycemic episodes. Most of these episodes occurred in the first half of pregnancy, peaking between the eighth and 14th week of pregnancy. Their recommendations for such women:

- frequent blood testing
- multiple injections of short-acting insulin
- intermediate insulin at bedtime
- rapid-acting insulins or a continuous infusion insulin pump
- frequent meals and snacks
- complete education of the patient.

After Delivery of the Baby

Once the child is safely delivered, it is checked for any signs of diabetes, respiratory difficulty, jaundice, and other possible medical problems. If the child was large, it is also checked for SHOULDER DYSTOCIA and other problems that might occur with a difficult childbirth. The child is also checked for symptoms of hypoglycemia. If the baby weighs over nine pounds, calcium and magnesium levels are checked to learn if the infant needs supplemental calcium or magnesium.

The mother is also checked thoroughly and often given insulin intravenously. Her glucose levels are taken and she is evaluated for hypoglycemia and any other medical problems that may have developed during the delivery.

At the American Diabetes Association meeting in 2001, Dr. Tom Buchanan presented his data on the prevention of the development of postpartum Type 2 diabetes among women who had had gestational diabetes. Nonpregnant, nondiabetic Hispanic women who had gestational diabetes within the past four years were studied. Based on past studies, it was predicted that these women would have a 70 percent chance of developing Type 2 diabetes within five years.

The patients were treated with troglitazone (a THIAZOLIDINEDIONE drug removed from the United States market in 2000). Of the women in the study, 121 were given a placebo and 114 were given troglitazone. Nineteen percent of the women on troglitazone subsequently developed Type 2 diabetes, while a much larger percentage, 53 percent, of the women receiving the placebo developed diabetes. Dr. Buchanan believed that the drug helped decrease the workload of the beta cells and preserved its function.

In summary, the two most important things to keep in mind about pregnant women who have diabetes are that (1) preconception planning and consulting with physicians prior to the pregnancy have enormous benefits to both mother and child, and (2) careful glycemic control, by working with medical experts and self-monitoring greatly increase the probability of having a healthy and normal child. (See also CHILDREN OF DIABETIC MOTHERS, FERTILITY, GENETIC RISKS, GESTATIONAL DIABETES, HYPOGLYCEMIA, INSULIN PUMP, OBESITY.)

Centers for Disease Control, "Diabetes During Pregnancy—United States, 1993–1995," *Morbidity and Mortality Weekly Report* 47, no. 20 (May 29, 1998): 408–414.

T. Cundy et al., "Perinatal Mortality in Type 2 Diabetes Mellitus," *Diabetic Medicine: A Journal of the British Diabetic Association* 17, no. 1 (January 2000): 33–39.

The Diabetes Control and Complications Trial Research Group, "Pregnancy Outcomes in the Diabetes Control and Complications Trial," *American Journal of Obstetrics & Gynecology* 174 (1996): 1343–1353.

Steven G. Gabbe, M.D., et al. "Benefits, Risks, Costs, and Patient Satisfaction Associated with Insulin Pump Therapy for the Pregnancy Complicated by Type 1 Diabetes Mellitus," *American Journal of Obstetrics and Gynecology* 182, no. 6 (June 2000): 1283–1291.

David R. Hadden, M.D., "How to Improve Prognosis in Type 1 Diabetic Pregnancy," *Diabetes Care* 21, Supp. 2 (March 1999): B104–B108.

David R. Hadden and David R. McCance, "Advances in Management of Type 1 Diabetes and Pregnancy," *Current Opinions in Obstetrics & Gynecology* 11, no. 6 (December 1999): 557–562.

Emily V. Holing, Ph.D., et al., "Why Don't Women with Diabetes Plan Their Pregnancies?" *Diabetes Care* 21, no. 6 (1998): 889–895.

M. B. Landon, "Obstetric Management of Pregnancies Complicated by Diabetes Mellitus," *Clinical Obstetrics & Gynecology* 43, no. 1 (March 2000): 65–74.

Finn Lauszus et al., "Diabetic Retinopathy in Pregnancy During Tight Metabolic Control," *Acta Obstetricia et Gynecologica Scandinavica* 79 (2000): 367–370.

Lynn L. Moore, M.D., et al., "A Prospective Study of the Risk of Congenital Defects Associated with Maternal Obesity and Diabetes Mellitus," *Epidemiology* 11, no. 6 (November 2000): 689–694.

E. Albert Reece, M.D., and Carol J. Homko, R.N., M.S., "Why Do Diabetic Women Deliver Malformed Infants?" *Clinical Obstetrics & Gynecology* 43, no. 1 (March 2000): 32–45.

Barak M. Rosenn and Menachem Miodovnik, "Glycemic Control in the Diabetic Pregnancy: Is Tighter Always Better?," *Journal of Maternal-Fetal Medicine* 9 (2000): 29–34.

B. M. Rosenn and M. Miodovnik, "Medical Complications of Diabetes Mellitus in Pregnancy," *Clinical Obstetrics & Gynecology* 43, no. 1 (March 2000): 17–31.

B. M. Sibai, "Risk Factors, Pregnancy Complications, and Prevention of Hypertensive Disorders in Women with Pregravid Diabetes Mellitus," *Journal of Maternal Fetal Medicine* 9, no. 1 (January–February 2000): 62–65.

Marja S. Vaarasmaki et al., "Factors Predicting Peri- and Neonatal Outcome in Diabetic Pregnancy," *Early Human Development* 59 (July 2000): 61–70.

prevention of diabetes   Actions to delay or altogether prevent the development of diabetes. Type 1 diabetes cannot be prevented (as of this writing), but many doctors believe that it is possible to delay its onset.

In the case of Type 2 diabetes, the illness may be prevented or at least delayed for years, particularly when those with a genetic predisposition for diabetes keep their weight down and exercise regularly. Among those individuals with impaired glucose tolerance who have not yet progressed to Type 2 diabetes, experts say there are a variety of lifestyle changes that individuals can make to avoid developing diabetes.

The Diabetes Prevention Program (which ended in 2001), of about 3,000 people with impaired glucose tolerance showed that 150 minutes of exercise per week plus a 5 to 7 percent decline in weight led to a 58 percent decrease in the development of diabetes. In another group in this study that used MET-FORMIN, subjects had a 33 percent decrease in the development of diabetes.

According to Dr. Tuomilehto et al., in their article for the *New England Journal of Medicine* in 2001, their study revealed that patients' success in changing their lifestyles had a direct inverse correlation with developing diabetes: the more successful they were, the less likely that diabetes would develop. The researchers studied 522 middle-aged overweight individuals with impaired glucose tolerance, assigning them to either the intervention group, which received individual counseling, or the control group.

The groups were evaluated for diabetes after one year and also four years later. The intervention group had a much lower percentage of diabetes and was able to decrease its risk for diabetes by 58 percent. Even four years after the study, the incidence of diabetes was only 11 percent in the intervention group compared to 23 percent in the control group.

The individuals who succeeded at preventing diabetes were those who decreased their consumption of fat, sugar, salt, and alcohol, and who increased their consumption of vegetables and fiber. They also decreased their weight and increased their exercise. The researchers said,

> Achieving a relatively conservative target of more than four hours of exercise per week was associated with a significant reduction in the risk of diabetes in the subjects who did not lose weight. It is likely that any type of physical activity—whether sports, household work, gardening, or work-related physical activity—is similarly beneficial in preventing diabetes.

PATIENTS WITH DIABETES WHO OBTAINED RECOMMENDED TESTS

State	Dilated Eye Examination %	Foot Examination %	SMBG[†] %	HbA1C[§] %
Alabama	53.6	42.4	41.0	16.9
Alaska	76.8	59.9	49.5	37.7
Arizona	60.5	45.3	42.2	20.8
Arkansas	47.0	49.0	38.4	21.0
California	58.2	51.1	37.2	29.0
Colorado	56.0	59.6	49.8	40.8
Connecticut	72.5	65.2	58.5	31.3
District of Columbia	68.1	57.9	33.5	20.7
Florida	53.5	51.7	48.1	18.8
Georgia	57.6	52.6	41.4	18.3
Hawaii	70.2	61.8	29.7	25.5
Idaho	59.6	51.4	52.7	27.8
Iowa	63.8	55.0	45.2	26.2
Kansas	57.4	49.8	39.3	17.1
Kentucky	58.6	60.1	45.7	24.1
Louisiana	66.9	52.7	41.2	22.0
Maine	76.0	69.4	47.9	42.4
Massachusetts	81.0	65.4	51.8	27.9
Michigan	58.0	45.8	36.3	22.1
Minnesota	61.8	58.0	58.3	31.6
Mississippi	52.5	52.9	34.1	18.1
Montana	66.4	63.3	65.5	39.9
Nebraska	55.9	58.4	55.1	38.2
Nevada	63.5	51.8	35.8	20.8
New Hampshire	60.5	53.6	47.2	31.1
New Jersey	63.6	58.6	47.5	25.6
New Mexico	62.3	59.3	45.2	25.1
North Carolina	67.3	54.6	42.9	23.8
North Dakota	71.5	67.8	53.7	35.7
Ohio	61.7	62.1	49.2	21.7
Pennsylvania	62.4	58.3	46.6	27.8
Rhode Island	68.4	58.7	45.4	30.2
Tennessee	51.7	53.2	57.4	17.2
Texas	55.3	53.1	41.7	17.9
Utah	63.9	65.4	54.3	31.4

State	Dilated Eye Examination %	Foot Examination %	SMBG[†] %	HbA1C[§] %
Vermont	71.9	50.8	36.2	35.8
Virginia	64.2	59.3	46.5	24.2
West Virginia	55.0	63.7	50.5	24.1
Wisconsin	64.6	62.9	55.3	27.7
Wyoming	56.5	48.0	50.8	30.2

* Estimates are age-adjusted to the 2000 U.S. adult population, 3-year averages. Data from the following states and territories were not included in the analysis: Delaware, Illinois, Indiana, Maryland, Missouri, New York, Oklahoma, Oregon, South Carolina, South Dakota, Washington, Puerto Rico, Guam, and the U.S. Virgin Islands.
† Self-monitoring of blood glucose.
§ Glycosylated hemoglobin.

Data from the Diabetes Prevention in Type 1 (DPT-1) study was negative. Relatives of patients with Type 1 diabetes who were at high risk for developing diabetes did develop diabetes despite prior treatment with low-dose insulin. Data from the oral treatment arm of the study has yet to be analyzed, as of this writing.

In 2001, British researchers performed research on newly diagnosed patients with Type 1 diabetes, using an experimental peptide known as Peptide p277 or Dia Pep 277. In the study, patients given the peptide needed less insulin to maintain the same level of glycemic control. Further research is needed but these results are promising. (See also DIABETES PREVENTION TRIALS.)

Morbidity and Mortality Weekly Report, "Levels of Diabetes-Related Preventive Care Practices—United States, 1997–1999," *Morbidity and Mortality Weekly Report* 49, no. 42 (October 27, 2000): 954–958.

Jaako Tuomilehto, M.D., Ph.D., et al., "Prevention of Type 2 Diabetes Mellitus by Changes in Lifestyle among Subjects with Impaired Glucose Tolerance," *New England Journal of Medicine* 344, no. 18 (May 3, 2001): 1343–1350.

prognosis Professional evaluation of the short- and long-term outcome of disease. When diabetes is diagnosed in the early stage, and when the patient is willing and able to comply with medical recommendations regarding medication, diet, and exercise, the prognosis for the future is good to excellent. However, when diagnosis occurs at a late stage and damage has already occurred to organs such as the eyes, kidneys, and other areas, the prognosis is less favorable.

proliferative retinopathy See DIABETIC RETINOPATHY.

prosthesis A device, such as an artificial leg or arm, that is used to replace a limb that has been amputated. The term may also refer to an implant of a hip, knee, or other body part. A prosthesis may also be a device used to supplement body functioning, such as a hearing aid. People with diabetes have a high rate of AMPUTATIONS, primarily due to foot ULCERS, which have progressed to GANGRENE.

After an amputation it is often critical that patients with diabetes work with a rehabilitation team to properly fit the prosthesis and to learn how to use it properly. This usually involves using the assistance of physical therapists and physical medicine medical doctors known as physiatrists, as well as prosthetists, specialists in prosthetic devices.

proteinuria Protein in the urine, which is usually a sign of kidney disease. (Exercise and fever can sometimes temporarily increase the protein levels in the urine.) When detected early enough, the underlying abnormality may be treated; however, when there are large amounts of proteinuria, this indicates that the person has a kidney or cardiovascular disease and may be in danger of kidney failure, stroke, or heart attack. The individual may also have diabetes, HYPERTENSION, or other illnesses (or the patient may have two or more illnesses, such as having both hypertension and diabetes or another combination of ailments).

Proteins are processed by the body and they are usually too large to pass through the kidney into the urine. As a result, they normally cannot be found in urinalysis. However, in the case of early damage to the kidneys, the two major types of proteins that may be found in the urine are albumin and globulins. Of these, albumin is smaller and more likely to be seen than are globulins.

When a person has either Type 1 or Type 2 diabetes, even a small amount of albumin in the urine (microalbuminuria) is an indication of early kidney malfunction.

Testing for Proteinuria

There are no specific symptoms that are experienced by those with proteinuria, and, consequently, the only way to tell if the problem exists is to test the urine. One such test is done with a urinary dipstick that tests for albumin. If the urine dipstick is negative, then the patient should have a yearly spot urine test for microalbumin by radioimmunoassay. This is a very sensitive test to detect tiny amounts of protein (30–300 mg protein/every 1,000 mg creatinine).

Another test for proteinuria is a 24-hour urine collection, in which urinary protein excretion is measured over a 24-hour period. Kidney function and protein loss can be quantified by a 24-hour collection. In general, the 24-hour test is used on adults and adolescents rather than on children, because it is usually more difficult to collect the child's urine for such a long timeframe and spot tests provide reasonable data.

If protein is found in the urine, then blood tests are usually ordered. The doctor will generally order a test for creatinine and urea nitrogen levels. The reason for this testing is that creatinine and urea nitrogen are normally removed from the blood by the kidneys. However, if there are high levels of creatinine and urea nitrogen in the blood, this is an indication that the kidneys are not functioning normally.

Physicians recommend that testing for proteinuria be done annually on people who have already been diagnosed with hypertension or with Type 1 or Type 2 diabetes. Others who fall into certain risk groups should receive periodic testing as well, according to the determination of the individual's physician.

Some groups of people are more likely than others to have proteinuria, including:

- people with diabetes (both Type 1 and Type 2)
- people with hypertension
- African Americans
- American Indians
- Hispanic Americans
- Pacific Islander Americans
- elderly individuals
- obese individuals
- those with a family history of kidney disease

Treatment of Proteinuria

After diagnosing proteinuria, the medical goal usually is to determine and treat the underlying cause. For example, if the primary problem is hypertension, the goal is to reduce the blood pressure. Some people do not have hypertension but they do have proteinuria. The doctor should work to determine the cause and treat the proteinuria. The person with diabetes should work to normalize blood pressure, improve glucose control, and adjust his or her diet.

The more copious the protein in the urine, the more important it is to bring blood pressure levels under control. For example, if the proteinuria exceeds 1 g per 24 hours, the National Heart, Lung, and Blood Institute recommends that the blood pressure be maintained below 125/75 mm Hg. **Note:** 125/75 is considered a normal and not hypertensive level, however, when the person has proteinuria that is caused by diabetes, then attaining an even lower blood pressure will work to improve the prognosis for the individual.

If diabetes is the main cause of the proteinuria rather than hypertension, then the goal will be to attain glycemic control. Doctors may also recommend dietary changes such as cutting back on salt and protein and may have other recommendations.

If the individual has both diabetes and hypertension, the doctor may prescribe a medication from the angiotensin-converting enzyme (ACE) inhibitor class of drugs, which are more protective of the kidneys than are other medications for blood pressure control.

ACE drugs should be used as soon as tests reveal that a person has microalbuminuria, a condition that precedes proteinuria. Normal levels of albumin in the urine are less than 30 mg/g creatinine. When the levels are 30–300 mg albumin/g creatinine, that is defined as microalbuminuria. An even greater problem is proteinuria, in which levels greater than 300 mg albumin/g creatinine. When the person receives medication when the problem is still at the microalbuminuria level, the protein levels may still be pushed back into the normal range. But if treatment does not occur until proteinuria is present, then medication can only diminish the rate of decline—rather than stopping the decline altogether, as can be done at earlier stages of the problem.

Some people cannot tolerate ACE drugs, and in that case, ANGIOTENSIN RECEPTOR BLOCKER (ARB) medications may be used as a good second choice. It should also be noted that either of these medications may also be used in a person who does not have hypertension, but who does have microalbuminuria or overt proteinuria.

For further information, contact the following organizations:

American Kidney Fund
6110 Executive Boulevard
Suite 1010
Rockville, MD 20852
(800) 638-8299 (toll-free) or (301) 881-3052
www.akfinc.org

National Kidney Foundation
30 East 33rd Street
New York, NY 10016
(800) 622-9010 (toll-free) or (212) 889-2210
www.kidney.org

Ronald J. Hogg, M.D., et al., "Evaluation and Management of Proteinuria and Nephrotic Syndrome in Children: Recommendations from a Pediatric Nephrology Panel Established at the National Kidney Foundation Conference on Proteinuria, Albuminuria, Risk, Assessment, Detection, and Elimination (PARADE)," *Pediatrics* 105, no. 6 (June 2000): 1242–1249.

National Kidney and Urologic Diseases Information Clearinghouse, "Proteinuria," NIH Pub. No. 01-4732, May 2000.

pruritis   A generalized constant itching of the skin. Pruritis may be a symptom of uncontrolled diabetes, although it is not a common symptom. Improvement may be found with skin moisturizers. People with diabetes may also need to use a humidifier during winter months, to avoid excessive drying of the skin. It's also important to drink plenty of fluids, especially water. (See also ITCHING SKIN, SKIN PROBLEMS.)

pumps   See IMPLANTABLE INSULIN PUMPS.

quality of life   In the context of diabetes, quality of life refers to the ability of interventions to prevent complications and suffering as well as ensuring that the interventions/treatments do not cause adverse effects. Most analyses of new medications and treatments now routinely assess the effect of the interventions in quality of life issues in addition to its effect on blood glucose, blood pressure, or whatever issues are being treated. (See also DEPRESSION, EMOTIONAL PROBLEMS.)

The Diabetes Control and Complications Trial Research Group, "Influence of Intensive Diabetes Treatment on Quality-of-Life Outcomes in the Diabetes Control and Complications Trial," *Diabetes Care* 19, no. 3 (March 1996): 195–203.

William H. Polonsky, Ph.D., C.D.E., "Understanding and Assessing Diabetes-Specific Quality of Life," from *Diabetes Spectrum* 13, no. 1 (1999), in *Annual Review of Diabetes 2000* (Alexandria, Va: American Diabetes Association, 2000): 230–237.

race/ethnicity Racial or ethnic background. Race and ethnicity are both significant factors in diabetes, primarily in TYPE 2 DIABETES. African Americans are more likely to suffer from Type 2 diabetes than are whites. Hispanics also have an elevated risk of Type 2 diabetes and Native Americans, especially PIMA INDIANS, have an extremely high rate of disease, with half of tribe members over age 35 being diagnosed with diabetes.

Type 1 diabetes appears to be far less linked to racial factors among non-white people, because white children have a higher rate of Type 1 diabetes than children of other races. (See also AFRICAN AMERICAN, ALASKA NATIVES, AMERICAN INDIAN/NATIVE AMERICAN, HISPANICS, PACIFIC ISLANDERS, PIMA INDIANS.)

reagent strips Chemically treated strips that change color when exposed to blood, urine, or other substances. People with diabetes use these reagent strips to test their blood glucose levels. The glucose levels in the patient's urine are rarely tested by the patient at home or the doctor in the clinic, because blood testing provides much more accurate information. The most common urine test for a patient with diabetes to check at home is for urinary KETONES. (See also SICK DAY RULES.)

Physicians use reagent strips in the office to test patients' urine for protein, blood, and signs of infection. More sophisticated reagent strips allow physicians and patients to test their own FRUCTOSAMINE levels at home as well as to test for ketones in their blood.

The reagent strips come with a color code to compare the used strip. The color code allows the person to determine their own levels and whether they are within the normal range or not.

One caution: reagent strips may be sensitive to extreme weather conditions. As a result, they should be stored in the airtight container that they come in unless they are individually foil wrapped. The expiration date on the bottle should be noted as well.

A diagnosis of diabetes should not be made *solely* on the results of a reagent strip analysis. Instead, the individual should also have a fasting blood glucose level or an ORAL GLUCOSE TOLERANCE TEST (OGTT). (See also DIAGNOSIS; HOME BLOOD GLUCOSE MONITORING.)

religion/spirituality Spiritual belief in a higher power, which may include practices in the rituals that are associated with an organized religious group, such as prayer, singing, or other religious practices. For the majority of Americans, religion plays an important part in their lives, and 62 percent attend religious services at least monthly. For many people in other countries, religion also plays a key role. Religion may enable people to cope more effectively with their illnesses, including diabetes.

Several studies have indicated that individuals who are regular attendees at their place of worship actually live longer. In one such study, 2,025 Marin County, California residents over age 55 were followed for five years. Researchers found that the best predictor for those who were still alive at the end of the study was weekly attendance at religious services.

The researchers attempted to determine the cause for the enhanced longevity of the religious attendees. They factored out chronic diseases such as diabetes, as well as sex, race, and other variables, but they still could not discover the reason for the increased life expectancy of the religious attendees. The authors said, "Even after controlling for six classes of potential confounding and intervening variables, we were unable to explain the protection against mortality offered by religious attendance."

Some experts believe that places of worship may also be an effective place to provide individuals with information on diabetes and even to offer screening to them. In an article published in the *American Journal of Health Studies* in 1998, researcher Michael Kelly reported on a study of individuals screened for diabetes at four Catholic churches on the West Texas/Mexico border. Many of the attendees were Hispanics, a group at high risk for diabetes. Many American Diabetes Association affiliates have formed relationships with African-American churches for the same purpose.

Kelly concluded, "Some churches are becoming more receptive to secondary health intervention, such as diabetes and heart disease screening. . . . Still more progressive churches are exploring the realm of primary health intervention, better known as health education and promotion."

When Faith and Medicine Clash

Sometimes a person's religious beliefs may interfere with what a physician believes to be medically best or even necessary. Confronted with such a conflict, the physician may discuss the situation in the context of the patient's spirituality or enlist the aid of a clergyperson. However, sometimes those options are not available or possible or they do not work.

In some cases, the courts or law enforcement may be drawn in. For example, in 1996, a 16-year-old girl with diabetes died at her home in Altoona, Pennsylvania, because her parents had refused to provide her with medical treatment and relied instead upon prayer. The girl, whose

blood sugar level was 18 times the norm, died and her parents were charged with manslaughter. The Pennsylvania Supreme Court upheld their conviction in 2000.

Associated Press, "Faith-Healing Parents Convicted of Manslaughter," *St. Louis Post-Dispatch,* November 29, 2000.
Michael P. Kelly, "Diabetes Screening and Health Education at Roman Catholic Churches Along the West Texas Mexico Border," *American Journal of Health Studies* 14, no. 1 (January 1998): 48.
David B. Larson, M.D., M.S.P.H., et al., "Patient Spirituality in Clinical Care: Clinical Assessment and Research Findings: Part One," *Primary Care Reports Archives* (October 2, 2000).
Douglas Oman, and Dwayne Reed, "Religion and Mortality among the Community-Dwelling Elderly," *American Journal of Public Health* 88, no. 10 (1998): 1469–1475.

renal replacement therapy Refers to dialysis (peritoneal at home or hemodialysis in a clinic) or kidney transplantation. The most severe complication of diabetic kidney damage is END-STAGE RENAL DISEASE (ESRD), a disease more common among people with diabetes than among nondiabetics.

repaglinide See MEGLITINIDES.

research See CLINICAL RESEARCH.

retinopathy See DIABETIC RETINOPATHY, EYE PROBLEMS.

risk factors Factors that increase the risk for the development or worsening of diabetes. There are a variety of racial/ethnic, genetic, and environmental factors that increase the probability of a person suffering from diabetes.

Genetics

The highest risk for diabetes occurs when both biological parents have the illness.

Environmental

Some researchers have found linkages between the onset of Type 1 diabetes and the individual's contracting of a virus, particularly the mumps or Coxsackie virus.

Obesity

Excessive weight or obesity is a risk factor for Type 2 diabetes in those who have a genetic predisposition to the illness. The majority of people with Type 2 diabetes are obese. Improvements or even complete remission may occur with weight loss.

RR intervals Refers to the time from one heartbeat to the next as measured by electrocardiogram. The "R" represents electrical activity from the ventricle. Normally, people have some variation in the R to R interval with normal breathing. If a patient with diabetes develops autonomic neuropathy, however, this variation is lost and indicates that the patient is at higher risk of arrhythmia and sudden death.

RR intervals can be measured by having the patient perform specific breathing maneuvers while being hooked up to an electrocardiogram.

Scandinavian Simvastatin Survival Study (4-S Study) A study of 4,444 patients ages 35–70 years who had prior CORONARY HEART DISEASE and high CHOLESTEROL levels. The subjects included people with and without diabetes. They were given either drug therapy with Zocor (Simvastatin) to lower their cholesterol levels or they were given a placebo. This study is significant for people with diabetes because of the high rate of heart disease that occurs among people with diabetes. Also, the data on the patients with diabetes were reported on as a subgroup and then compared to the total group.

The subjects were followed for about five years. The medication was extremely effective and reduced the risk of death from coronary heart disease among patients with previous MYOCARDIAL INFARCTION. The drug also reduced the risk of major coronary events (fatal and near fatal myocardial infarctions).

The patients with diabetes showed even more dramatic improvements than nondiabetic coronary heart patients. The patients with diabetes reduced their cholesterol levels and also showed a 54 percent risk reduction in major coronary events. In contrast, patients without diabetes had only a 32 percent risk reduction. This study proved the importance of cholesterol levels to the person with diabetes as well as the effectiveness of medication to counteract high levels of cholesterol. (See also HDL, LDL.)

T. R. Pedersen et al., "Baseline Serum Cholesterol and Treatment Effect in the Scandinavian Simvastatin Survival Study," *The Lancet* 345, no. 8960 (May 20, 1995): 1274–1275.

T. R. Pedersen et al., "Safety and Tolerability of Cholesterol Lowering with Simvastatin During 5 Years in the Scandinavian Simvastatin Survival Study," *Archives of Internal Medicine* 156 (October 14, 1996): 2085–2092.

school Educational institution. Attendance at a school is required by most cultures for a given period of time. Some individuals with diabetes have experienced problems in the school environment, almost always those with Type 1 diabetes who must self-inject insulin. It is hoped that the AMERICANS WITH DISABILITIES ACT has or will resolve most of these problems; however, reports of problems continue to crop up.

Another law that affects children with diabetes is Section 504 of the Rehabilitation Act of 1973, still in force in the United States. This law protects students from discrimination when they have a "physical or mental impairment that substantially limits one or more of major life activities." This law applies to all public schools and any private schools that receive federal dollars.

Parents can request that the accommodation needed by the child be placed in the child's school record. However, since many teachers do not review student records, individual teachers should also be informed about the child's diabetes and what is needed.

According to the American Diabetes Association, some types of accommodations the school may be expected to make under Section 504 are:

- allowing a child to self-test glucose levels and act on the results

- permitting children to eat when they need to and have enough time to eat
- allowing extra bathroom trips as well as trips to the water fountain
- planning for where the child's insulin will be tested and insulin given

Missed Days at School

According to the 1994 National Health Survey, children with diabetes have a higher rate of missing school than children who do not have diabetes. In a two-week period, about 14 percent of children with diabetes missed one or more days of school, compared to 8 percent of nondiabetic children. It is unclear why the children missed these days, although illness is assumed.

Difficulties to Anticipate and Resolve

Children with Type 1 diabetes have an additional burden to overcome in school, because they require insulin to live. Yet many schools have been reluctant to either allow children to test their own blood and administer insulin themselves, or to provide other individuals who will perform these functions if children cannot (or are not allowed to) perform these necessary tasks for their continued health and life.

The Americans with Disabilities Act requires accommodations for a disabled individual at school as well as in the workplace, and the AMERICAN DIABETES ASSOCIATION and others have successfully prevailed in lawsuits where school boards attempted to block children from needed care. In some cases, parents have sued and prevailed because they wanted the school to be prepared to administer emergency GLUCAGON in the event of an incident of HYPOGLYCEMIA.

If the child is old enough and is allowed to test his or her blood and administer insulin, the child needs a place and time to accomplish this in the school, as well as privacy.

Even something as mundane as eating lunch in the cafeteria can present a problem for children with diabetes, if the typical fare is heavily laden with carbohydrates and non-nutritious foods. In addition, if children in school are rewarded with candy and sweets, this presents yet another problem for the child with diabetes. First, the child generally would like to eat the candy. Second, children may feel singled out if they refuse candy. In addition, unaware adults often press candy on children, telling them that it is all right, one piece of cake won't hurt and so forth. For these reasons, it is important for parents and children to inform teachers about the child's diabetes and to repeat the information as needed. (See also DISCRIMINATION.)

Shereen Arent, National Director of Legal Advocacy, American Diabetes Association, "Major Federal Education Laws Affecting Children with Diabetes," April 2000. (Available at: www.Diabetes.org/advocacy/schoollaw.asp.)

William L. Clarke, M.D., "Advocating for the Child with Diabetes," *Diabetes Spectrum* 12, no. 4 (1999): 230–235.

screening for diabetes Testing of an individual to determine if he or she may have diabetes (or another illness). According to the AMERICAN DIABETES ASSOCIATION, the prevalence of diabetes among American adults was about 7.4 percent in 1995. That prevalence was expected to increase to about 9 percent by 2025.

Screening for diabetes may be indicated in patients who have close family members with diabetes, especially if they have risk factors, such as OBESITY. This is particularly true if they are displaying any prominent symptoms, such as extreme thirst or hunger or constant urination. If a person is diagnosed and treated for diabetes in the early stages, often many COMPLICATIONS of diabetes can be avoided in the future, assuming that the person performs HOME BLOOD GLUCOSE MONITORING, takes prescribed medications, and works to maintain a normal weight.

Generally, it is more apparent that an individual has Type 1 diabetes than Type 2 diabetes. The individual with Type 1 diabetes has usually had a weight loss, is not obese, and is often experiencing extreme symptoms.

During PREGNANCY, many obstetricians screen for diabetes because the disease can have a profound effect on both the mother and her fetus. With good prenatal care and adherence to medical guidelines, most women with diabetes can have a healthy normal child.

Screening for Type 2 Diabetes: Risk Factors

Some subgroups within the population have a greater risk for diabetes than others. For example, AFRICAN AMERICANS, HISPANICS, and NATIVE AMERICANS are at high risk for Type 2 diabetes. The risk for developing Type 2 diabetes also rises with increasing age as well as with other factors, such as OBESITY, HYPERTENSION or a physically inactive lifestyle. A family history of diabetes is another risk factor. Physicians take such factors into account when determining whether screening for diabetes should occur in an individual case. A woman who has delivered a very large baby (over nine pounds) or who has had GESTATIONAL DIABETES is also at risk for developing Type 2 diabetes.

Because impaired glucose tolerance is common and about 10 percent of patients per year will progress to diabetes, screening is important.

Testing for Diabetes

Physicians usually use the FASTING PLASMA GLUCOSE (FPG) TEST or the ORAL GLUCOSE TOLERANCE TEST (OGTT) to test an individual for either Type 1 or Type 2 diabetes. The American Diabetes Association recommends the FPG test because it is easier and faster and it is less expensive than the OGTT.

If the FPG test is given, and the results are equal to or greater than 125 mg/dL, this is an indicator of diabetes and the test is usually done again to confirm the diagnosis. Normal glucose levels for the FPG are less than 110. If the FPG is between 110–125, this is called impaired fasting glucose. If the FPG is less than 126 but the physician is still suspicious of diabetes, he may choose to order an OGTT. If the glucose level in the OGTT after two hours is greater than or equal to 200 mg/dL, this is positive for diabetes. (See also DIAGNOSIS, SYMPTOMS.)

American Diabetes Association, "Screening for Diabetes," Diabetes Care 24, Supp. 1 (2001): 521–524.
Michael M. Engelgau, M.D., M.S., et al. "Screening for Type 2 Diabetes," *Diabetes Care,* 23, no. 10 (October 2000): 1563–1580.

secondary diabetes Diabetes that is either caused by conditions stemming from another illness such as excessive growth hormone found in ACROMEGALY, or by excessive iron found in hemochromatosis or excessive cortisol found in CUSHING'S DISEASE/SYNDROME. Diabetes may also be induced by medications or chemicals, such as the excessive use of steroid drugs, pentamidine, or diuretic drugs. Physicians seek to find the underlying cause in order to eliminate the diabetes or to make it less severe.

self-care/self-monitoring Personal management of a medical problem, such as diabetes. Although physicians, diabetes nurse educators, and other experts can provide a great deal of advice and information, the reality is that people with diabetes must take charge of their own self-care. This includes periodic blood testing, monitoring the diet, often taking prescribed medication and visiting their physician on a regular basis. Both patient and doctor need to perform monitoring for any signs or symptoms that the diabetes has gone beyond the normal range. However, patients must do most monitoring themselves.

Such monitoring is extremely important and often can mean the difference between relative stability as well as the avoidance of serious complications.

The failure to adequately monitor glucose levels can ultimately lead to a variety of very severe conditions such as blindness, amputation of limbs, kidney and heart disease, and even death. It may also lead to DIABETIC KETOACIDOSIS (DKA), a very dangerous condition requiring hospitalization.

Because of the importance of self-care among people with diabetes, experts say that physicians must take on much more of a partnership role, and one that is very different from what they may be used to maintaining with their other patients. According to a manual called "Basic Practice Guidelines for Diabetes Mellitus," jointly prepared by the South Dakota Diabetes Control Program and the South Dakota Diabetes Advisory Council in 1999,

> This represents a major paradigm shift in which new roles are required from both the patient and provider. Patients need to understand and accept that diabetes care is their personal responsibility. In addition, professionals need to assume their 'new' role as consultant and view the patient as the decision maker.

The physician must also help patients develop strategies to work out changes themselves, rather than depending on flat directives issued by their doctors. The South Dakota experts said,

> The tendency to solve problems for the patients rather than helping them work through a problem is another barrier. If the person is in need of technical expertise, for instance, making the glucose meter work, such behavior is warranted. On the contrary, most challenges facing people are more psychosocially based than technical, for example, 'it is very hard for me to cut back on fat in my diet, when my family insists on eating fried foods all of the time.' In this situation, the solution needs to be addressed by the patient, with selected input from the provider. It is the process of helping the patient discover the capacity to creatively think and find solutions to their work problems. This empowerment creates and reinforces their self-efficacy and responsibility for the treatment of their diabetes.
>
> In order for the professionals to use the empowerment approach with success, patients need to believe that they are viewed as the 'driver' in the diabetes care process.

South Dakota Diabetes Control Program and South Dakota Diabetes Advisory Council, "Basic Practice Guidelines for Diabetes Mellitus," February 1999.

sexuality and sexual problems   The impact of diabetes on sexual desire or sexual problems experienced by men and women. Adults with diabetes may experience a variety of sexual problems that stem from their illness, although according to the AMERICAN DIABETES ASSOCIATION, the topic of sexual problems is often avoided by both patients with diabetes and their physicians. The subject may embarrass them or the patient may believe that there is nothing that can be done. However, in many cases, doctors do (or should) know about ways to assist patients struggling with sexual problems related to their diabetes.

The most prominent sexual problem that men with diabetes may suffer from is ERECTILE DYSFUNCTION. Both men and women with diabetes may also experience a lack of sexual desire.

WOMEN WITH DIABETES may have problems with vaginal lubrication or pain that occurs during sex (dyspareunia) because of dryness or another reason. The doctor may recommend a vaginal lubricant and may also advise the woman to try Kegel exercises, which are muscle-tightening exercises in the pelvic area.

Women with diabetes may also suffer from NEUROGENIC BLADDER, or bladder spasms and leakage of urine. Doctors may advise women with such problems to urinate before and then again after having sex. This practice will also help the woman to prevent vaginal and bladder infections, which is important, since many women with diabetes are prone to such infections. (See also IMPOTENCE.)

shoes, therapeutic   Special shoes to help a person with a medical problem. The MEDICARE THERAPEUTIC SHOE ACT, passed in 1993, provides for the coverage of special shoes and shoe modifications for patients who have diabetes and other conditions, such as recurrent foot ulcers, neuropathy, a partial or total foot amputation and other conditions. In addition, many private health insurance companies also provide coverage for special shoes for individuals with diabetes, particularly those with Type 1 diabetes who are at risk for DIABETIC NEUROPATHY. Despite this coverage, research indicates that only a minority of older patients with diabetes are purchasing therapeutic shoes. (See also FOOT CARE.)

shoulder dystocia   A birthing crisis in which the baby's shoulder and arm are trapped on the pelvic bone of the mother. This can harm the baby's neck and cause paralysis in one or both arms. This injury is referred to as a "brachial plexus injury." The baby may also suffer from ERB'S PALSY.

Mothers with diabetes or GESTATIONAL DIA-BETES are at risk for having a baby with shoulder dystocia. Other risk factors are:

* having a large baby (nine pounds or more)
* obesity of the mother
* excessive weight gain of the mother during pregnancy (over 35 pounds)
* a baby that is overdue: more than 40 weeks in gestation

To decrease the risk of the baby experiencing shoulder dystocia, pregnant women should work with their obstetricians and their diabetes specialists, such as endocrinologists, registered dietitians, and nurses. The physician may also suggest an implantable pump for better glycemic control. (See also GESTATIONAL DIABETES, PREGNANCY.)

sick day rules   Encompasses the general management concepts to use during illness which physicians/nurses/dietitians teach patients who have diabetes. These concepts will help them when they are sick with other illnesses in addition to diabetes, such as a severe cold, the flu, or another ailment that makes it difficult to eat or drink or to take normal care of themselves.

Some people think that when people with diabetes are ill, they need not worry about their diet or fluid intake. This is not true because sickness can cause blood sugar to rise due to a lack of food or fluid intake. It is also very important for the sick person to continue to take diabetes medication as well as to test blood sugars and write down the results, so that the information can be reported to the doctor. Ill people with diabetes are at risk for the extremes of either HYPOGLYCEMIA or DIABETIC KETOACIDOSIS (DKA)/HYPEROSMOLAR COMA, both of which can be life-threatening conditions.

It is almost inevitable that at some point, the person with diabetes will develop an illness. As a result, it is important to develop a plan for what to do *before* the person becomes sick. A written checklist may be helpful, because many people do not think as clearly as normal when they are feeling ill. If they can instead refer to a simple checklist, it is more likely that they will be able to follow it. If the patient wishes to develop such a list, it should be reviewed with their physician. (A very simplified list of basic "to do" items are included in this essay.)

Principles Underlying Sick Day Rules

Patients with diabetes need a basic understanding of the fact that when people are sick, they are also under stress from their own bodies, in response to the bacteria, virus or other medical problem they are experiencing.

An illness is a form of physiological stress (mental or physical, or both) that will induce the release of stress hormones. Some examples of these stress hormones are adrenaline (epinephrine), noradrenaline (norepinephrine), cortisol, growth hormones, and GLUCAGON. Stress hormones are also released when a person becomes ill and/or feverish.

Avoiding risk of ketone buildup   If stress levels continue to increase (i.e. an increase in insulin resistance or decrease in insulin sensitivity), the body becomes less able to utilize glucose and to store fatty acids in fat and instead, begins to break down fat into fuel for the body. The breakdown product of these fats is ketone bodies or ketoacids. As a result, when a person with diabetes is ill, he or she needs to test their urine for KETONES to avoid further complications such as DIABETIC KETOACIDOSIS or HYPEROSMOLAR COMA. Over-the-counter REAGENT STRIPS can measure these ketone levels.

If a significant amount of ketones is found in the urine, then the person who takes insulin needs more insulin. If the person is unable to eat or drink because of nausea and vomiting, and glucose levels are falling because the person has injected insulin, then he or she needs to go to a hospital emergency room for an intravenous infusion of both insulin and glucose.

If the Patient Takes Insulin

Unfortunately for the person with diabetes who uses insulin, all of these stress hormones counteract the effects of INSULIN. They either cause insulin to work less well than usual or they cause more glucose to enter the circulation from where it was stored in the liver. Either way, the glucose in the system tends to increase. Even if a person has not eaten anything and may have been vomiting and/or had diarrhea, blood glucose levels tend to increase.

As mentioned, many people think that if they are not eating anything, then they don't have to worry about coping with their diabetes. This is a serious mistake that could lead to acute diabetic complications necessitating emergency room visit or hospitalization. In fact, when a person is sick, he or she may need *more* than their normal dose of insulin, even when not eating.

If the Patient Is on Oral Medications

Even if a person with diabetes does not need insulin, it is still important to establish Sick Day Rules. The effect of the illness can throw the system off and put the patient at risk for a more serious illness than whatever temporary medical problem he or she is experiencing.

Avoiding Dehydration Is Important

Another problem that may occur when a person with diabetes is ill is that as glucose levels rise, the person may develop GLYCOSURIA (glucose in the urine) and experience DEHYDRATION. This dehydration will worsen rising glucose levels. As a result, a second principle for patients with diabetes is that when they are sick, they need to push themselves to drink fluids in order to stay well hydrated. Most patients who are sick are told to drink plenty of fluids, whether they have diabetes or not. But this advice is even more important for people with diabetes. The ill person should drink 6–8 ounces of fluid every waking hour. Recommended fluids include: water, diet ginger ale, broth or decaffeinated tea. If the ill person cannot eat, nondiet liquids should be consumed every other hour, such as 4 ounces of apple juice or Gatorade.

If the Ill Person Cannot Follow Meal Plans or Cannot Eat At All

When people with diabetes cannot follow their normal meal plans, experts say that they may replace the carbohydrate portion of meals by eating items such as orange juice ($1/2$ cup), regular yogurt with fruit ($1/3$ cup), regular ice cream ($1/2$ cup) and honey (1 tablespoon). One or two of these items can be eaten every one to two hours.

Contacting the Physician Right Away

People with diabetes who are sick should call their doctor right away if any of the following conditions are present:

- diarrhea for more than 24 hours
- blood sugar levels above 300 in two or more tests
- low blood sugar
- vomiting or inability to keep any fluids down for two to three hours

If a Patient Cannot Comply with Sick Day Rules

If the patient is so sick that he or she cannot comply with these recommendations, then another family member or other person should provide such care. If sick day rules are not followed, the person with diabetes may need hospitalization, depending on how long the sickness lasts, how severe it is and how debilitated the patient was before the illness.

Summarizing the Basics

In summary, the patient with diabetes who is also sick with another illness that makes them unable to perform their normal activities, such as illnesses that cause nausea and vomiting, should:

- Check glucose levels every one to three hours, depending upon the situation and severity of illness.
- Check and recheck urine ketones until they are negative and the person is feeling much better.
- Continue taking insulin, preferably short-acting insulin.
- Push fluids, drinking as much as tolerated to avoid lightheadedness/dizziness. Patients often may need to drink high calorie beverages that they typically avoid in order to take in some nutrition at this time.
- Contact the physician for diagnosis and advice on how to treat the underlying illness as well as advice on any recommended variations of the insulin dosage and or oral medications.

Joslin Diabetes Center affiliate at New Britain General Hospital, New Britain, Connecticut and Joslin Diabetes Clinic, Boston, Massachusetts, "Sick Day Guidelines Nutrition Management," 1995.

Singapore   Asian country whose residents have a very high rate of diabetes. According to the World Health Organization in 2000, nearly one-third of Singapore residents (27 percent) ages 30–69 have diabetes. The rise in diabetes in Singapore was primarily attributed to both affluence and an aging population.

Parliamentary Secretary for Health Chan Soo Sen noted that it was important to encourage healthy lifestyles and exercise. He added, "A good management programme calls for a high degree of continued selfcare and discipline on the part of patients."

skilled nursing facilities (SNFs, nursing homes) Refers to long-term care facilities for the aged and disabled. Some nursing facilities also offer temporary rehabilitative services to those who are not ill enough to remain in the hospital but who are too sick to return home. Many skilled nursing facilities receive payments for their residents from MEDICARE or MEDICAID. The rules for who may be admitted to a SNF under Medicare or Medicaid rules vary, as well as the rules on how long individuals may stay in a facility.

Because diabetes is a very common ailment among older people, SNF staffs need to be aware of the symptoms of diabetes, glucose testing, and symptoms of an individual who may be in danger. They also should be very knowledgeable about the medications used by people with diabetes as well as side effects and differences in reactions that older individuals may have to medications.

Many older people have problems with slow stomach emptying (GASTROPARESIS) and many also have more than one illness, such as the combination of HYPERTENSION and diabetes. It is important for the staff to be very aware of these illnesses as well as problems with medication interactions. (See also ASSISTED LIVING FACILITIES, ELDERLY.)

skin problems   Pain or itching of the skin. Some individuals with diabetes have a serious problem with dry and itchy skin and, consequently, need to use skin moisturizers on a regular basis. It's also important for people with diabetes to perform regular checks of their feet because they are more prone to developing problems, which can become very serious, particularly if the person suffers from DIABETIC NEUROPATHY and/or PERIPHERAL VASCULAR DISEASE.

Some examples of skin problems that may occur in people with diabetes are:

- acanthosis nigricans
- acquired perforating dermatosis (a condition of small dome-shaped papules (flat lesions) or nodules (small bumps) with a crust-filled center)
- diabetic bullae (blisters)
- granuloma annulare (fleshy red papules or plaques arranged like pearls on strings in a semicircle. Center is unaffected and borders are raised. Most commonly seen on backs of hands or on feet or legs)
- xerosis (very dry skin)
- fungal infections, such as Tinea pedis (feet), Tinea cruris (groin), and Tinea capitis (scalp)

One uncommon form of skin disorder in some people with diabetes is necrobiosis lipoidica diabeticorum. This disease was first described in 1929 and is strongly associated with Type 1 diabetes. The disease is four times more common in women than men. Sixty percent of those with the disorder have diabetes and most of the remaining patients have impaired glucose tolerance or impaired fasting glucose levels. In 10–20 percent of the cases, the problem resolves on its own. No therapies are effective.

Scleroderma diabeticorum is another skin condition associated with diabetes. It slowly evolves without preceding infection or trauma. It typically starts as a nonpitting thickening in the neck area and can involve the neck, back, trunk, and even legs. It is four times more common in men, usually those with long-term diabetes. It is usually not painful and there is no known treatment. The cause is unknown. (See also FOOT CARE, PRURITIS.)

smoking Use of tobacco products that are smoked. An estimated 27 percent of all Americans smoke, despite widespread disapproval among many groups, and the nearly universal acceptance that smoking is bad for everyone. Smoking is especially unhealthy for people with diabetes and may exacerbate many complications of the disease. Smoking is also very dangerous for women and, in fact, more American women die of lung cancer than of breast cancer.

In the United States, the percentage of people smoking varies greatly from state to state. For example, in 1998, the lowest rate (14 percent) was in Utah and the highest rate (31 percent) was in Kentucky. People from many other countries are also heavy smokers and, as a result, suffer similar health problems as American smokers.

Studies of cigarette smokers reveal that in about half the cases of death (52 percent of men and 43 percent of women), the cause of the deaths was attributed to smoking. Millions of people worldwide smoke, making them at risk for a broad array of severe ailments, including CARDIOVASCULAR DISEASES, cancer, respiratory ailments, DIABETIC RETINOPATHY, NEUROPATHY, and other illnesses.

According to an article in a 2000 issue of *Diabetes Care*, "Smoking cessation is one of the few interventions that can safely and cost-effectively be recommended for all patients and has been identified as a gold standard against which other preventive behaviors should be evaluated."

In a study of 1,266 middle-aged men (35–59 years old) in Japan reported in the *Annals of Internal Medicine* in 2000, the number of cigarettes smoked per day and the number of packs smoked per year were positively associated with the risk of developing impaired fasting glucose and Type 2 diabetes.

Diabetic Smokers

It is problematic when people with diabetes smoke because in addition to the well-known health risks for the average person, smoking further increases an already elevated risk for the person with diabetes in developing heart and/or kidney disease. It also raises the probability of the individual ultimately suffering from BLINDNESS, cancer, heart attacks, STROKES, amputations of limbs, and a broad array of other ailments.

Yet, according to the previously alluded to issue of *Diabetes Care,* only about half of all smokers with diabetes are advised by their own physicians that they should quit smoking to avoid the likely health consequences. It is unclear whether physicians feel they do not have enough time to emphasize smoking cessation or if doctors believe patients would not listen. There may be other reasons for failing to stress to diabetic patients that they should stop smoking. Some experts believe that if diabetic smokers were made aware of the full severity of the possible consequences of continued smoking, then many of them would stop smoking.

Sometimes the mere act of being diagnosed with diabetes is apparently sufficient to motivate a person to quit smoking. Presumably at least part of the impetus for this motivation is that, upon initial diagnosis, a physician would usually urge a newly diagnosed person with diabetes to end their smoking habit immediately to avoid future severe health risks.

A study, performed at the University of Michigan and reported at the annual meeting of the American Diabetes Association in 2000, found that in a sample of smokers, those diagnosed with diabetes between 1992 and 1994 were twice as likely to stop smoking by 1996 than other smokers.

Researcher Linda Wray, Ph.D. concluded, "It seems that a big medical shock is what it takes to scare some Americans out of their tobacco habits, and some keep smoking despite the increased risk that the combination of their disease and smoking poses."

Interestingly, smokers with diabetes who were also obese in this study were also significantly more likely to stop smoking.

In looking at the demographics of smokers, they tend to be of lower income and are less educated than the general population. Individu-als with less than a high school education are more likely to be smokers and there is an inverse relationship between years of education and smoking. That is, college graduates are less likely to smoke than high school graduates. Individuals with diabetes appear to smoke at about the same level as people who don't have diabetes, although, as mentioned, smoking is even more dangerous for people who are diabetic.

Smoking as a Possible Cause of Diabetes

Some studies seem to indicate that smoking may be a cause or trigger of the development of Type 2 diabetes in individuals who have a genetic predisposition to the illness. In one study of nearly 42,000 men in the United States who were followed for six years, the men who smoked more than 25 cigarettes per day developed diabetes at about twice (1.94) the rate of nonsmokers. A study of about 2,000 Japanese men reported similar results.

In a study of about 114,000 women smokers who were followed for eight years, about 2,000 of the women subsequently developed Type 2 diabetes. In this study, women who smoked more than 25 cigarettes daily had a moderately greater risk (1.42) of developing diabetes than nonsmokers.

Some researchers have also found that prediabetic insulin resistance was much higher among smokers.

Smoking Cessation Medications

There are a variety of medications that smokers may use to withdraw from cigarettes. Nicotine is available in the form of gum, nasal spray, patch, or inhaler. Good success has also been found with medications such as bupropion (Zyban). In a study of the sustained-release form of bupropion, the following smoking cessation results were found, drawn from the researchers' data. As can be seen from these results, even the lowest dose of the medication produced cessation results that were better than placebo.

Placebo (sugar pill) group	100 mg bupropion	150 mg	300 mg
12.4%	19.6%	22.9%	23.1%

Other Cessation Treatments

In addition to nicotine replacement therapy and Zyban, some smokers find success with hypnotherapy or group or individual psychotherapy. One breakthrough treatment that is undergoing clinical trials is an antismoking vaccine (NicVAX) that physicians hope will radically diminish the amount of nicotine that will reach the brain. Clinical results on rats indicate that the vaccine induced the development of antibodies which then acted to neutralize nicotine in the blood and reduce the level that reached the brain by 65 percent.

The theory is (if the vaccine is approved in humans), when smokers receive this one-time injection, afterwards, if they smoke, they will experience only a diminished nicotine surge to the brain. Thus, it should be easier to quit smoking. At this time, it is unknown if or when the vaccine will be available to the public.

"Smoking and Diabetes," *Diabetes Care* 24, no. 1, supplement 1 (2001): S64–S65.
Debra Haire-Joshu, Ph.D., "Smoking and Diabetes," *Diabetes Care* 22, no. 11 (1999): 1887–1898.
N. Nakanishi et al., "Cigarette Smoking and Risk for Impaired Fasting Glucose and Type 2 Diabetes in Middle-Aged Japanese Men," *Annals of Internal Medicine* 133 (2000): 183–191.
Barbara Shine, "Nicotine Vaccine Moves toward Clinical Trials," *NIDA Notes* 15, no. 5 (2000).

Social Security Disability Disability payment that is usually accompanied by MEDICARE coverage for eligible individuals. For example, if a person has been employed in the past and has now become disabled due to BLINDNESS or another disability, then he or she may be eligible for a Social Security disability payment prior to attaining retirement age. Some adults younger than age 65 are eligible for SSA dis-

ability as are some widowed individuals. The person must formally apply for this disability and provide documentation to support the claim.

According to the Social Security Administration, 82,106 people with diabetes received Social Security disability as of December 2000, including 76,496 disabled workers, 5,247 widowed people, and 363 adult children. (See also DISABILITY, MEDICAID, MEDICARE.)

sorbitol A sugar alcohol that is produced by the body and that may contribute to tissue damage found in the nerves, eyes, and kidneys. An alternative definition is that of an artificial sweetener that is primarily used in diet foods. If an excess amount is ingested, it will cause diarrhea. Sorbitol is not calorie free.

SSI (Supplemental Security Insurance) A public assistance program for indigent and disabled individuals. Launched in 1974, SSI is funded by federal and state funds and provides the individual with a monthly check and MEDICAID benefits as well. The amount of payments is based on the individual's income in a formula that is used by the Social Security Administration. As of December 2000, there were 39,996 people with diabetes receiving SSI benefits, according to statistics provided by the Social Security Administration.

Most SSI recipients are disabled (79 percent). Twenty percent are aged and 1 percent are blind. Most recipients (56 percent) are between the ages of 18 and 64, followed by 31 percent who are ages 65 or older and 13 percent who are under age 18. Most SSI recipients (59 percent) are females. Disabled individuals receiving SSI benefits are re-evaluated at least every three years to verify that they are still disabled and poor. (See also DISABILITY, MEDICAID.)

Electronic communication between Christine Adamec and Social Security Administration officials on May 16, 2001.

Starlix See PHENYLALANINE DERIVATIVES.

stiff man syndrome A very rare neurological syndrome wherein patients develop progressive rigidity due to abnormal gamma amino butyric acid (GABA) neurotransmission. The GAD antibody was first described in this syndrome. GAD is the enzyme needed to synthesize GAA. About one third of these patients have Type 1 diabetes.

stress Increased emotional strain due to family, personal or work problems (or a combination of all of them). Stress can make individuals with diabetes feel much worse, because they may be less likely to monitor their symptoms carefully and because stress can exacerbate already-existing symptoms. It can also make it more difficult to maintain GLYCEMIC CONTROL. Stress may also refer to a physical strain on the body, such as that caused by illness and which induces the release of stress hormones such as EPINEPHRINE.

Some researchers have hypothesized that psychological stress and/or DEPRESSION can in some cases lead to the onset of Type 2 diabetes, particularly if a person has an underlying genetic predisposition to develop diabetes with insulin resistance.

"Dutch Study Finds Stress Increases Risk of Diabetes," *Diabetes Management Archives* (May 1, 2000) n.p.

stress tests/exercise tolerance tests Tests that are administered on a treadmill and other devices and which help determine a person's overall physical stamina and the heart's response to exercise. Before people with diabetes undergo an EXERCISE regimen, their physicians may recommend a stress test to ensure they are healthy enough to undergo the type of exercise they have chosen. This is particularly true if they have or are at risk for CARDIOVASCULAR DISEASE.

People who are able to walk may have a simple treadmill test, with monitoring of the heart, blood pressure, and pulse. For those unable to walk well or for as long as six to 12 minutes, the cardiologist may administer a nuclear stress test with thallium or sestamibi to take pictures of the heart. In addition, medications such as dipyridamole and dobutamine may be given to artificially "stress" the heart.

stroke A sudden and life-threatening loss of blood flow to a part of the brain that results in damage or death of brain cells and may be fatal. Also known as a "brain attack." People with diabetes have a greater risk for stroke, particularly those with DIABETIC NEPHROPATHY and HYPERTENSION. They also have at least twice the risk of death from stroke compared to nondiabetics.

Very prompt medical attention often means the difference between life and death for the person who has had a stroke. If patients receive medical attention within one to three hours of a stroke, their chances of survival are much greater because the patient may be given a medication that dissolves the blood clots that obstruct arteries, a common cause of a stroke. Immediate medical attention may also improve the prognosis for later health and decrease the severity of problems with long-term disability that many stroke patients suffer.

A stroke may cause the following medical consequences:

- temporary or permanent paralysis
- cognitive (thinking) problems
- language deficits
- pain
- emotional problems
- death: about 15 percent of stroke victims die soon after the stroke and stroke is the third leading cause of death in the United States

Important Precautions for People with Diabetes

Because of the risks related to stroke, it is very important for everyone who has diabetes to maintain excellent glycemic control and also to work to attain as near to normal as possible blood pressure (less than 135/85 mm Hg) levels. Tobacco products should be avoided altogether because tobacco increases the risk of stroke. It is also important to keep lipids at goal levels set by the physician, in order to avoid a first stroke as well as to decrease the later probability of another stroke.

Symptoms of Stroke

According to the National Institute of Neurological Disorders and Stroke in Bethesda, Maryland, if a person has one or more of any of the following symptoms, they should seek immediate emergency attention. In the United States, the individual or others should call 911 for emergency assistance. The patient should not drive, nor should others take the person to the hospital. Instead, in most cases, an ambulance is best.

The danger symptoms of stroke are:

- sudden confusion in understanding speech or in speaking
- sudden numbness in the face, leg, or arm, especially if it is on one side of the body only
- sudden blindness or difficulty seeing in one or both eyes
- sudden inability or a severe difficulty in walking

Risk Factors for Stroke

As mentioned, people with diabetes are at a greater risk for experiencing a stroke than the general population. Other risk factors for stroke include:

- hypertension (high blood pressure)
- history of heart disease, particularly atrial fibrillation or irregular heartbeat in the left upper chamber of the heart
- history of transient ischemic attacks (TIAs), or mini-strokes
- cigarette smoking: heavy smokers are at greatest risk
- obesity

- race: African Americans have a risk of stroke that is nearly twice that of Caucasians. In addition, African Americans who are between the ages of 45–55 years and who have a stroke face a five to six times greater risk of dying from a stroke than a white American of the same age who has had a stroke
- age greater than 65 years old
- high count of low-density lipoprotein (LDL) cholesterol count (in patients with diabetes the goal is less than 100 mg/dl)
- high consumption of alcohol
- use of illegal drugs, especially ones that can elevate blood pressure, cause irregular heart rhythms, or cause blood vessels to constrict such as cocaine and amphetamines

Diagnosis of Stroke

When an individual has possible stroke symptoms, doctors generally use radiologic methods to verify whether the person has actually had a stroke and, if a stroke has occurred, to determine the degree of severity. Physicians may use computed tomography (CT) scans of the brain to determine if an acute stroke has occurred. Another diagnostic device is the magnetic resonance imaging (MRI) scan, which can detect the tiny after effects of a stroke, such as an increase in the water content of the brain tissue, also called cytotoxic edema.

Physicians may use ultrasound to image the carotid arteries. These images will assist the doctor in identifying blockages or clots. Magnetic resonance angiography (MRA) is rapidly replacing conventional angiography as a technique to look for blockages in blood vessels in the brain, including blockages of both the carotid arteries (anterior) and the vertebral arteries (posterior). The MRA is a way of using MRI (magnetic resonance imaging) to look at a blood vessel but without the traditional intravenous "dye" contrast that can potentially damage the kidneys in a patient with diabetes.

Treatment of Stroke

The stroke victim requires hospitalization and stabilization of his or her vital signs, especially of blood pressure. Medications such as antiplatelet agents and anticoagulants are often prescribed. Two common anticoagulants, as of this writing, are warfarin and heparin. Neuroprotectant medications may also be prescribed, such as calcium channel blocker medications as well as newer medications that are in development as of this writing.

If the patient is over age 50, after stabilization, his or her physician may choose to place the patient on long-term ASPIRIN therapy to reduce the risk of further strokes. If the patient was already on aspirin prior to the stroke, he or she may be changed to another drug plus the aspirin, such as clopidogrel or dipyridamole.

In rare cases, the stroke patient may require surgery to treat an acute stroke or to repair damage that has already occurred. This is generally required only with intracranial bleeds and is performed to relieve the pressure on the brain.

Rehabilitation Therapy Is Usually Needed

Many patients will require at least some degree of rehabilitation, including physical therapy, occupational therapy and speech therapy. Psychological help may also be needed to help the patient cope with anxiety and depression.

Physical therapists can assist the patient in regaining lost abilities in such basic skills as walking, sitting, ambulating from one position to another, and similar important daily skills.

Occupational therapists may be needed to help the stroke victim relearn a variety of tasks, ranging from reading and writing to bathing, dressing and other daily life activities that were formerly mastered long ago and now must be mastered yet again.

Speech therapists can often help the patient who can think rationally but who has difficulty in physically getting the words to come out right or enunciating them (dysarthria). Some patients also have mental rather than physical trouble understanding verbal language (aphasia). These therapists also help patients relearn swallowing and how to avoid aspiration if that is necessary.

Psychological counseling may help a patient deal with anxiety, anger, frustration and the other emotions that accompany the trauma of recovering from a stroke. Many patients require antidepressants.

Lifestyle Changes

If the stroke victim was a smoker, physicians will urge him or her to stop smoking immediately and permanently, in order to reduce the risk of further strokes. A broad array of other lifestyle recommendations may be made, depending on the individual needs of the patient.

In addition, good blood pressure control is also critically important. Generally, blood pressure can be lowered to normal. A large drop in blood pressure may potentially worsen the decreased blood flow to the damaged area.

Ongoing Research

A number of studies have revealed that patients with diabetes whose glucose levels are controlled in the 100–180 mg/dL range tend to have better outcomes. Thus, a patient with diabetes who is hospitalized with a stroke should have frequent glucose testing and also be given rapid or short-acting insulin in order to keep glucose as near to normal as possible if needed.

As of this writing, some clinical research indicates that vasodilator medications may be helpful in the rehabilitation of stroke patients. There are a variety of clinical studies that seek to find the answers to preventing stroke or, when it occurs, enabling the person to recover as fully as possible. Some animal studies are examining the impact of lowered body temperature (hypothermia) on delaying brain damage. Other studies are looking at the impact of transcranial magnetic stimulation (TMS) of specific parts of the brain in rehabilitating the victims of strokes.

For further information, contact:

American Heart Association/American Stroke Association
7272 Greenville Avenue
Dallas, TX 75231-4596
(800) AHA-USA1 (242-8721; toll-free)
www.americanheart.org

National Rehabilitation Information Center
1010 Wayne Avenue
Suite 800
Silver Spring, MD 20910-5633
(800) 346-2742
www.naric.com

National Stroke Association
9707 East Easter Lane
Englewood, CO 80112-3747
(303) 649-9299 or 800-STROKES (toll-free)
www.stroke.org

Stroke Clubs International
805 12th Street
Galveston, TX 77550
(409) 762-1022

(See also ASPIRIN, CEREBRAL VASCULAR DISEASES, CHOLESTEROL, DEATH, DEPRESSION, ELDERLY, HYPERTENSION, SMOKING.)

Adria Arboix, M.D., Ph.D., "Diabetes Is an Independent Risk Factor for In-Hospital Mortality from Acute Spontaneous Intracerebral Hemorrhage," *Diabetes Care* 23, no. 10 (2000): 1527–1532.
Robert S. Lindsay, Ph.D., et al., "Diabetic Nephropathy Is Associated with an Increased Familial Risk of Stroke," *Diabetes Care* 22, no. 3 (March 1999): 422–425.

sugar   A form of carbohydrate. Sugar in and of itself is not bad for people with diabetes although generally the diet must be carefully controlled. Instead, it is the blood glucose levels that are problematic. Excessive amounts of sugar raise the glucose level of the blood. Table sugar is sucrose. Milk sugar is lactose.

The term "sugar" is used colloquially to mean blood glucose, as in "My sugar [blood glucose] is high."

sugar alcohols   Sugar substitutes, such as sorbitol, xylitol, and mannitol. They may have fewer acute effects on blood glucose levels, but these substances still contain calories. An excessive intake can cause diarrhea.

sulfonylureas   A class of oral medications used to treat some individuals with Type 2 diabetes. The drugs in this class promote the pancreatic secretion of insulin and thus lower blood glucose levels. They are also known as "secretagogues" along with medications in the meglitinide and phenylalanine classes. All three classes of drugs directly stimulate the pancreatic beta cell to secrete insulin. About 5 percent of patients treated with sulfonylureas each year fail to respond to the medication (secondary failure).

Sulfonylureas do NOT cause the pancreas to lose its ability to secrete insulin any sooner nor do they protect the beta cell. Patients in the UNITED KINGDOM PROSPECTIVE DIABETES STUDY (UKPDS) who were treated with sulfonylureas gained an average of six pounds. Although there is a theoretical concern that sulfonylureas can increase the risk of heart attack, no increased risk was seen in the UKPDS study subjects.

These medications are broken down into first generation agents and second generation agent sulfonylureas. The first four drugs in this class were Diabinese (chlorpropamide), Tolinase (tolazamide), Orinase (tolbutamide), and Dymelor (acetohexamide). These drugs are rarely used today. The first-generation agents are generally less potent, have a wider side-effect profile, and have a slightly greater risk of interactions with other medications that the patient may be taking.

Second-generation agents, which are used more frequently today, include glyburide (with brand names of DiaBeta, Glynase PresTab, and Micronase), glipizide (Glucotrol), glipizide-GITS (Glucotrol XL), and glimepiride (Amaryl).

All sulfonylurea drugs have the common side effect of potentially causing HYPOGLYCEMIA. They

MOST COMMONLY USED SULFONYLUREA MEDICATIONS

Name	How Supplied	Starting Dose	Max	Dosing
Glyburide	1.25, 1.5, 2.5, 3.0, 5.0, 6.0, 10 mg	Usu 2.5–5.0	20 mg	Gen daily
Glipizde	2.5, 5.0, 10.0	Usu 2.5–5.0	40 mg/day	Usu 2x/day
Glimepiride	1.0, 2, 4	0.5–2.0	8 mg/day	Daily

may also cause weight gain, stomach upset, and skin rash or itching. Hypoglycemia is most common with glyburide and chlorpropamide, due to their long half-lives (which means, they remain in the body for a long time) and active metabolites. The ingestion of alcohol with sulfonylureas can lead to a flushing Antabuse-like reaction. (Antabuse is a drug given to alcoholics, which induces vomiting if the alcoholic person consumes any alcohol.)

Sulfonylureas can cause weight gain and the average weight gain over the course of a year is 4 to 6 pounds. These drugs provide 80 to 90 percent of their maximal effect at 50 percent of their maximal dose.

These drugs should absolutely not be used by patients who have Type 1 diabetes, because, by definition, they have no beta cell function, and thus cannot cause increased secretion of insulin from the pancreas.

The UNITED KINGDOM PROSPECTIVE DIABETES STUDY (UKPDS) showed that the use of sulfonylureas did not increase cardiovascular morbidity (illness) and mortality (death).

These drugs should not be used in women who are pregnant or in people who have Type 1 diabetes. They should also be avoided by patients who are allergic to sulfa drugs. Patients with some liver failure or with kidney disease should also avoid them.

Sulfonylureas lower glucose levels within two to three days and lower HbA1C by 1 to 2 percent. The most common side effect is hypoglycemia, found more frequently with chlorpropamide and glyburide. These are older "first generation" drugs that are not commonly used. Second-generation drugs are less likely to cause hypoglycemia, although it can occur. Another effect that can occur if the patient also consumes alcohol is a flushing syndrome. Alcohol consumption is not recommended with this class of drugs.

sweating, gustatory An unusual form of diabetic autonomic NEUROPATHY that causes affected persons to perspire profusely when eating. It is annoying but not dangerous. There are no treatments at this time.

symptoms of diabetes Physical indicators of either Type 1 or Type 2 diabetes. There are specific symptoms that are commonly found in many people who have diabetes. If a person has such symptoms, he or she should check with a medical doctor to find out if diabetes is present. A person may have some but not all of these symptoms. It is also possible to have Type 2 diabetes and experience few or no symptoms. In addition, it is also possible to have some or all of the following symptoms and yet the person does not have diabetes.

Common symptoms of diabetes include:

- blurred vision
- constant thirst
- frequent skin or other infections
- frequent urination
- increased hunger
- excessive fatigue for no apparent reason
- unexplained weight loss is a symptom of Type 1 diabetes

When some or all of the above symptoms are seen in a person along with other characteristics that are found among many people with diabetes, the physician is even more suspicious of diabetes. For example, OBESITY is a very common factor found among people with Type 2 diabetes. In addition, people who are of AFRICAN-AMERICAN or NATIVE AMERICAN descent are more likely to have Type 2 diabetes than are people of other races. Age is another factor: individuals who are over age 65 have a much greater risk of developing diabetes than do people of younger ages. (See also POLYDIPSIA/POLYPHAGIA/POLYURIA.)

Syndrome X   A cluster of symptoms that can result in severe health problems, particularly cardiovascular ailments and diabetes, if untreated. Stanford University professor of medicine Gerald Reaven coined the term in 1988. Also known as "metabolic syndrome" or INSULIN RESISTANCE SYNDROME or "cardiac dysmetabolic syndrome."

Syndrome X by definition is INSULIN RESISTANCE and may also include HYPERTENSION, abnormal GLUCOSE levels, high TRIGLYCERIDE levels, and low levels of HDL cholesterol or "good" cholesterol. It remains uncertain as to whether insulin resistance causes these other medical problems or is merely associated with them. Many people with Syndrome X are also obese. This medical problem may be present for as long as 10 years before the symptoms become distinct enough for diagnosis.

Syndrome X can lead to ATHEROSCLEROSIS, kidney disease (DIABETIC NEPHROPATHY), TYPE 2 DIABETES, CARDIOVASCULAR DISEASE, and other severe medical problems.

Individuals with Syndrome X have low levels of HDL cholesterol (good cholesterol) and high levels of TRIGLYCERIDES.

syringe   Device used to inject liquid medications into the body. The syringe is a hollow device with a plunger inside and it may include an attached needle. The medicine is placed into the syringe. When the syringe includes a needle and the plunger is depressed, the needle forces the insulin into the body. All people with Type 1 diabetes and some people with Type 2 diabetes need to inject insulin to control their blood glucose levels.

Nearly all syringes are made from plastic and are disposable. They are manufactured in three typical sizes, 0.3 cc, 0.5 cc, and 1.0 cc, and hold a maximum of 30, 50, and 100 units of insulin respectively. All insulin on the market is U-100, which means there are 100 units per one cc. If a patient needs U-500 insulin, it must be specially ordered.

The needles attached to the syringes have become ever sharper and smaller and most now are 29-, 30-, and 31-gauge (the larger the number, the smaller the needle). Needles are also silicon-coated to allow them to pass through the skin almost painlessly. Experts advise patients against wiping the needle with alcohol because this may remove the silicon coating.

Reuse of Needles

Many patients reuse their syringes and needles in order to save money. Although it is not recommended, this practice can work for some patients when they are very cautious and are sure to keep their skin very clean, and recap the needle after each usage.

Disposal of Syringes and Needles

There is no standard approach to the disposal of needles and syringes. The traditional teaching has been to have patients fill an old plastic bleach bottle with syringes and needles, and when it was full, to recap the bottle, tape it up, and place it in a standard trash container. It should be labeled "non-recyclable." There are also devices available on the market that can safely remove the needle from the syringe and prevent any inadvertent needle sticks as well as prevent someone else from reusing the needle.

Many patients prefer prefilled insulin PEN DEVICES, because dosing is easier and more accurate. The needles on the pen devices tend to cause far less discomfort, because the insulin is already inside the syringe. As a result, the patient does not need to push the needle through a rubber stopper on an insulin bottle to draw up insulin; this very act decreases the sharpness of the needle. A duller needle causes more pain upon injection.

systolic blood pressure   Refers to the peak pressure generated by the left ventricle as the heart contracts. Systolic pressure is the numerator (top number) that is reported when blood pressure results are given. For example, if the blood pressure were 120/80, the 120 would be the systolic pressure. The lower number is the diastolic pressure. The heart spends about $2/3$ of its time in diastole (at rest, i.e., between beats) and $1/3$ in systole.

Individuals with both Type 1 and especially Type 2 diabetes are at high risk for developing high levels of both diastolic and systolic blood pressure, or HYPERTENSION. People with diabetes are more likely to suffer from hypertension. The combination of diabetes and hypertension can directly lead to or exacerbate both microvascular and macrovascular complications.

The microvascular complications that clearly are affected by hypertension include DIABETIC RETINOPATHY and DIABETIC NEPHROPATHY, while the macrovascular complications include myocardial infarction (heart attack), STROKE, ERECTILE DYSFUNCTION, and peripheral vascular disease (clinical syndrome of intermittent claudication, i.e., pain in the legs or buttocks with walking).

In the recent past, it was felt that the systolic blood pressure was *less* important than the diastolic blood pressure. This assumption is now known to be incorrect. Increased systolic blood pressure correlates better with a risk of stroke. Increased diastolic blood pressure actually correlates better with a risk for heart attack. Both measures are important.

Isolated systolic hypertension (ISH) in the elderly is common and should be treated. Studies such as the SHEP (Systolic Hypertension in the Elderly Program) trial have demonstrated that the treatment of ISH in patients who are over age 65 dramatically lowers complications these individuals experience. (See also DIASTOLIC BLOOD PRESSURE.)

Taiwan An Asian country whose elderly population has a high rate of Type 2 diabetes. Although individuals of Asian descent often have lower than usual rates of diabetes, a study reported in the 2000 issue of the *Journal of Gerontology* found that of 586 Taiwanese subjects ages 65 and over, about 20 percent of the men and 21 percent of the women were found to have HYPER-GLYCEMIA, i.e., impaired fasting glucose levels.

The study authors also noted that significant risk factors for hyperglycemia/diabetes were obesity, high systolic blood pressure, and high trigylceride levels. These are risk factors for most ethnicities and also are all related to SYNDROME X or "insulin resistance syndrome."

Shih-Wei Lai, Ehe-Keong Tan, and Kim-Choy Ng, "Epidemiology of Hyperglycemia in Elderly Persons," *Journal of Gerontology* 55A, no. 5 (2000): M257–M259.

team management of diabetes The concept of using a group of medical experts that assists an individual with diabetes in managing diabetes. This concept was developed by Dr. Joslin in the early 20th century and is still considered very important today by leading diabetes experts. Unfortunately, due to managed care and cost constraints, it may be difficult for patients to receive treatment from an entire team. Yet good team treatment is essentially cost-effective because it can prevent severe and costly consequences such as AMPUTATIONS, STROKES, and other complications of diabetes.

As a result, most medical experts believe that, whenever possible, individuals with diabetes should be treated by a team of medical experts, including a physician, registered dietitian, certified diabetes educator, and other diabetes practitioners. Other possible members of the healthcare team may be NEUROLOGISTS, NEPHROLOGISTS, podiatrists, social workers, psychologists, exercise physiologists, and OPHTHALMOLOGISTS. Also, if a woman with diabetes becomes pregnant, she needs to coordinate the care provided by her obstetrician with the expertise that her other "team members" provide.

Some research has indicated that team management provided to people with diabetes results in lower costs due to less frequent hospitalizations. (See HMOs.)

thiazolidinediones (TZDs) The newest class of oral medications used to treat people with Type 2 diabetes. These drugs only work in patients who still make some insulin. TZDs make the body more sensitive to existing insulin, allowing it to move glucose from the bloodstream into the cells more effectively and giving the body more energy. The drug takes 12 to 16 weeks to reach its maximal effects. When used as monotherapy (one drug), TZDs can lower glucose levels by about 1 to 2 percent.

Examples of drugs in this class are Avandia (rosiglitazone) and Actos (pioglitazone). Rezulin (troglitazone) was a drug in this class but the Food and Drug Administration (FDA) removed it from the market in 2000 after reports of liver toxicity in some patients. TZDs work to directly improve the problem of INSULIN RESISTANCE. Thus, TZDs do not cause a greater output of insulin but instead enable the body to more efficiently use the insulin that is produced.

TZDs can cause weight gain (four to eight pounds), anemia (mild and dilutional, due to fluid retention) and EDEMA (swelling) in the legs and the ankles. They can also interact with BIRTH CONTROL pills, making them less efficacious and are not often used with women taking birth control pills.

Sometimes thiazolidinedione drugs are taken in combination with other medications for diabetes, such as METFORMIN or insulin.

Although the FDA and the manufacturers recommend testing the liver prior to the use of TZDs, and every two months for the first year of use, there has been *no* significant evidence of liver toxicity with the remaining two drugs in this class that are still on the market.

These drugs should not be used in patients with coronary heart disease but can be used in patients with kidney failure.

These drugs may have other beneficial effects in addition to the effect on glucose; for example, they may slow ATHEROSCLEROSIS and thus, prevent heart attack (MYOCARDIAL INFARCTION) and STROKE.

TZD drugs have also been used to treat women with POLYCYSTIC OVARIAN SYNDROME, in order to treat excessive hairiness (hirsutism) and to improve fertility. These are not FDA-approved indications.

thirst Excessive thirst and a constant need for fluids is one symptom of diabetes and any person experiencing such a chronic problem should be sure to report this symptom to his or her physician. (See also DEHYDRATION, SYMPTOMS.)

thrush A fungal mouth infection (Candida). The key symptom of thrush is white patches on the skin of the inside of the mouth. When a person with diabetes has thrush, it may be caused by high glucose levels, which enable the thrush infection to proliferate. It may also be seen after the use of antibiotics for the treatment of a bacterial infection. On occasion, thrush may also cause the tongue to become discolored, becoming either black or brown.

Thrush may be treated with antifungal medications given as a liquid suspension, an oral suppository, or a pill. (See also INFECTIONS, SKIN PROBLEMS, YEAST.)

thyroid disease An abnormality of the thyroid, which is a butterfly-shaped gland that is located in the neck. The key thyroid disorders are hyperthyroidism, which is an excess of thyroid hormone and hypothyroidism, which is due to insufficient thyroid hormone. Hypothyroidism is more common among people with diabetes. Graves' disease, an autoimmune disorder, is the most common cause of hyperthyroidism.

About 6 percent of the nondiabetic population has a thyroid disorder and the risk further increases to 10 percent for people with diabetes. According to Patricia Wu, M.D., in her 2001 article for *Diabetes Self-Management*, the risk further increases to 30 percent for WOMEN WITH DIABETES.

Others who are at risk to develop thyroid disorders include:

- women (who develop hypothyroidism about five times as often as men)
- those with other family members with thyroid disease
- people over age 50 (aging brings an increased risk of hypothyroidism)
- those who take medications that can decrease thyroid levels, such as lithium
- Existence of another autoimmune disorder such as Type 1 diabetes, pernicious anemia, vitiligo, Addison's disease

Causes of Thyroid Disease

Many thyroid diseases are autoimmune disorders, which means that the body mistakenly attacks the thyroid as it would a foreign invader. In fewer cases, the body may react to medications such as lithium (for manic depression), or amiodarone (for some heart conditions), which may trigger hypothyroidism. Much more rarely, a disorder of the hypothalamus or the pituitary gland may cause hypothyroidism.

Symptoms of Hyperthyroidism

Hyperthyroidism may be detected by a physician when a patient has some or all of the following symptoms below. **Note:** these symptoms may also indicate many other diseases and thus, only an experienced physician can perform the diagnosis.

- elevated heart rate (pulse) of over 100 beats per minute
- enlarged thyroid
- increased requirement for insulin and worsening of blood glucose levels, if the person has diabetes
- insomnia/nightmares
- weight loss despite a greater appetite
- heavy sweating
- extreme nervousness and irritability/anxiety
- heat intolerance
- shaking hands
- decreased menstruation or no menstruation, prior to menopause or surgical removal of the uterus

Symptoms of Hypothyroidism

There are basic symptoms common to many people whose thyroid levels are low. However, these symptoms may also indicate other diseases. Common symptoms of hypothyroidism are:

- chronic constipation
- puffy face, especially under the eyes
- dry and itchy skin, doughy skin
- depression/lack of energy/apathy
- sensitivity to cold temperatures

- decreased need for insulin in those who have diabetes
- heavier menstruation
- muscle cramps and aches
- more frequent bowel movements (although not diarrhea)

The most common form of hypothyroidism is Hashimoto's thyroiditis. This is an autoimmune condition in which the body mistakenly makes antibodies (proteins) against the enzyme in the thyroid. Initially, it can cause hyperthyroidism because excess thyroid hormone is released from the damaged thyroid cells (Hashitoxicosis). More frequently, however, it will cause hypothyroidism. This is due to ongoing damage to the thyroid gland.

Diagnosis of Thyroid Disease

If the doctor believes a person has thyroid disease based on the symptoms displayed, then he or she will usually order a blood test known as a thyroid stimulating hormone (TSH) assay. This will determine if levels are high, low or in the normal range. The lower the TSH outside the normal range, the more hyperthyroid a person is. The higher the TSH outside the normal range, the more hypothyroid the person is.

Treating Thyroid Disease

The treatment depends on the cause. Treatment may be very simple, such as prescribing supplemental thyroid hormone to the hypothyroid patient and following up with periodic blood tests to ensure the blood levels of thyroid are in the normal range. Conversely, if the person has excessive levels of thyroid, the physician may attempt to suppress thyroid function through various means, such as with prescribing antithyroid pills or radioactive iodine. In some cases, surgery will become necessary. The primary test used to diagnose thyroid disease, the TSH (thyroid-stimulating hormone) has numerical levels that are inversely related to thyroid function. This means that numbers that are high indicate hypothyroidism and numbers that are very low indicate hyperthyroidism.

When the person with thyroid disease also has diabetes, then blood glucose levels must be monitored even more carefully than usual until the doctor believes the patient has achieved a stable level of thyroid function. After that point, regular glucose monitoring should continue. Glucose levels are more unstable with hyperthyroidism than with hypothyroidism.

If people with diabetes are hypothyroid, however, this increases the risk for LIPID abnormalities, such as an increase in low-density lipoproteins, otherwise known as "bad cholesterol." Therefore, patients with elevated levels of cholesterol should be screened for hypothyroidism.

Patricia Wu, M.D., F.A.C.E., F.R.C.P., "Thyroid Disease and Diabetes," *Diabetes Self-Management* 18, no. 3 (Winter 2000): 6–12.

transplant (of islet cells) (See ISLET CELL TRANSPLANTATION.)

travel Leaving home to go to another site, usually for a day or more and for business or pleasure. Many people with diabetes enjoy traveling. The importance of GLYCEMIC CONTROL, however, does not take a holiday and is still an issue for people with both Type 1 and Type 2 diabetes.

According to Davida F. Kruger, author of *The Diabetes Travel Guide: How to Travel with Diabetes—Anywhere in the World,* it's important for people with diabetes to see their physicians at least four to six weeks before a trip. This will enable the person with diabetes to have a physical examination and receive advice from the physician. It is also a good idea to obtain a letter from the doctor that states the person has diabetes and what medications the person takes.

Medication Preparation

The person with diabetes should bring sufficient medication for the duration of the trip. Kruger says it's also a good idea to ask the doctor to write a prescription for generic medication, in case the patient needs but is unable to obtain the specific usual form of medication at the travel site. It is unlikely that it will be possible to fill a prescription in a foreign country; however, the prescription will enable a physician in that country to write a prescription, if necessary.

It is not advisable to check luggage that has medication packed inside it because luggage may be misplaced or lost. Instead, if traveling by plane, it is best to bring medication in a carry-on bag or in another container that will fit under the seat.

It is also a good idea to buy and wear a medical identification necklace, bracelet, or anklet that includes key information about the person with diabetes, such as that he or she has diabetes and what medication is taken. ID cards inserted into wallets are not useful in emergencies because they are often not searched immediately when a person becomes seriously ill. A medical ID, in contrast, will reveal important information immediately to emergency medical experts and others.

People with diabetes who need injected insulin should consider a plan to dispose of their syringes and medications, such as a personal size disposal box. It can be dangerous and even illegal to dispose of syringes and lancets by throwing them in a public trash can.

Food Snacks

Regardless of how well an individual with diabetes manages the illness, it is still a good idea to bring some basic snacks along on a trip, to avoid any possibility of HYPOGLYCEMIA. These items should be placed in sealable plastic bags to decrease the probability of spoilage. People with diabetes should not assume that airlines will have nutritious snacks. (Individuals with diabetes may request a diabetic meal two to three days before the flight.)

Emergency Medical Assistance

If the person with diabetes becomes ill when faraway from home or in another country, he or she should ask the hotel concierge for assistance, being sure to explain that he or she has diabetes. If in a foreign country, the ill individual may also need to contact the consul office for their country. U.S. citizens can obtain a list of consulates by calling the U.S. State Department ahead of time or visiting their website: http://travel.state.gov.

Whether in the country or out of the country, it is important for all people with diabetes to wear EMERGENCY MEDICAL IDENTIFICATION, so that treatment can occur quickly if it is needed.

M. J. Dendinger, "Traveling with Diabetes: Business as Usual," *Diabetes Self-Management* 15, no. 3 (1998): 7–8, 11–13.

Davida F. Kruger, M.S.N., R.N., C.S., C.D.E., *The Diabetes Travel Guide: How to Travel with Diabetes—Anywhere in the World* (Alexandria, Va: American Diabetes Association, 2000).

V. Peragallo-Dittko, "Planes, Trains, and Diabetes: A Guide to Safe Travel," *Diabetes Self-Management* 14, no. 3 (1997): 32–33, 35, 38–40.

"Traveling with Diabetes," *Postgraduate Medicine* 105, no. 2 (1999): 233–234.

triglyceride   A form of fat that is found in the blood. Insulin helps store fat and when diabetes is well-controlled, triglycerides are efficiently removed. When diabetes is not controlled, triglyceride levels increase and the individual has an increased risk for developing vascular diseases and pancreatitis. (Pancreatitis is a significant risk if triglycerides exceed 1,000 mg/dl.) Additionally, when a person's triglyceride level increases, low density lipoprotein (LDL, or "bad cholesterol") levels tend to become more atherogenic (more likely to cause clots or breakages).

Other forms of fats are high density lipoproteins (HDLs). (See also FATS, HDL, LDL, LIPIDS.)

Type 1 diabetes   One of the two prevailing forms of diabetes and far less common than Type 2 diabetes. Formerly known as "insulin-dependent diabetes mellitus" or "juvenile-onset diabetes." This type was renamed Type 1 diabetes because the disease may be diagnosed in adults as well as in children. In addition, children diagnosed with Type 1 diabetes continue to have the illness into adulthood and throughout their lives.

Individuals with Type 1 diabetes constitute an estimated 5–10 percent of all cases of diabetes found in North America. In the United States, there are about 900,000 children and adults who have Type 1 diabetes and an estimated 13,000 new cases are diagnosed each year.

Type 1 diabetes is generally considered an autoimmune disease in which the afflicted individual's own immune system destroys the beta cells in the pancreas. These are the cells that make insulin. As a result, people with Type 1 diabetes must take INSULIN in order to survive.

The delivery of insulin may be by injection via standard syringes, a "pen" device, or an insulin pump. It is also critically important that people with Type 1 diabetes carefully monitor their blood glucose levels at least several times daily, depending on the advice provided by their physicians. They also need to monitor their diets and may need to do CARBOHYDRATE COUNTING.

Many studies, most prominently the DIABETES CONTROL AND COMPLICATIONS TRIAL (DCCT) have proven that glucose levels that are as close to normal as possible will greatly reduce the risk for an individual with Type 1 diabetes to develop one or more of the serious COMPLICATIONS of diabetes. Some examples of such complications are:

- amputations
- blindness
- cardiovascular disease
- death
- diabetic nephropathy
- diabetic neuropathy
- diabetic retinopathy
- stroke

Women with Type 1 diabetes who experience PREGNANCY should consult with their physicians for the best ways to keep themselves and their unborn babies healthy. Studies also indicate that preconception planning is a critical course of action for women with diabetes and will greatly reduce the risk of miscarriage and fetal abnormalities.

Type 2 diabetes　The more common form of diabetes, accounting for at least 90 percent of all cases of diabetes in the United States. Formerly called non-insulin dependent (NIDDM) diabetes, or adult onset diabetes mellitus (AODM) the illness was renamed "Type 2 diabetes" in the latter part of the 20th century because researchers felt that the name of the illness should not depend on the treatment or age at diagnosis, as it is now being diagnosed in children and adolescents. In addition, some individuals who have Type 2 diabetes may need to use insulin. In the United States about 7.4 percent of adults had Type 2 diabetes in 1995, and the prevalence was expected to increase to about 9 percent by 2025.

Type 2 diabetes is most common among certain racial groups, such as AFRICAN AMERICANS and NATIVE AMERICANS. The risk for developing Type 2 diabetes also rises with advancing age. Certain conditions, such as OBESITY and lack of physical activity, are associated with the development of Type 2 diabetes. In addition, diet and nutrition play a role as well; for example, the PIMA INDIANS in Arizona have very high rates of Type 2 diabetes; however, Pima Indians in Mexico have very low rates. The Mexican Pima Indians are generally slender and very active in contrast to the obese and sedentary Pima of Arizona.

Some women are at risk for developing Type 2 diabetes, including women who have had GESTATIONAL DIABETES MELLITUS (GDM) or women who have had polycystic ovary syndrome. Men and women with HYPERTENSION, DYSLIPIDEMIA, or IMPAIRED GLUCOSE TOLERANCE (IGT) have an increased risk of developing Type 2 diabetes.

Genetics is another factor in the development of Type 2 diabetes and the disease clearly "runs in" families. If a parent or sibling has the disease, the risk is heightened for other family members. However, environmental constraints also play a role. For example, the parent or sibling with Type 2 diabetes may eat a very high carbohydrate and high calorie diet, which diet is shared by other family members.

Type 2 diabetes is on the rise among affluent populations and is also increasingly found among adolescents and even children in developed and affluent societies where inactivity is the rule and food is plentiful. As of this writing, the only approved treatment for diabetes in children is the use of INSULIN or METFORMIN (Glucophage).

GLYCEMIC CONTROL is important for any person with diabetes and affected individuals should test their blood at least once daily and make adjustments based on the results. Study after study has demonstrated that glycemic control can reduce the risk for serious complications of diabetes such as DIABETIC RETINOPATHY, DIABETIC NEPHROPATHY, or DIABETIC NEUROPATHY. The most prominent and largest study of this nature was the UNITED KINGDOM PROSPECTIVE DIABETES STUDY (UKPDS).

Many people with diabetes suffer from HYPERTENSION, and the combination of hypertension and diabetes causes a greatly increased risk for CARDIOVASCULAR DISEASE.

People with diabetes should see a physician on a regular basis. They should also check their feet on a daily basis for any damage. In addition, an annual dilated-eye examination will help detect any serious eye diseases before it is too late and avoid BLINDNESS.

ulcer A break or sore in the skin, which may become infected if untreated. People with diabetes are at greater risk for developing ulcers of the foot or legs that result from skin that is accidentally abraded in minor scrapes. The most common risk factor is neuropathy leading to loss of sensation. In the worst cases, an untreated ulcer may lead to GANGRENE and the subsequent need for AMPUTATION of the affected limb.

Regular FOOT CARE can prevent the many cases of ulcers that lead to infection and HOSPITALIZATION each year. For example, patients with diabetes should remove their shoes and socks every time they see their doctor before he arrives in the room. This will help the doctor to remember to check the feet.

People with diabetes should never go barefoot, even in the house, lest they step on an object that harms their feet. They should also examine their own feet carefully every day.

Ultralente insulin Long-acting form of insulin. There are also short and medium-acting forms of insulin. Ultralente insulin action does not work until about four to six hours after injection. It continues to work for about 24 to 28 hours. It has lower peak activity than NPH insulin or Lente insulin, and thus, may bring less of a risk for hypoglycemia. However, Ultralente insulin may also be a bit more variable in its absorption rates.

When it was available in the past as animal insulin, Ultralente insulin was often used once per day as a "basal" insulin and then regular insulin was used to cover meals. Now Ultralente insulin is available only as recombinant human insulin. It may still be used once per day but it is also often used two to three times per day and combined with rapid or short-acting insulin. (See also INSULIN.)

ultrasound Noninvasive radiologic imaging test that is used to diagnose a variety of illnesses including DIGESTIVE DISORDERS, DIABETIC NEPHROPATHY, DIABETIC NEUROPATHY, and blockages in the carotid arteries. It is also used during the PREGNANCY of a women with diabetes to determine the status of the fetus and whether the child has any malformations or is unusually large or small. No radiation is used and there are no known adverse effects.

unit of insulin Refers to how insulin is measured. Now all insulin used in the United States is U-100, which means its concentration is 100 units of insulin per milliliter (mL) or per cubic centimeter (cc).

United Kingdom Area in Europe comprised of England, Scotland, Northern Ireland, and Wales. According to reviews of services to people with diabetes in the United Kingdom performed by the National Health Service in 2000, about 1.5 million people in England and Wales were diagnosed with diabetes; however, the number was projected to double by 2010 to 3 million. The primary reason for the increase was the aging and obese population.

According to the organization Diabetes UK (the former British Diabetic Association), of those who have been diagnosed, 75 to 90 percent have Type 2 diabetes. Asians and African Caribbeans in the United Kingdom have a three to five times greater risk of developing diabetes than other racial groups.

It is also believed that there are an additional 1 million more people in the United Kingdom who have yet to be diagnosed.

Scotland and Diabetes

About 100,000 people in Scotland, 2 percent of the Scottish population, have diabetes and this disease is estimated to use 5 percent or more of the National Health Service budget. Most of these individuals have Type 2 diabetes. In 2000, the Health Department in Scotland asked all local Health Boards to create diabetes registries for patients in their care and to submit information for a nationwide survey of patients with diabetes.

For more information, contact:

Diabetes UK
10 Queen Anne Street
London, W1G 9LH
England
(020) 7323 1531
www.diabetes.org.uk

Roger Dobson, "Number of UK Diabetic Patients Set to Double by 2010," *British Medical Journal* 320 (April 15, 2000): 1029.

United Kingdom Prospective Diabetes Study (UKPDS)   A massive study performed in the United Kingdom of over 5,000 patients recently diagnosed with Type 2 diabetes in 23 centers within the United Kingdom. The average patient was followed for 10 years. This study definitively proved that control of hyperglycemia and hypertension among people with diabetes dramatically reduced the subjects' risk for a variety of common complications faced by people with diabetes, such as DIABETIC RETINOPATHY, DIABETIC NEPHROPATHY, heart attack, STROKE, and death.

The study concentrated on the impact of tight glucose control on individuals with Type 2 diabetes and whether intensive medication therapy using insulin, metformin, glibenclamide (such as glyburide) and chlorpropamide would provide clinical benefits. In a substudy, patients with high blood pressure also received either an ACE inhibitor drug or a beta-blocker medication.

The study definitively proved that tight control greatly decreased the likelihood of later complications from diabetes, such as DIABETIC RETINOPATHY and DIABETIC NEPHROPATHY. The study also showed that for every percentage point decrease in $HgbA_{1C}$, there was a corresponding decrease in deaths and fatal or nonfatal MYOCARDIAL INFARCTIONS. In addition, the study proved that decreased hypertension was significantly correlated with a corresponding decreased risk for STROKE, death related to diabetes, heart failure, BLINDNESS, and other COMPLICATIONS of diabetes.

Hypertension risks   Followup studies of smaller subsets of the UKPDS group also revealed significant findings. For example, in a study of 1,148 male newly diagnosed hypertensive patients drawn from the UKPDS group, reported in a 1998 issue of the *British Medical Journal,* one group was assigned to the "tight" blood pressure control group and achieved an average pressure of 144/82 mmHg. The standard treatment group achieved an average pressure of 154/87 mmHg. Subjects were treated with beta blockers and ACE drugs as well as others as clinically needed.

Compared to the standard group, the tight control group had marked reduction in deaths from diabetes (down 32 percent), strokes (down 44 percent), and DIABETIC RETINOPATHY (34 percent). The tight control group had a risk of 3.6 risk events per 1,000 patient years for heart failure, compared to 8.1 for the less tight control group. The risk of death from kidney failure was lower for the tight control group, whose members had a risk of 0.3 of death from kidney failure, compared to 1.0 for the nontight group. The tight control group had a lower risk of fatal stroke (1.5) versus 3.6 for the nontight group. The tight group had a lower risk of fatal MYOCARDIAL INFARCTION (heart attack), at 9.8 versus 13.8 for the less controlled group.

Clearly, control of HYPERTENSION among patients with diabetes is crucial to their continued lives and health.

American Diabetes Association, "Implications of the United Kingdom Prospective Diabetes Study," *Diabetes Care* 21 (1998): 2180–2184.

R. C. Turner et al., "Risk Factors for Coronary Artery Disease in Non-Insulin Dependent Diabetes Mellitus: United Kingdom Prospective Diabetes Study (UKPDS): 23," *British Medical Journal* 316 (March 14, 1998): 823–828.

UK Prospective Diabetes Study Group, "Tight Blood Pressure Control and Risk of Macrovascular and Microvascular Complications in Type 2 Diabetes: UKPDS 38," *British Medical Journal* 317 (September 12, 1998): 703–713.

urinary tract infection (UTI) A commonly used generic term which may indicate several different urological problems, including pyelonephritis (inflammation of the kidney), CYSTITIS (inflammation of the bladder) or urethritis (inflammation of the urethra, the tube leading from the bladder and through which urine travels to be voided). However, the most common use of the phrase "urinary tract infection" is to indicate bladder IN-FECTIONS. These infections are often caused by *E. coli* bacteria or other organisms that are known to be associated with infections of the bladder.

Urinary tract infections are common problems experienced by people with diabetes, especially women. (Women in general are more prone to UTIs than men, primarily because of the shortness of the urethra, which is the tube that leads to the bladder.)

Cultures of the urine can determine what type of bacteria are present and can also indicate what antibiotics would be most effective to eliminate the infection. However, often doctors prescribe medications the first time for infrequent UTIs, without ordering cultures or seeing results based on a urinalysis alone. The reason for this action is that doctors know there are specific bacteria that are commonly found in the urinary tract and the physician may assume that the bacteria causing the current infection is one of these. However, in people who have recurrent UTIs, a urine culture should be done.

Urologists advise people with recurrent UTIs to drink plenty of fluid, especially water, every day. Some urologists also advise women who are prone to UTIs to urinate before and again after having sexual intercourse. Women may also be given medications that are bladder anesthetics in addition to antibiotics. The reasons for this is it may take several days before the antibiotic alleviates the symptoms. It is important for the entire course of medication to be taken to avoid recurrences.

Risk Factors for Recurrent UTIs Among Women with Diabetes

In a study reported in a 2000 issue of *Diabetes Care*, researchers studied women with both Type 1 and Type 2 diabetes. Among the women with Type 1 diabetes, 115 women or 20 percent of the total population, developed a urinary tract infection and many patients developed repeated infections.

For the women with Type 1 diabetes, 34 of the 241 women (14 percent) developed UTIs. Researchers found that the most common risk factor for the development of urinary tract infections was having had sexual intercourse the week before the study. A lesser risk factor was the use of oral contraceptives.

Of the women with Type 2 diabetes, 81 of the 348 women, or 23 percent, developed a urinary tract infection. For these women, the only significant risk was the existence of asymptomatic bacteria that was present in their urine when they joined the study. The authors concluded, "The risk factors for UTI development in diabetic women are the same as those reported for women without diabetes."

Suzanne E. Geerlings, M.D., Ph.D., et al., "Risk Factors for Symptomatic Urinary Tract Infection in Women with Diabetes," *Diabetes Care* 23, no. 12 (December 2000): 1737–1741.

urine testing   Laboratory testing of urine for diabetes, infection or other purposes. In the past, physicians tested individuals for diabetes by urinalysis, using REAGENT STRIPS. The problem with relying upon urinalysis for diagnosis is that an individual with diabetes may have fairly severe hyperglycemia well before any evidence actually appears in the person's urine. As a result, blood testing is far more reliable and is considered the "gold standard" for those with diabetes. However, urine testing is still an essential part of SICK DAY RULE management and is also essential if the physician suspects DIABETIC KETOACIDOSIS (DKA), a potentially fatal condition. KETONES are easily tested for in the urine.

Urine testing can be done for other purposes as well. For example, a urinalysis or urine culture is commonly performed to determine if a person has a URINARY TRACT INFECTION (the physician will test for red blood cells, white blood cells, and the presence of nitrates, an enzyme that will indicate the presence of bacteria). Sometimes, because of problems with DIABETIC NEUROPATHY (see NEUROGENIC BLADDER), a person with diabetes who has a UTI may not have the common problems of pain and urgency that would be felt by a person without diabetes.

Urine testing is frequently done on patients with diabetes at office visits to test for protein in the urine (PROTEINURIA or MICROALBUMINURIA). If a routine urine reagent strip is used and it does not reveal the presence of proteins, then the physician may do a second test in the urine to screen for very tiny amounts of protein in the urine (microalbuminuria). Many times, a sample of urine will then be sent to the laboratory to quantitatively measure the very small amounts of protein, using a method called radioimmunoassay. This test can be followed serially by the physician to determine whether or not the patient's renal function is improving, stabilizing, or worsening.

vaginitis Infection in the vaginal area, often a fungal infection. In about 85–90 percent of the cases caused by yeast, the infection is caused by *Candida albicans*. In recurrent or complicated cases of fungal vaginitis, the problem may be caused by *C. glabrata*. WOMEN WITH DIABETES are more likely to develop vaginal infections than are nondiabetics because of their elevated glucose levels. It is not uncommon for a gynecologist to diagnose women who have recurrent vaginal infections with diabetes.

Tight glycemic control is critical for the woman with diabetes who has frequent bouts of vaginitis. Without it, infections are likely to recur.

Should the woman be pregnant, the physician needs to be given this information, because it will affect the decision on what to prescribe; for example, oral antifungal medications could be dangerous during pregnancy.

Symptoms of Vaginitis

Some common symptoms of vaginal infection are:

- Unusual discharge (which, if yeast, often is characterized by a white or cottage cheese appearance to the discharge)
- Pain with urination (this may also be a symptom of a URINARY TRACT INFECTION)
- Pain with sexual intercourse (dyspareunia)
- Itching in the vaginal area
- Unusual odor in the vaginal area

Other Vaginal Diseases

It is also possible that a vaginal discharge or other symptom associated with a common form of vaginitis could instead be a sign of a sexually transmitted disease. For this reason, it's very important for the woman who has symptoms of vaginitis to be examined by a medical doctor rather than attempting to self-medicate with over-the-counter drugs.

Treatment of Vaginitis

Treatment depends on the cause. If the physician believes the cause of the vaginitis is fungal, then he or she will prescribe an antifungal medication such as fluconazole (Diflucan), nystatin, clotrimazole, or miconazole. The medication may come in the form of a cream or suppository to be inserted into the vaginal area or it may be an oral medication that is prescribed to eradicate a systemic fungal infection. One oral dose may be sufficient or a longer course may be needed. Some antivaginitis medications may be purchased over the counter.

If the woman has recurrent fungal infections, after treating the most recent infection, the physician may prescribe low-dose preventive oral antifungal medications for as long as six months.

"Drugs for Vulvovaginal Candidiasis," *The Medical Letter* 43, no. 1095 (January 8, 2001): 3–4.

veterans (military) According to the Department of Veterans Affairs within the U.S. Veterans Administration, diabetes is more prevalent among military veterans than in the general population. This may be because many military veterans are older/retired men. An estimated 16 percent of military veterans, or about 500,000, have diabetes, versus about 6 percent of the general public. In addition, of the 5,900 AMPUTATIONS performed by the VA in 1999, 75 percent were performed on patients with diabetes. About 98 percent of these veterans were male and most were over age 65. (Most older military veterans are male.)

Veterans who developed or were diagnosed with diabetes during their military service or within one year after leaving the military may be eligible for additional compensation. Also, special rules apply to Vietnam veterans who have developed Type 2 diabetes since their discharge from military service.

Vietnam Veterans

Some evidence from the Institute of Medicine (IOM) has indicated a possible linkage between an exposure to Agent Orange and other herbicides that were used during the Vietnam War, and the subsequent development of Type 2 diabetes in veterans who served in Vietnam. The IOM report also noted that traditional risk factors for diabetes, such as OBESITY, sedentary lifestyle, and other factors common to the veterans, outweighed the Agent Orange–induced risk for diabetes.

However, as a result of the report, in November of 2000, the U.S. Department of Veterans Affairs (VA) ruled that military veterans who had served in Vietnam and were since diagnosed with Type 2 diabetes may be eligible to apply for disability compensation. According to VA estimates, an estimated 178,000 veterans may be eligible for this compensation.

In addition to Type 2 diabetes, the VA considers other conditions as service-connected for veterans who served in Vietnam, including prostate and respiratory cancers, acute or subacute PERIPHERAL NEUROPATHY (associated with diabetes), and other illnesses.

For further information, contact the local office of the Veterans Administration or the national office at its toll-free number, (800) 827-1000. Or visit the website at www.va.gov.

visiting nurse Nurse who works for a home health care agency that provides nursing services to individuals who are too ill to go to a clinic or physician's office. This service enables people to recover from surgery or an injury at home and also helps people who have chronic health problems that need periodic attention. The service is often covered by MEDICARE or MEDICAID or by state agencies, although donations may be accepted as well.

For further information, contact:

Visiting Nurse Associations of America
11 Beacon Street
Suite 910
Boston, MA 02108
(617) 523-4042 or (888) 866-8773 (toll-free)
www.vnaa.org

vitamins Fat or water soluble organic compounds that are required in very small amounts for normal cellular function and growth. Some vitamins, such as vitamin E, may cause an improvement in diabetic symptoms or in symptoms related to problems that stem from diabetes. However, clinical studies are ongoing and definitive health benefits are yet to be proven.

Vitamin B_1 and B_6 have been occasionally helpful in treating DIABETIC NEUROPATHY. Epidemiological data suggest that an increased intake of antioxidants can decrease cardiovascular disease risk. Patients with diabetes seem to have more oxidative damage. Thus, many patients and medical doctors use antioxidant vitamins such as vitamin C and vitamin E for patients with diabetes, although there is no long-term care data showing that these antioxidants clearly decrease hard endpoints such as heart attack or stroke.

waist to hip ratio (WHR) A comparison of waist size to hip size and a measure of obesity. The waist equals midway between the iliac crest, which is the top part of the pelvic bone, and the lowest rib. The hips are measured at the widest point.

Many studies have measured abdominal fat by comparing the waist size to the hip measurements. However, waist circumference alone appears to be a better measure of both abdominal fat and the risk of developing Type 2 diabetes than the WHR. People who have an "apple" shape (with enlarged abdomens) are at greater risk for health problems than overweight or obese people with "pear" shapes (who carry their fat in the hip area rather than the abdomen). Acceptable values are 0.8 to 1.0 for men and 0.7 to 85 for women.

Studies have found that when obese people with diabetes lose weight and consequently have a decrease in their abdominal fat, such people also show a related improvement in both glucose tolerance and insulin action. (See also BMI, EATING DISORDERS, OBESITY.)

warning signs of diabetes Physical indicators of diabetes. An estimated 800,000 Americans who have diabetes have not yet been diagnosed. Individuals who experience the following warning signs should be evaluated by their physician for possible diabetes:

- constant and excessive thirst
- frequent urination
- extreme tiredness

- sudden weight loss (characteristic of Type 1 diabetes and not Type 2 diabetes)
- blurred vision
- slowly healing wounds

(See also DIAGNOSIS, SYMPTOMS.)

weight Body weight is a factor in Type 2 diabetes, because about 80 percent of people with this illness are obese. In the majority of cases, weight loss may lead to marked improvement of glucose levels and insulin tolerance. (See also BODY MASS INDEX, EATING DISORDERS, EXERCISE, OBESITY, WAIST TO HIP RATIO.)

whole grain foods Foods that contain items such as oats and whole wheat. Some research has indicated that eating whole grain foods such as oatmeal and whole grain breads can significantly reduce the risk for developing Type 2 diabetes. In a 2000 study in the *American Journal of Public Health,* conducted by researchers at Harvard University on the diets of more than 75,000 women over 10 years, researchers found that one serving of cooked oatmeal eaten two to four times per week was linked to a 16 percent reduction in the risk for developing Type 2 diabetes. In addition, the study also revealed that consuming one serving of oatmeal five or six times per week was linked to a 39 percent reduction in risk.

The researchers said, "The overall protective effect of whole grains (on risk for Type 2 Diabetes) was observed for individual whole-grain foods, including dark bread, whole grain breakfast cereal, popcorn, oatmeal, brown rice, wheat germ, bran and other grains."

Whole grain contains FIBER, which may be another reason why it has healthful preventive effects against Type 2 diabetes. (See also CARBO-HYDRATES, CARBOHYDRATE COUNTING, DIET, FIBER.)

Liu et al. "A Prospective Study of Whole-Grain Intake and Risk of Type 2 Diabetes Mellitus in U.S. Women," *American Journal of Public Health* 90, no. 9 (2000): 409–415.

Wisconsin Diabetic Retinopathy Study (WESDR) A study that occurred between July 1979 and June 1980 on patients with diabetes in Wisconsin, with the purpose of identifying risk factors for the development of DIABETIC RETINOPATHY. The researchers also looked at the number of patients who required CATARACT surgery at a later date.

The WESDR study divided patients into two groups. One group of 1,210 patients, the "younger-onset" group, were diagnosed with diabetes before the age of 30 and were also using insulin. The other group was comprised of 1,770 patients who were diagnosed after age 30, the "older-onset" group. In the older group, 824 patients were using insulin and 956 patients were not. The subjects were followed four years later and then again, ten years later. (Not all subjects participated in followups. Some had died or relocated or were not interested in participating.)

Cataract surgery Over a 10-year period, the researchers found that 27 percent of the people with diabetes in the "younger-onset" group (who were 45 years or older at followup) needed cataract surgery. They also found that 44 percent of the "older-onset" group who were age 75 or older had already had cataract surgery.

Factors associated with needing cataract surgery were as follows among the younger-onset group:

- severity of diabetic retinopathy
- high systolic blood pressure

- proteinuria (equal to or less than 0.30 g)
- use of thiazide diuretics
- use of central antiadrenergic agents

Among the older-onset patients with diabetes, the primary associated factor for requiring cataract surgery was the use of thiazide diuretics.

Study Findings

The WESDR demonstrated that increased levels of cholesterol were associated with an increased severity of retinal hard exudates (a leakage of fat and protein into the retina). Epidemiological followup data revealed that 90 percent of the patients with Type 1 diabetes who were diagnosed at over 30 years old had retinopathy after 10–15 years of diabetes. Proliferative retinopathy was seen in 25 percent of Type 1 patients after 10–15 years.

For patients over 30 years old who were diagnosed with Type 2 diabetes, they had been diagnosed less than five years ago. Forty percent of the patients who were taking insulin and 24 percent who were taking oral medication had retinopathy.

Aspirin use in patients with proliferative retinopathy did not increase the risk of vitreous hemorrhage and was associated with a 17 percent decrease in cardiovascular disease and death. Therefore, the existence of proliferative retinopathy is not a contraindication for aspirin.

The study also showed that high cholesterol levels were associated with an increased risk of retinopathy. In addition, it showed that early laser therapy in older patients with severe nonproliferative and early proliferative retinopathy was effective at reducing vision loss.

In addition, the study demonstrated that laser therapy was beneficial for patients who had macular edema involving or threatening to involve the center of the macula. (See also CATARACTS, DIABETIC RETINOPATHY, DIURETICS, EYE PROBLEMS.)

The Diabetes Control and Complications Trial Research Group, "A Comparison of the Study Populations in the Diabetes Control and Complications Trial and the Wisconsin Epidemiologic Study of Diabetic Retinopathy," *Archives of Internal Medicine* 155 (April 10, 1995): 745–754.

Barbara E. K. Klein, "Incidence of Cataract Surgery in the Wisconsin Epidemiologic Study of Diabetic Retinopathy," *American Journal of Ophthalmology* 119, no. 3 (March 1995): 295–301.

women with diabetes   Females with Type 1 or Type 2 diabetes. About 8 million women in the United States have diabetes, although at least one third of them have not yet been diagnosed. Of these, about 90–95 percent have Type 2 diabetes.

Generally, females with Type 1 diabetes have an onset of the disease during their childhood or adolescence, while the onset of Type 2 diabetes often occurs during adulthood. However, it is possible for Type 1 diabetes to appear in adulthood. It is also true that increasing numbers of adolescent girls (and boys) in the United States and other developed countries are being diagnosed with Type 2 diabetes. Generally, the teenagers with Type 2 diabetes are adolescents who are obese and inactive and they also have a family history of diabetes.

Diabetes affects both genders, but women are affected in several unique ways. For example, women with diabetes are at much greater risk of death from CORONARY HEART DISEASE than nondiabetic men or women. The risk for diabetic women is even greater than for diabetic men, the reverse of the situation for nondiabetics, where men have the higher risk. The death risks are highest for females with diabetes. As a result, the risks for coronary heart disease and/or death are as follows:

Risks for Coronary Heart Disease/Death (Highest to Lowest)

women with diabetes
men with diabetes
nondiabetic men
nondiabetic women

Women with diabetes also have a greater risk for developing HYPERTENSION than nondiabetic people as well as men with diabetes. Women with diabetes are also at higher risk of dying from CARDIOVASCULAR DISEASE than nondiabetics or men with diabetes. What is most shocking is that, as death rates from heart disease have dropped for most groups, including nondiabetics and diabetic males, they have actually *increased* by 24 percent for women with diabetes.

As might be expected, women with diabetes have a shorter life expectancy than nondiabetic women. In addition, women with diabetes have a greater risk for BLINDNESS than nondiabetics and a greater risk than men with diabetes.

Women with diabetes require careful monitoring during PREGNANCY to avoid harm to the fetus and to themselves. In addition, some women who have not previously experienced diabetes may have GESTATIONAL DIABETES MELLITUS (GDM) during pregnancy only. This illness should be carefully monitored by the patient and her physician because of serious potential harm that may come to both mother and child if glucose levels are not kept under control.

Women with diabetes are more prone to developing a variety of medical problems that nondiabetic women face at a much lower rate, such as VAGINITIS or INFECTIONS. Women with diabetes also have a risk of developing DIABETIC KETOACIDOSIS (DKA) that is 50 percent greater than the risk faced by men. They are also nearly eight times more likely to suffer from peripheral vascular disease (diminished blood and oxygen flow to the feet and lungs, causing pain) than are men.

The risk of STROKE that women with diabetes face is four times greater than the risk found among men with diabetes.

Women with Type 2 Diabetes Compared to Nondiabetic Women

Researchers have reported on sociodemographic differences among women ages 45–64 with Type 2 diabetes versus nondiabetic women in 1989 and that data is still useful today. (See Table 1.)

Women with diabetes are more likely to have low income compared to nondiabetic women. The majority (51.5 percent) of women with diabetes had family incomes of less than $20,000. Among the nondiabetic women, only 30.5 percent had family incomes at this level. Women with diabetes were also less likely to have graduated from high school or to be employed.

Racial differences Black women have an increased risk of suffering from Type 2 diabetes and this risk increases with age. In addition, African American women who have diabetes have an even greater risk for developing heart disease and other complications that stem from diabetes. About 28 percent of black women over age 50 have diabetes compared to about 19 percent of black males over 50 years. Hispanic women are also at high risk for Type 2 diabetes. American Indian women have a very high risk of developing Type 2 diabetes, and in some tribes, such as the PIMA INDIANS, the majority of women have diabetes.

Diabetes ranks third among causes of death for American Indian females and fourth for Hispanics and blacks. It is not among the top five causes of death for white females. However, all women with diabetes are at an increased risk of death from cardiovascular disease.

Characteristics of Women with Diabetes

There are also common traits among women with diabetes, and many of these can be seen at different life stages, such as adolescence, during childbearing years, and after menopause. These were the general times of life used by the CDC in their 2001 report, *Diabetes and Women's Health Across the Life Stages: A Public Health Perspective.*

Adolescent females Most female adolescents who have diabetes have Type 1 diabetes although some, particularly those who are obese and who have a family history for the disease, have Type 2 diabetes. According to the CENTERS FOR DISEASE CONTROL AND PREVENTION (CDC), adolescent girls with diabetes have a five times greater risk of death than nondiabetic teenagers.

An estimated 61,500 adolescent girls in the United States have Type 1 diabetes, according to the CDC. Of these, 92 percent are white, 4 percent are black and 4 percent are either Hispanic or Asian American. This racial makeup is very different from that found among teenagers who have Type 2 diabetes, in which case the majority of those with the disease are African American or Hispanic.

Diabetic ketoacidosis (DKA) is a common problem among adolescent girls with Type 1 diabetes, as is HYPOGLYCEMIA. In one study of girls ages nine to 16 who were followed for eight years, described by the CDC in their 2002 report on diabetes and women's health, 30 percent had one or more incidents of DKA and 21 percent had at least one episode of hypoglycemia. According to the CDC, research has indicated that adolescent girls of all races who have diabetes have a greater risk of HOSPITALIZATION for DKA than boys. This may be because teenage girls generally have a poorer record of glycemic control than adolescent males.

The CDC reports that nearly 22 percent of all adolescents with diabetes already have some form of ALBUMINURIA, a predictor for kidney disease. Some studies indicate that adolescent girls have a greater risk for microalbuminuria than adolescent boys, although other studies find that the risks are about the same.

Teenage girls with diabetes are at risk for emotional problems such as DEPRESSION and anxiety. Several studies have found that girls with diabetes believe that their illness has a greater negative impact on their lives than what is reported by teenage boys with diabetes.

Research also indicates that adolescent girls with diabetes may be at greater risk of suffering from EATING DISORDERS than nondiabetic girls. In a study of 356 Canadian girls with Type 1 diabetes who were ages 12–19 years and who were compared to nondiabetic adolescents, the researchers found that the girls with diabetes had about twice the number of eating disorders as the nondiabetic girls.

This is of special concern because some adolescent girls with diabetes may withhold their insulin or cut back on their doses in order to manipulate their weight. Such behavior could result in serious long-term or short-term health consequences, such as DIABETIC RETINOPATHY, DIABETIC NEPHROPATHY, DIABETIC NEUROPATHY, or even death.

Smoking is a risk behavior that increases the risk of cardiovascular disease among the already high-risk females with diabetes. Yet many adolescents and young adults smoke and some research indicates that people with diabetes are more likely to smoke than nondiabetics.

Adolescents are notoriously poor at maintaining good GLYCEMIC CONTROL, including testing their blood or administering sufficient insulin frequently enough. However, according to the CDC, some research has indicated that when adolescents with diabetes interact with adults who also have diabetes, their attitude about the illness improves. With this improved attitude may come a stronger belief that it is important to monitor diet and blood levels and to take medication. Belief may then be followed by action, including regular blood checks, following medication regimens, and monitoring of diets.

Women in childbearing years (18–44) An estimated 1.85 million women between the ages of 18 and 44 have diabetes and about 500,000 have not yet been diagnosed. Most of these women have Type 2 diabetes. In addition, an estimated 3–4 percent of women who are pregnant develop gestational diabetes mellitus (GDM). This is a form of diabetes that remits when the pregnancy ends, although the woman has an increased risk to develop Type 2 diabetes later in life. Over the period 1990 to 1998, the diabetes rate increased 70 percent among women between the ages of 30 and 39 years. The death rates for women with diabetes 25–44 are over three times higher than for nondiabetic women of the same ages.

Pregnancy can be very difficult for the woman with diabetes, and she needs strong support from her obstetrician, endocrinologist, dietitian, and other members of the medical profession who help her manage her illness.

Women with diabetes are less likely to be employed than nondiabetics. According to the CDC information, about 71 percent of women without diabetes were employed, compared to about 52 percent of women who had diabetes. Educational levels also differed. Women with diabetes had less education than nondiabetic women. About 13 percent of diabetic women had a college education, compared to 20 percent of nondiabetic women.

Diabetic mastopathy, or painless lumpy breasts, is another problem some scientists have found among women with Type 1 diabetes, usually women who are in their late thirties and who were diagnosed with diabetes as a child. In addition, women with diabetic mastopathy are also more likely to have diabetic retinopathy as well. This condition causes breast tissue to be denser than normal and can make reading of mammograms difficult. It does not appear to be related to any increased risk of breast cancer, however, suspicious nodules must be investigated anyway.

Women with diabetes and INSULIN RESISTANCE have a greater risk for developing POLYCYSTIC OVARIAN SYNDROME (PCOS).

Middle-aged women (ages 45–64) According to the National Institutes of Health, the number of women in their midlife years in the United States who have diabetes will increase from 27 million in 2001 to about 41 million by 2010. Almost all of these women have or will develop Type 2 diabetes. (See Table 2.)

Minority women in their midlife years are most likely to have Type 2 diabetes. Among women who are ages 50 to 59 years, race is a strong predictor for developing diabetes. For example, 24 percent of Mexican Americans and 23 percent for African Americans have diabetes, compared to 9.7 percent for Caucasians. The risk is higher for African American women. Black women are 2.4 times more likely to have diabetes than white women, while black men are 1.5 times more likely to have diabetes than white males.

However, Native American women pass everyone when it comes to risk for developing diabetes. For example, the Pima Indians are at very high risk for diabetes and the majority (70 percent) of middle aged women have diabetes. About 41 percent of middle-aged Navajo women have diabetes.

Middle-aged women with diabetes also have a risk of dying from coronary heart disease that is three to seven times greater than that for nondiabetic women.

Obesity is another factor that is very common to many women with diabetes, with some differences among races. For example, according to the CDC, research studies have shown that among women ages 45–64 with Type 2 diabetes, nearly half (49 percent) of Mexican American women with diabetes were obese in terms of their BODY MASS INDEX. About half (51 percent) of white women were obese. The percentage was much higher for black women with diabetes: about 70 percent were obese.

Older women   According to the CDC, about 4.5 million women ages 60 and over have diabetes and most have Type 2 diabetes. The risk for developing Type 2 diabetes increases with age. Experts predict that the number of older women with diabetes will increase from 20 million in 1995 to 23 million by 2010.

	Non-Hispanic White		Non-Hispanic Black		Total	
Characteristic	**Diabetes**	**No Diabetes**	**Diabetes**	**No Diabetes**	**Diabetes**	**No Diabetes**
Marital status						
Married	70.4	67.2	59.9	37.0	65.6	62.7
Widowed	1.0	0.6	3.6	1.5	2.1	0.7
Divorced or separated	13.6	10.5	21.8	17.7	19.0	11.4
Never married	15.0	22.2	14.7	43.8	13.2	25.2
Living Arrangements						
Alone	5.7	8.7	9.3	8.2	6.1	8.3
Nonrelative only	1.4	3.4	2.4	0.9	1.9	2.9
Spouse	69.7	66.7	59.9	35.1	65.3	61.8
Other relative only	23.2	21.2	28.5	55.8	26.8	27.0
Household Size						
1	7.0	12.1	11.7	9.2	8.0	11.3
2	24.6	20.8	23.1	20.6	22.4	20.2
3	31.0	24.3	6.1	23.4	25.9	23.9
≥4	37.3	42.8	59.2	46.7	43.8	44.6
Years of education						
<9	2.6	1.8	6.3	3.0	6.9	3.6
9–12	62.9	49.7	63.5	61.3	62.3	50.8
>12	34.6	48.4	30.2	35.7	30.8	45.6
≥16	17.3	22.3	4.8	10.8	12.8	20.0
Family income (thousands)						
<$10	21.0	8.7	30.5	28.6	25.7	12.2
$10≤$20	23.0	16.8	46.9	24.9	27.2	18.5
$20≤$40	36.2	37.7	8.6	31.5	29.6	36.5
≥$40	19.9	36.8	14.1	15.0	17.5	32.8
Employment status						
Employed	56.2	73.3	37.4	65.1	52.1	70.8
Unemployed	8.9	3.0	13.6	6.9	9.0	3.5
Not in labor force	34.9	23.7	49.0	28.0	38.9	25.7

TABLE 1   SOCIODEMOGRAPHIC CHARACTERISTICS OF WOMEN AGED 18–44 WITH TYPE 2 DIABETES—UNITED STATES, 1989

Most older women with Type 2 diabetes are obese and 70 percent of them are 20 percent or more over their desired weight. Physical inactivity is another risk factor for Type 2 diabetes and many older people have significantly decreased levels of physical activity. Diabetes is also the cause of death or related to the cause of death for many women ages 65 and over.

Some studies indicate that older women with diabetes are at greater risk for cognitive difficul-

ties than other aging women who are nondiabetic. (See also BIRTH CONTROL, ELDERLY, HORMONE REPLACEMENT THERAPY (HRT), MENOPAUSE, MENSTRUATION, URINARY TRACT INFECTIONS, VAGINITIS, YEAST.)

Gloria L.A. Beckles, and Patricia E. Thompson-Reid, eds, *Diabetes and Women's Health Across the Life Stages: A Public Health Perspective.* Conference Edition. Atlanta: U.S. Department of Health and Human Services, Centers for Disease Control and Preven-

TABLE 2 SOCIODEMOGRAPHIC CHARACTERISTICS OF WOMEN AGED 45–64 YEARS WITH AND WITHOUT TYPE 2 DIABETES, BY RACE/ETHNICITY—UNITED STATES, 1989

Characteristic	All Racial and ethnic groups		Non-Hispanic White		Non-Hispanic Black	
	Type 2	Nondiabetic	Type 2	Nondiabetic	Type 2	Nondiabetic
	%	%	%	%	%	%
Marital status						
Married	58.3	72.2	63.0	76.1	44.3	46.9
Widowed	15.6	9.4	15.7	8.2	17.8	20.6
Divorced/Separated	19.3	14.5	16.2	12.4	27.7	25.7
Never married	6.8	3.9	5.1	3.3	10.1	6.9
Living Arrangements						
Alone	18.4	13.4	19.0	13.3	21.8	17.4
Nonrelative only	1.0	1.2	1.6	1.2	0.0	1.2
Spouse	57.6	71.5	63.0	75.7	43.0	44.7
Other relative only	23.0	14.0	16.4	9.9	35.2	36.7
Household Size						
1	19.4	14.6	20.6	14.5	21.8	18.6
2	39.0	46.4	44.1	49.7	25.0	31.1
3	20.5	20.0	20.8	20.0	21.3	16.7
≥4	21.0	19.0	14.6	15.8	31.9	33.6
Years of education						
<9	22.7	9.7	13.8	5.6	22.7	21.8
9–12	60.4	58.6	67.7	60.9	59.5	53.6
>12	16.9	31.7	18.5	33.6	17.9	24.7
>16	6.7	14.5	7.7	14.9	6.6	10.8
Family income (thousands)						
<$10	28.5	11.3	24.6	8.3	37.8	31.7
$10≤$20	26.0	19.2	26.2	17.8	23.3	25.3
$20≤$40	26.5	33.5	27.7	34.5	24.9	23.7
≥$40	19.0	36.0	21.5	39.4	14.0	19.3
Employment status						
Employed	38.3	58.4	41.4	59.2	40.1	59.2
Unemployed	1.8	2.1	1.4	1.9	3.0	2.7
Not in labor force	59.9	39.5	57.2	38.9	56.9	38.2

Source: Cowie, C.C., Eberhardt, M.S. Sociodemographic characteristics of persons with diabetes. In: National Diabetes Data Group, editors. *Diabetes in America.* 2nd ed. Bethesda, Md.: National Institutes of Health, 1995:85–116. (NIH Publication No. 98-1468)

tion, National Center for Chronic Disease Pretension and Health Promotion, Division of Diabetes Translation, 2001.

Jennifer M. Jones et al., "Eating Disorders in Adolescent Females with an Without Type 1 Diabetes: Cross Sectional Study," *British Medical Journal* 320, (June 10, 2000): 1563–1566.

Warren L. Lee, M.D., et al., "Impact of Diabetes on Coronary Artery Disease in Men and Women," *Diabetes Care* 23 no. 7 (July 2000): 962–968.

Laurinda M. Poirier, M.P.H., R.N., C.D.E., and Katharine M. Coburn, M.P.H., *Women & Diabetes: Staying Healthy in Body, Mind, and Spirit* (Alexandria, Va.: American Diabetes Association, 2000).

work See EMPLOYMENT.

World Diabetes Day Sponsored by the World Health Organization and the International Diabetes Federation, World Diabetes Day is on November 14th of each year, in honor of the birthday of Sir Frederick Banting of Canada, the key discoverer of insulin in 1921. The first World Diabetes Day was in 1991 and continues to be observed annually, as of this writing. November is National Diabetes Month.

World Health Organization (WHO) A global health organization. Formed in 1948, the World Health Organization is based in Geneva, Switzerland, and is an organization that tracks diseases such as diabetes and other ailments as well as mortality (death) rates throughout the globe. WHO has 191 members, all also members of the United Nations or whose application for membership has been approved by the World Health Assembly.

Diabetes throughout the World

WHO produces global estimates of diabetes and publishes publications and articles on worldwide diabetes as well as the projected risk for the population of a country to develop diabetes. The organization estimates that there will be more than 300 million cases of diabetes worldwide by

2025, nearly double that of the estimated 154 million people who had diabetes in 2000.

Some parts of the world are expected to experience a very rapid growth of diabetes. For example, experts estimate that about 4 million people in Africa had diabetes in 2000. This number is projected to more than double to about 9.8 million by 2025. In the WHO Region of the Americas (region countries are listed at the end of this essay), the World Health Organization estimates that the number of cases of diabetes will increase from about 34.8 million in 2000 to 64.5 million by 2025. These findings, as well as those for other countries, are summarized in the chart that follows.

WORLD HEALTH ORGANIZATION ESTIMATES FOR GLOBAL DIABETES, 1995–2025				
Number of Cases (in thousands)	1995	1997	2000	2025
WHO Region of Africa	3,363	3,617	3,997	9,783
WHO Region of the Americas	30,711	32,344	34,795	63,526
WHO Region of the Eastern Mediterranean	13,803	14,964	16,706	42,857
WHO Region of Europe	33,002	33,989	35,469	47,761
WHO Region of South East Asia	27,642	29,652	32,667	79,517
WHO Region of Western Pacific	26,391	27,972	30,343	55,911
World	135,286	142,538	154,392	299,974

Source: Derived from information supplied by the World Health Organization, 2000.

WHO member countries, as of this writing, include as follows:

Regional office for Africa Algeria, Angola, Benin, Botswana, Burkina Fasto, Burundi, Cameroon, Cape Verde, Central African Republic, Chad, Comoros, Congo, Ivory Coast, Equatorial Guinea, Eritrea, Ethiopia, Gabon, Gambia, Ghana, Guinea, Guinea-Bissau, Kenya, Lesotho, Liberia, Madagascar, Malwai, Mali, Mauritania, Mauritius, Mozambique, Namibia, Niger, Nigeria, Rwanda, Sao Tome-Principe, Senegal, Seychelles, Sierra Leone, South Africa, Swaziland, Togo, Uganda, United Republic of Tanzania, Zaire, Zambia, Zimbabwe.

Regional office for Americas (PAHO) Antigua and Barbuda, Argentina, Bahamas, Barbados, Belize, Bolivia, Brazil, Canada, Chile, Columbia, Costa Rica, Cuba, Dominica, Dominican Republic, Ecuador, El Salvador, Grenada, Guatemala, Guyana, Haiti, Honduras, Jamaica, Mexico, Nicaragua, Panama, Paraguay, Peru, Puerto Rico (Associate Member), Saint Kitts and Nevis, Saint Lucia, Saint Vincent and the Grenadines, Suriname, Trinidad and Tobago, United States of America, Uruguay, Venezuela.

Regional office for Southeast Asia (SEARO) Bangladesh, Bhutan, Democratic People's Republic of Korea, India, Indonesia, Maldives, Myanmar, Nepal, Sri Lanka, Thailand.

Regional office for Europe (EURO) Albania, Andorra, Armenia, Austria, Azerbaijan, Belarus, Belgium, Bosnia and Herzegovina, Bulgaria, Croatia, Czech Republic, Denmark, Estonia, Finland, France, Georgia, Germany, Greece, Hungary, Iceland, Ireland, Israel, Italy, Kazakhstan, Kyrgyzstan, Latvia, Lithuania, Luxembourg, Malta, Monaco, Netherlands, Norway, Poland, Portugal, Republic of Moldova, Romania, Russian Federation, San Marino, Slovakia, Slovenia, Spain, Sweden, Switzerland, Tajikistan, The Former Yugoslav Republic of Macedonia, Turkey, Turkmenistan, Ukraine, United Kingdom of Great Britain and Northern Ireland, Uzbekistan, Yugoslavia.

Regional office for the Eastern Mediterranean (EMRO) Afghanistan, Bahrain, Cyprus, Djibouti, Egypt, Islamic Republic of Iran, Jordan, Kuwait, Lebanon, Libyan Arab Jamahiriya, Morocco, Oman, Pakistan, Qatar, Saudi Arabia, Somalia, Sudan, Syrian Arab Republic, Tunisia, United Arab Emirates, Yemen.

Regional office for the Western Pacific (WPRO) Australia, Brunei, Darussalam, Cambodia, China, Cook Islands, Fiji, Japan, Kiribati, Lao People's Democratic Republic, Malaysia, Marshall Islands, Federated States of Micronesia, Mongolia, Nauru, New Zealand, Niue, Palau, Papua New Guinea, Philippines, Republic of Korea, Singapore, Solomon Islands, Tokelau (Associate Member), Tonga, Tuvalu, Vanuatu, Vietnam, Western Samoa.

xerosis A condition of very dry skin experienced by many people with diabetes. Skin lotion, both over the counter and prescribed, can improve the condition. (See also DRY SKIN.)

yeast infections Fungal infections, usually of the genitals or the mouth, but which can also be found in other parts of the body. People with diabetes are more susceptible to yeast infections than are nondiabetics. WOMEN WITH DIABETES are more likely than nondiabetics to develop vaginal yeast infections. Individuals who have been on antibiotic regimens are also susceptible to developing a yeast infection, particularly when they have been on more than one course of antibiotics.

These infections are treated with prescribed or over-the-counter antifungal creams, suppositories, or oral medications. Sometimes infections are also treated with ALTERNATIVE MEDICINE such as acidophilus tablets, which may also be used as a preventive remedy in some cases.

The most common forms of yeast infections are THRUSH, esophageal yeast infection, Candida BALANITIS and Candida VAGINITIS. Thrush is an oral infection, characterized by a white or black tongue and throat. The key symptom of an esophageal yeast infection is painful swallowing. Candida balanitis is an infection of the foreskin of the penis. Candida vaginitis is a yeast infection of the vaginal area.

Z

zinc   A trace element needed by humans and usually obtained through food. Individuals with diabetes, particularly those who are elderly, may experience a deficiency of zinc. Zinc aids in the healing of wounds and a deficiency could lead to an increased probability of pressure ulcers, particularly in homebound individuals or those confined to their beds. Experts recommend that individuals with diabetes who are experiencing pressure ulcers should be supplied with supplemental zinc.

When people with diabetes develop low zinc levels, it has often been felt to be secondary to either poor intake or increased excretion associated with poor glycemic control. Improvement in glycemic control can help improve zinc levels.

APPENDIXES

APPENDIX I
IMPORTANT ORGANIZATIONS

AARP
601 E Street, NW
Washington, DC 20049
(202) 434-2277
www.aarp.org

Administration on Aging
Department of Health and
    Human Services
330 Independence Avenue, SW
Washington, DC 20201
(202) 619-7586
www.aoa.gov

Alzheimer's Association
919 North Michigan Avenue
Suite 1100
Chicago, IL 60611-1676
(800) 272-3900 or (312) 335-
    8700
www.alz.org

American Academy of
    Ophthalmology
655 Beach Street
San Francisco, CA 94109
(415) 561-8500
www.wyenet.org

American Academy of
    Optometry
6110 Executive Boulevard
Suite 506
Rockville, MD 20852
(301) 984-1441
www.aaopt.org

American Academy of Pediatrics
601 13th Street, NW
Suite 400 North
Washington, DC 20005
www.aap.org

American Amputee Foundation
P.O. Box 250218
Little Rock, AR 72225
(501) 666-2523

American Association of
    Clinical Endocrinologists
    (AACE)
1000 Riverside Avenue
Suite 205
Jacksonville, FL 32304
(904) 353-7878
www.aace.com

American Association for
    Marriage and Family Therapy
1133 15th Street, NW
Suite 300
Washington, DC 20005-2710

American Association of Diabetes
    Educators (AADE)
444 N. Michigan Avenue
Suite 1240
Chicago, IL 60611
(800) 338-3633 or
    (312) 644-2233

American Association of Sex
    Educators, Councilors and
    Therapists
P.O. Box 238
Mount Vernon, IA 52314-0238

American Bar Association
    Commission on Mental and
    Physical Disability Law
740 15th Street, NW
Washington, DC 20005-1009
(202) 666-1570
www.abanet.org/disability

American Board of Medical
    Specialties
47 Perimeter Center East
Suite 500
Atlanta, GA 36346
(800) 776-2378

American Board of Pediatric
    Surgery
1601 Dolores Street
San Francisco, CA 94110
(415) 826-3200

American Chronic Pain
    Association
P.O. Box 850
Rocklin, CA 95677-0850
(916) 632-0922
www.theacpa.org

The American College of Foot
    and Ankle Surgeons
    (ACFAS)
515 Busse Highway
Park Ridge, IL 60068
(847) 292-2237
www.acfas.org

American College of Sports
    Medicine
P.O. Box 1440
Indianapolis, IN 46206-1440
(317) 637-9200
www.ascm.org/sportsmed

American Council of the Blind
1155 15th Street, NW
Suite 720
Washington, DC 20005
(202) 467-5081 or
    (800) 424-8666

American Diabetes Association (ADA)
ADA National Service Center
1660 Duke Street
Alexandria, VA 22314
(800) 232-3472 or
  (703) 549-1500
www.diabetes.org

American Dietetic Association
216 W. Jackson Boulevard
Chicago, IL 60606-6995
(312) 899-0040
www.eatright.org

American Foundation for
  the Blind
11 Penn Plaza
Suite 300
New York, NY 10001
(212) 502-7634
www.afb.org

American Foundation for
  Urologic Disease, Inc. (AFUD)
1128 North Charles Street
Baltimore, MD 21201
(800) 242-2383 or
  (410) 468-1800
www.afud.org

American Heart Association/
  American Stroke Association
7272 Greenville Avenue
Dallas, TX 75231-4596
(800) AHA-USA1 (242-8721)
www.americanheart.org

American Medical Association
515 North State Street
Chicago, IL 60610
(312) 464-5000
www.ama-assn.org

American Optometric Association
1505 Prince Street
Suite 300
Alexandria, VA 22314
(703) 739-9200
www.aoanet.org

American Pharmaceutical
  Association
2215 Constitution Avenue, NW
Washington, DC 20037-2985
(202) 628-4410
www.aphanet.org

American Podiatric Medical
  Association (APMA)
9311 Old Georgetown Road
Bethesda, MD 20814-1698
(301) 571-9200
www.apma.org

American Printing House for
  the Blind
1039 Frankfurt Avenue
P.O. Box 6085
Louisville, KY 40206
(502) 895-2405 or (800) 223-1839

American Psychiatric Association
1400 K Street, NW
Washington, DC 20005
(202) 682-6000
www.psych.org

American Psychological
  Association
750 First Street, NE
Washington, DC 20002-4242
(202) 336-5500
www.apa.org

American Society of Human
  Genetics
9650 Rockville Pike
Bethesda, MD 20814
(301) 571-1825
www.Faseb.org/genetics

American Society of Nephrology
  (ASN)
1200 19th Street, NW
Suite 300
Washington, DC 20039
(202) 857-1190
www.asn-online.com

American Urological Association
  (AUA)
1120 North Charles Street
Baltimore, MD 21201
(410) 727-1100
www.auanet.org

Association of American Indian
  Physicians
1235 Sovereign Row
Suite C-9
Oklahoma City, OK 73108
(405) 946-7651

Association for Glycogen Storage
  Disease
P.O. Box 896
Durant, IA 52747
(319) 785-6038

Association of Asian Pacific Community Health Organizations
1440 Broadway, #510
Oakland, CA 94612
(510) 272-9536
www.aapcho.org

Centers for Disease Control and
  Prevention (CDC)
Division of Diabetes Translation
National Center for Chronic
  Disease Prevention and
  Health Promotion
Mail Stop K-10
4770 Buford Highway, NE
Atlanta, GA 30341-3717
(877) CDC-DIAB
www.cdc.gov/diabetes

Centers for Medicare and
  Medicaid Services (formerly
  the Health Care Financing
  Administration)
6325 Security Boulevard
Baltimore, MD 21207
(410) 786-3000
www.hcfa.gov

Diabetes Action Research and
  Education Foundation
426 C Street, NE
Washington, DC 20002
(202) 333-4520
www.diabetesaction.org

Diabetes Exercise and Sports
  Association (DESA)
1647 West Bathany Home Road
#B
Phoenix, AZ 85015
(800) 898-4322
www.diabetes-exercise.org

Disability Rights Education and
  Defense Fund, Inc.
2212 6th Street
Berkeley, CA 94710
(510) 644-2555 (voice and TDD)
  or (800) 466-4232

Eldercare Locator
National Association of Area
  Agencies on Aging
15th Street, NW
6th Floor
Washington, DC 20005
(800) 677-1116
www.aoa.dhhs.gov/elderpage/
  locator.html

Endocrine Society
4350 East West Highway
Suite 500
Bethesda, MD 20814-4410
(301) 941-0200
www.endo-society.org

Equal Employment Opportunity
  Commission (EEOC)
1801 L Street, NW
Washington, DC 20502
(202) 663-4900

Family Caregiver Alliance
690 Market Street
Suite 600
San Francisco, CA 94104
(415) 434-3388
www.caregiver.org

Food and Nutrition Information
  Center
National Agricultural
  Library/USDA
10301 Baltimore Boulevard
Room 304
Beltsville, MD 20705-2351
(301) 504-5719

The Genetic Alliance
4301 Connecticut Avenue, NW
Suite 40
Washington, DC 20008-2304
(202) 966-5557
www.geneticalliance.org

The Glaucoma Foundation
116 John Street
Suite 1605
New York, NY 10038
(800) GLAUCOMA or
  (212) 651-1900
www.glaucoma-foundation.org

Hypoglycemia Support
  Foundation, Inc.
3822 NW 122nd Terrace
Sunrise, FL 33323
(954) 742-3098
www.hypoglycemia.org

Impotence World Association
10400 Little Patayent Parkway
Suite 485
Columbia, MD 21044
(410) 715-9609 or
  (800) 669-1603

Indian Health Service
  Headquarters
Diabetes Program
5300 Homestead Road, NE
Albuquerque, NM 87110
(505) 248-4182
www.his.gov/MedicalPrograms/
  Diabetes

International Association for
  Medical Assistance to Travelers
417 Center Street
Lewiston, NY 14092
(716) 754-4883

International Diabetic Athletes
  Association (IDAA)
1647 West Bethany Home Road
#B
Phoenix, AZ 85015
(800) 898-4322
www.diabetes-exercise.org

Juvenile Diabetes Research
  Foundation (JDF) International
120 Wall Street
19th Floor
New York, NY 10005
(800) 223-1138 or
  (212) 889-7575
www.jdf.org

Medic Alert Foundation
P.O. Box 1009
Turlock, CA 95381-1009
(209) 668-3331
www.medicalert.org

National Amputation Foundation
38-40 Church Street
Malverne, NY 11565
(516) 887-3600

National Alliance for Hispanic
  Health
1501 16th Street, NW
Washington, DC 20036
(202) 387-5000
www.hispanichealth.org

National Association for
  Visually Handicapped
  (East Coast)
22 West 21st Street
New York, NY 10010
(212) 889-3141
www.navh.org

National Association for Visually
  Handicapped (West)
3201 Balboa Street
San Francisco, CA 94121
(415) 221-3201

National Chronic Pain Outreach
  Association
P.O. Box 274
Millboro, CA 24460
(540) 997-5004

National Council on Aging
409 3rd Street, NW
2nd Floor
Washington, DC 20024
(202) 479-1200 or
  (800) 424-9046

National Diabetes Information
  Clearinghouse (NDIC)
1 Information Way
Bethesda, MD 20892-3560
(301) 654-3327
www.niddk.nih.gov/health/
  diabetes.ndic.htm

National Easter Seal Society
230 West Monroe Street
Suite 1800
Chicago, Ill 60606-4802
(800) 221-6827
www.easter-seals.org

National Eye Institute (NEI)
National Eye Health Education
  Program
P.O. Box 20/20
Bethesda, MD 20892-3655
(301) 496-5248
www.nei.nih.gov

National Family Caregivers
    Association
10400 Connecticut Avenue
Suite 500
Kensington, MD 20895-3944
(301) 942-6430 or
    (800) 896-3650
www.nfcacares.org

National Federation of the Blind
1800 Johnson Street
Baltimore, MD 21230
(410) 659-9314 or
    (800) 638-7518
www.nfb.org

National Heart, Lung and Blood
    Institute
Information Center
P.O. Box 30105
Bethesda, MD 20824-0105
(301) 592-8573
www.nhlbi.nih.gov

National Information Center for
    Children and Youth with
    Disabilities (NICHCY)
P.O. Box 1492
Washington, DC 20013
(800) 695-0285
www.nichcy.org

National Institute on Aging
Building 31, Room 5C27
31 Center Drive
MSC 2292
Bethesda, MD 20892
(301) 496-1752
www.hih.gov/nia

National Institute of Diabetes and
    Digestive and Kidney Diseases
National Institutes of Health
Building 31, Room 9A04
31 Center Drive
MSC 2560
Bethesda, MD 20892-2560
(301) 496-3583
www.niddk.nih.gov

National Institute on Aging
National Institutes of Health
Building 31, Room 5C27
31 Center Drive
MSC 2292
Bethesda, MD 20892-2292

(301) 496-1752
www.nih.gov/nia

National Kidney and Urologic
    Diseases Information Clearing-
    house (NKUDIC)
3 Information Way
Bethesda, MD 20892-3580
(800) 891-5390 or
    (301) 654-4415
www.niddk.nih.gov/health/
    kidney/kidney.htm

National Kidney Foundation, Inc.
30 East 33rd Street
New York, NY 10016
(800) 622-9010 or
    (212) 889-2210
www.kidney.org

National Library Service for the
    Blind and Physically Handi-
    capped
Library of Congress
1291 Taylor Street, NW
Washington, DC 20542
(202) 707-5100 or
    (202) 707-0744 TDD

National Oral Health Information
    Clearinghouse (NOHIC)
1 NOHIC Way
Bethesda, MD 20892-3500
(301) 402-3500
www.nohic.nidcr.nih.gov

National Organization for Rare
    Disorders
P.O. Box 8923
New Fairfield, CT 06812-8923
(203) 746-6518

National Osteoporosis Foundation
1150 17th Street, NW
Suite 500
Washington, DC 20036-4603
(202) 223-2226
www.nof.org

National Rehabilitation
    Information Center
1010 Wayne Avenue
Suite 800
Silver Spring, MD 20910
(800) 346-2742
www.naric.com

National Stroke Association
9707 East Easter Lane
Englewood, CO 80112-3747
(303) 649-9299 or (800)
    STROKES
www.stroke.org

Nursing Home Information Service
c/o National Council of Senior
    Citizens
8403 Colesville Road
Suite 1200
Silver Spring, MD 20910
(301) 578-8800, ext. 8834

Office of Minority Health
    Resource Center
P.O. Box 37337
Washington, DC 20013
(800) 444-6472
www.omhrc.gov

Pedorthic Footwear Association
    (PFA)
7150 Columbia Gateway Drive
Suite G
Columbia, MD 21046
(410) 381-7278 or
    (800) 673-8447
www.pedorthics.org

President's Council on Physical
    Fitness and Sports
701 Pennsylvania Avenue, NW
Suite 250
Washington, DC 20004
(202) 272-3421
www.surgeongeneral.gov

Prevent Blindness America
500 East Remington Road
Schaumburg, IL 60173-4557
(800) 331-2020
www.preventblindness.org

Recording for the Blind and
    Dyslexic
20 Riszel Road
Princeton, NJ 08540
(609) 452-0606 or
    (800) 221-4792
www.rfhd.org

The Seeing Eye Inc.
P.O. Box 375
Morristown, NJ 07943-0375

(201) 539-4425
www.seeingeye.org

Society of American Indian Dentists
P.O. Box 15107
Phoenix, AZ 85060
(602) 954-5160

Transplant Recipient International
Organization (TRIO)
1000 16th Street, NW
Washington, DC 10036
(202) 293-0980
www.transweb.org

United Network for Organ
Sharing (UNOS)
1100 Boulders Parkway
Suite 500
P.O. Box 13770
Richmond, VA 23225
(804) 330-8500
www.unos.org

Veterans Health Administration
Program Chief, Diabetes
810 Vermont Avenue, NW
Washington, DC 20420
(202) 273-8490

Weight-Control Information
Network
1 Win Way
Bethesda, MD 20892-3665
(800) WIN-8098
www.niddk.nih.gov/health/nutrit
/winbro/winbrol.html

APPENDIX II
DIABETES PERIODICALS

Clinical Diabetes
American Diabetes Association
1701 N. Beauregard Street
Alexandria, VA 22311
(800) 806-7801

Diabetes
American Diabetes Association
1701 N. Beauregard Street
Alexandria, VA 22311
(800) 806-7801

Diabetes Care
American Diabetes Association
1701 N. Beauregard Street
Alexandria, VA 22311
(800) 806-7801

Diabetes Forecast
American Diabetes Association
1701 N. Beauregard Street
Alexandria, VA 22311
(800) 806-7801

Diabetes Interview
Kings Publishing, Inc.
6 School Street
#160
Fairfax, CA 94930
(800) 488-8468
www.diabetesinterview.com

Diabetes Self-Management
R.A. Rapaport Publishing, Inc.
150 West 22nd Street
New York, NY 10011
(800) 234-0923

Diabetes Spectrum
American Diabetes Association
1701 N. Beauregard Street
Alexandria, VA 22311
(800) 342-2383

APPENDIX III
DIABETES RESEARCH AND TRAINING CENTERS (DRTCS)

The National Institute of Diabetes and Digestive and Kidney Diseases (NIDDK) supports the research, seminars, and training materials of six diabetes research and training centers nationwide.

Albert Einstein DRTC
Belfer Building 701
1300 Morris Park Avenue
Bronx, NY 10461
(718) 430-3345

Indiana University DRTC
Regenstrief Institute
1050 Wishard Boulevard
RG 6

The National Institute for Fitness and Sport
Indianapolis, IN 46202
(317) 630-6499

Michigan DRTC
University of Michigan Medical School
1500 East Medical Center Drive
3920 Taubman Center
Box 0354
Ann Arbor, MI 48109
(734) 936-8279

University of Chicago DRTC
Howard Hughes Medical Institute
University of Chicago

5841 S. Maryland Avenue
Chicago, IL 60637
(773) 702-1334

Vanderbilt University DRTC
Vanderbilt University School of Medicine
707 Light Hall
1211 Nashville, TN 37232
(615) 322-7004

Washington University DRTC
Washington University School of Medicine
Metabolism Division
P.O. Box 8127
St. Louis, MO 63110
(314) 362-8680

APPENDIX IV
DIABETES ENDOCRINOLOGY RESEARCH CENTERS (DERCS)

Joslin Diabetes Center DERC
One Joslin Place
Boston, MA 02215
(617) 732-2635
www.joslin.harvard.edu

Massachusetts General Hospital
DERC
Diabetes Unit
Department of Molecular Biology
Wellman 8
50 Blossom Street
Boston, MA 02114
(617) 726-6909

University of Colorado DERC
Barbara Davis Center for
Childhood Diabetes
4200 East 9th Avenue
Box B-140
Denver, CO 80262
(303) 315-8796
www.uchsc.edu/misc/diabetes/
bdc.html

University of Iowa DERC
Department of Internal
Medicine
3-E 19 VA Medical Center
Iowa City, IA 52246
(319) 338-0581, ext. 7625
www.uiderc.icva.gov

University of Massachusetts
Medical School DERC
373 Plantation Street
Suite 218
Worcester, MA 01605
(508) 856-3800
www.umassmed.edu/diabetes

University of Pennsylvania
DERC
Division of Endocrinology
Diabetes and Metabolism
611 Clinical Research Building
415 Curie Boulevard
Philadelphia, PA 19104-6149
(215) 898-0198

www.english.upenn.edu/
%7Emorgan/research/centers.
html

University of Washington DERC
P.O. Box 358285
DVA Puget Sound Health Care
System
1660 S. Columbian Way
Seattle, WA 98108
(206) 764-2688
www.depts.washington.edu/
diabetes/index.html

Yale University School of
Medicine DERC
P.O. Box 208020
333 Cedar Street, Fitikiin 1
Department of Endocrinology
New Haven, CT 06520
(203) 785-4183
www.info.med.yale.edu/intmed/
endocrin/research_progr.html

APPENDIX V

DIABETES CONTROL PROGRAMS IN U.S. STATES AND TERRITORIES

ALABAMA

Diabetes Control Program
   Coordinator
Diabetes Program, RSA Tower
Suite 1464
Alabama Department of Public
   Health
201 Monroe Street
P.O. Box 303017
Montgomery, AL 36130-3017
(334) 206-2060

ALASKA

Diabetes Control Program
   Coordinator
Alaska Diabetes Control
   Program
Section of Epidemiology
3601 "C" Street
Suite 540
P.O. Box 240249
Anchorage, AK 99524-0249
(907) 269-8035

ARIZONA

Diabetes Control Program
   Coordinator
Arizona Department of Health
   Services
2700 N. 3rd Street
Suite 4050
Phoenix, AZ 85004
(602) 542-7515
www.hs.state.az.us/diabetes

ARKANSAS

Diabetes Control Program
   Coordinator
Arkansas Department of Health

4815 W. Markham
Slot #3
Little Rock, AR 72205
(501) 661-2093

CALIFORNIA

Diabetes Control Program
   Coordinator
Department of Health Services
601 N. Seventh Street, MS 725
P.O. Box 942732
Sacramento, CA 94234-7320
(916) 327-3053
www.dhs.ca.gov/diabetes/html/
   a_main.html

COLORADO

Diabetes Control Program
   Coordinator
Colorado Department of Public
   Health and Environment
4300 Cherry Creek Drive
   South
Denver, CO 80222-2505
(303) 692-2505
www.state.co.us/gov_dir/
   cdphe_dir/pp/dcphom.html

CONNECTICUT

Diabetes Control Program
   Coordinator
Connecticut Department of
   Public Health
410 Capitol Avenue
MS# 11HLS
P.O. Box 340308
Hartford, CT 06134-0308
(860) 509-7802

DELAWARE

Diabetes Control Program
   Coordinator
Delaware Division of Public
   Health
Federal and Water Streets
P.O. Box 637
Dover, DE 19903
(302) 739-4754

DISTRICT OF COLUMBIA

District of Columbia Diabetes
   Control Program
825 North Capitol Street, NE
3rd Floor
Washington, DC 20002
(202) 442-5911

FLORIDA

Diabetes Control Program
   Coordinator
Florida Department of Health
Bureau of Chronic Disease
4025 Esplinade Way
Tallahassee, FL 32399
(850) 487-2772
www.doh.state.fl.us/family/dcp/
   default.html

GEORGIA

Diabetes Control Program
   Coordinator
Community Health Branch, DHR
2 Peachtree Street
16th Floor
Atlanta, GA 30303
(404) 657-6629
www.ph.dhr.state.ga.us/
   programs/cardio/diabetes.shtml

HAWAII

Diabetes Control Program
  Coordinator
838 South Beretania Street
Suite 204
Honolulu, HI 96713
(808) 587-3900

IDAHO

Diabetes Control Program
  Coordinator
Bureau of Health Promotion,
  Division of Health
Department of Health and
  Welfare
450 West State Street
Boise, ID 83720-0036
(208) 334-4928

ILLINOIS

Diabetes Control Program
  Coordinator
Illinois Department of Human
  Services
Illinois Diabetes Control Program
535 West Jefferson
Springfield, IL 62761
(217) 782-2166
www.state.il.us/agency/dhs/
  diabetes/dhome3.htm

INDIANA

Diabetes Control Program
  Coordinator
2 North Meridian
6th Floor
Indianapolis, IN 46204
(317) 233-7793

IOWA

Diabetes Control Program
  Coordinator
Bureau of Health Promotion
Diabetes Control Program
Iowa Department of Public Health
Lucas State Office Building
321 East 12th Street
Des Moines, IA 50319-0075
(515) 281-7739
www.idph.state.ia.us/sa/hprom/
  dp-cp.htm

KANSAS

Diabetes Control Program
  Coordinator
Bureau of Health Promotion
Kansas Department of Health and
  Environment
Landon State Office Building
Suite 901 N
900 SW Jackson
Topeka, KS 66612-1220
(785) 291-3739
www.kdhe.state.ks.us/diabetes/

KENTUCKY

Diabetes Control Program
  Coordinator
Kentucky Department for Public
  Health
275 East Main Street
HSIC-B
Frankfort, KY 40621
(502) 564-7996

LOUISIANA

Diabetes Control Program
  Coordinator
Chronic Disease Control
Office of Public Health
325 Loyola Avenue
Room 414
New Orleans, LA 70112
(504) 568-7210

MAINE

Diabetes Control Program
  Coordinator
Division of Community and
  Family Health, Bureau of
  Health
Department of Human Services
151 Capitol Street
11 State House Station
Augusta, ME 04333
(207) 287-5180

MARYLAND

Diabetes Control Program
  Coordinator
Maryland Department of Health
  and Mental Hygiene
201 West Preston Street
Baltimore, MD 21201
(410) 225-6774

MASSACHUSETTS

Diabetes Control Program
  Coordinator
Massachusetts Department of
  Public Health
Bureau of Family & Community
  Health
Diabetes Control Program
250 Washington Street
4th Floor
Boston, MA 02108
(617) 624-5403
www.state.ma.us/dph/dphhome.
  htm

MICHIGAN

Diabetes Control Program
  Coordinator
Chief, Diabetes and Other
  Chronic Disabling Condition
  Section
Michigan Department of
  Community Health
P.O. Box 30195
3423 N. Martin Luther King, Jr.
  Boulevard
Lansing, MI 48906
(517) 335-8445
www.mdch.state.mi.us/pha/
  diabetes/index.htm

MINNESOTA

Diabetes Control Program
  Coordinator
Minnesota Department of Health
P.O. Box 64882
St. Paul, MN 55440
(651) 281-9842
www.health.state.mm.us/divs/fh/
  chp/diabmiss.htm

MISSISSIPPI

Diabetes Control Program
  Coordinator
Mississippi State Department of
  Health
570 East Woodrow Wilson
P.O. Box 1700
Jackson, MS 39216-1700
(601) 576-7781
www.msdh.stae.ms.us/
  promotion/chronic.htm

MISSOURI

Diabetes Control Program
    Coordinator
Bureau of High Risk Intervention
920 Wildwood Drive
P.O. Box 570
Jefferson City, MO 65102-0570
(573) 522-2875

MONTANA

Diabetes Control Program
    Coordinator
Montana Department of Public
    Health and Human Services
Chronic Disease Prevention and
    Health Promotion Programs
Cogswell Building
Room C-317
P.O. Box 202951
Helena, MT 59620-2951
(406) 444-0593
www.dphhs.state.mt.us/hpsd/
    pubheal/disease/diabetes/
    index.htm

NEBRASKA

Diabetes Control Program
    Coordinator
Nebraska Department of Health
301 Centennial Mall South
P.O. Box 95044
Lincoln, NE 68509-5044
(402) 471-0194

NEVADA

Diabetes Control Program
    Coordinator
State of Nevada, Department of
    Human Resources and Health
    Division
505 East King Street
Room 103
Carson City, NV 89701-4774
(775) 684-5949

NEW HAMPSHIRE

Diabetes Control Program
    Coordinator
New Hampshire Department of
    Health and Human Services
Office of Community and
    Public Health

New Hampshire Diabetes
    Education Program
6 Hazen Drive
Concord, NH 03301-6527
(603) 271-5172

NEW JERSEY

Diabetes Control Program
    Coordinator
New Jersey Department of
    Health
Division of Family Health
    Services
Health Promotion Program
CN 364
Trenton, NJ 08625-0364
(609) 292-5037
www.state.nj.us/health/fhs/
    scdiab.htm

NEW MEXICO

Diabetes Control Program
    Coordinator
New Mexico Department of
    Health
Harold Runnels building
1190 Saint Francis Drive
P.O. Box 26110
Santa Fe, NM 87502-6110
(505) 827-2953

NEW YORK

Diabetes Control Program
    Coordinator
Bureau of Chronic Disease
    Services
New York State Department of
    Health
Empire State Plaza Tower
Room 780
Albany, NY 12237-0678
(518) 474-1222
www.health.state.ny.us/nysdoh/
    consumer/diabetes/condiab.htm

NORTH CAROLINA

Diabetes Control Program
    Coordinator
Department of Health and Human
    Services
Division of Public Health
Diabetes Prevention and Control
    Unit

Mail Services Center 1915
Raleigh, NC 27699-1915
(919) 715-3355

NORTH DAKOTA

Diabetes Control Program
    Coordinator
North Dakota Department of
    Health
Division of Disease Control
600 East Boulevard
Bismarck, ND 58505-0200
(701) 328-2698
www.ehs.health.state.nd.us/NDH
    D/prevent/disease/diabetes/
    project.asp

OHIO

Diabetes Control Program
    Coordinator
Ohio Department of Health
Diabetes Unit
8th Floor
246 North High Street
Columbus, OH 43266-0588
(614) 466-2144

OKLAHOMA

Diabetes Control Program
    Coordinator
Chronic Disease Service
Oklahoma State Department
    of Health
1000 Northeast 10th Street
Oklahoma City, OK 73117-1299
(405) 271-4072

OREGON

Diabetes Control Program
    Coordinator
800 NE Oregon Street
Suite 730
Portland, OR 97232
(503) 731-4273

PENNSYLVANIA

Diabetes Control Program
    Coordinator
Pennsylvania Department
    of Health
Division of Disease Intervention
P.O. Box 90
Harrisburg, PA 17108
(717) 787-5876

RHODE ISLAND

Diabetes Control Program
   Coordinator
Rhode Island Department
   of Health
Disease Control and Prevention
3 Capitol Hill
Room 109
Providence, RI 02908
(401) 222-3442

SOUTH CAROLINA

Diabetes Control Program
   Coordinator
South Carolina Diabetes Control
   Program
Center for Health Promotion
South Carolina Department of
   Health and Environmental
   Control
2600 Bull Street
Columbia, SC 29201
(804) 737-4129

SOUTH DAKOTA

Diabetes Control Program
   Coordinator
South Dakota Department of
   Health
615 East 4th Street
c/o 500 East Capitol Avenue
Pierre, SD 57501-1700
(605) 773-6189
www.state.sd.us/doh/Disease2/
   diabetes.htm

TENNESSEE

Diabetes Control Program
   Coordinator
Tennessee Department of Health
425 5th Avenue North
6th Floor, Cordell Hull Building
Nashville, TN 37247-5210
(615) 741-7366

TEXAS

Diabetes Control Program
   Coordinator
Texas Diabetes Program/Diabetes
   Council
Bureau of Chronic Disease
   Prevention and Control

Texas Department of Health
1100 West 49th Street
Austin, TX 78756
(512) 458-7490

UTAH

Diabetes Control Program
   Coordinator
Utah Department of Health
Chronic Disease Control
Division of Community and
   Family Health Services
288 North 1460 West
P.O. Box 142107
Salt Lake City, UT 84114-2107
(801) 538-6141
www.utahdiabetes.org/

VERMONT

Diabetes Control Program
   Coordinator
Vermont Department of Health
P.O. Box 70
Burlington, VT 05402-0070
(802) 865-7708

VIRGINIA

Diabetes Control Program
   Coordinator
Virginia Department of Health
Chronic Disease Control Program
P.O. Box 2448, Room 132
Richmond, VA 23218-2448
(804) 786-5420
www.vahealth.org/diabetes/
   index.htm

WASHINGTON

Diabetes Control Program
   Coordinator
Washington Department of
   Health
Airdustrial Park, Building 11
MS 7836
Olympia, WA 98504-7836
(360) 664-9086

WEST VIRGINIA

Diabetes Control Program
   Coordinator
Bureau for Public Health
Office of Epidemiology and
   Health Promotion

350 Capitol Street
Room 319
Charleston, WV 25301-3717
(304) 558-0644

WISCONSIN

Diabetes Control Program
   Coordinator
Wisconsin Department of Health
1 West Wilson Street
Room 218
Madison, WI 453701-2659
(608) 261-6871
www.dhfs.state.wi.us/health/
   diabetes/Dbindex.HTM

WYOMING

Diabetes Control Program
   Coordinator
Division of Preventive Medicine
Hathaway Building
4th Floor
Cheyenne, WY 82002
(307) 777-3579
http://wdhfs.state.wy.us/
   diabetes

AMERICAN SAMOA

Diabetes Control Program
   Coordinator
Department of Health Services
American Samoa Government
Pago Pago, American Samoa
   96799
(684) 633-4606

**FEDERATED STATE OF
MICRONESIA**

Diabetes Control Program
   Coordinator
Department of Health, Education
   & Social Affairs
P.O. Box PS 70
FMS National Government
Palikir, Pohnpei, Federate State of
   Micronesia 96941
(0-11-691) 320-2619

GUAM

Diabetes Control Program
   Coordinator
Department of Public Health and
   Social Services

P.O. Box 2816
Agana, Guam 96910
(0-11-671) 475-0282

**REPUBLIC OF THE
MARSHALL ISLANDS**

Diabetes Control Program
  Coordinator
Ministry of Health Services
P.O. Box 16
Republic of the Marshall Islands
Majuro, Marshall Islands 96960
(0-11-692) 625-3355

NORTHERN MARIANA ISLANDS

Diabetes Control Program
  Coordinator
Department of Public Health
Government of Northern Mariana
  Islands

P.O. Box 409 CK
Saipan, Commonwealth Northern
  Mariana Islands 96950
(0-11-670) 234-8950, ext. 2005

REPUBLIC OF PALAU

Diabetes Control Program
  Coordinator
Chief of Public Health
Ministry of Health
Koror, Palau PW 96940
(0-11-680) 488-1757

PUERTO RICO

Diabetes Control Program
  Coordinator
Puerto Rico Department of
  Health
Secretaria Auxiliar de Promocion
  y Protecion de la Salud

Division de Prevencion y Control
  de Enfermedades Transmisibles
P.O. Box 70184
San Juan, Puerto Rico 00936
(787) 274-5634

VIRGIN ISLANDS

Director, Health Promotion &
  Disease Prevention and
  Project Director, Virgin Islands
  Diabetes Control Program

Virgin Islands Department of
  Health
Charles Harwood Complex
3500 Estate Richmond
Christiansted, Virgin Islands
  00820-4370
(340) 773-1311, ext. 3145

APPENDIX VI

WORLD HEALTH ORGANIZATION DIABETES COLLABORATING CENTERS WORLDWIDE

AFRICA

SENEGAL

Professor A. M. Sow
WHO Collaborating Centre for
  Control and Prevention of
  Diabetes Mellitus
Hôpital communal Abase Mdao
B.P. 6054
Dakar, Senegal
(221) 215-110

AMERICAS

ARGENTINA

Dr. Juan José Gagliardino
WHO Collaborating Centre for
  Diabetes Research, Education
  and Care
Centro de Endocrinologia
  Experimental y Aplicada
  (CENEXA)
Facultad de Ciencias Medicas
Universidad Nacional de la Pata
Calle 67 y 620
1900 La Plata
Argentina
(54-221) 483-6303

CANADA

Dr. George Steiner
WHO Collaborating Centre for
  the Study of Atherosclerosis in
  Diabetes
WHO Collaborating Centre &
  DAIS Project Office
Toronto Hospital
University of Toronto

200 Elizabeth Street, NUW 9-112
Toronto, Ontario M5G 2C4
Canada
(416) 340-4538

CUBA

Dr. Oscar Mateo De Acosta
WHO Collaborating Centre for
  Integrated Medical Care
  Services in Diabetes
Instituto Nacional de
  Endocrinologia y
  Enfermedades Metabolicas
Ministry of Public Health
Hospital Cmdte. Fajardo
La Havana 4
Cuba
(53-7) 329-707/327-275

USA

Dr. Frank Vinicor
WHO Collaborating Centre for
  the Development of Integrated
  Primary Care Programme for
  Community Practice
Division of Diabetes
Centers for Disease Control and
  Prevention (K 10)
1600 Clifton Road
Atlanta, GA 30333
(770) 488-5000

Dr. Maureen Harris
WHO Collaborating Centre for
  Diabetes Research, Information
  and Education
National Diabetes Data Group
National Institute of Diabetes
  and Digestive and Kidney
  Diseases

National Institute of Health
Natcher Building, Room 5AN24
45 Center Drive, MSC 6600
Bethesda, MD 20892-6600
(301) 594-8801

Dr. Donnell D. Etzwiller
WHO Collaborating Centre for
  Diabetes Education, Translation
  and Computer Technology
International Diabetes Center
Park Nicollet Medical Foundation
5000 West 39th Street
Minneapolis, MN 55416
(512) 927-3393

Dr. Peter H. Bennett
WHO Collaborating Centre for
  the Design, Methodology and
  Analysis of Epidemiological
  and Clinical Investigations in
  Diabetes
Phoenix Epidemiology and
  Clinical Research Branch
National Institute of Diabetes, and
  Digestive and Kidney Diseases
1550 East Indian School Road
Phoenix, AZ 85014
(602) 263-1600

Dr. Ronald Laporte
WHO Collaborating Centre for
  Diabetes Registries and Training
Department of Epidemiology
Graduate School of Public Health
University of Pittsburgh
Diabetes Research Center
3460 Fifth Avenue
5th Floor
Pittsburgh, PA 15213
(412) 692-5200

EASTERN MEDITERRANEAN

JORDAN

Professor Kamel Ajlouni
WHO Collaborating Centre for
   Diabetes Research, Education
   and Primary Health Care
National Centre for Diabetes,
   Endocrine and Inherited
   Diseases
P.O. Box 86
Amman, Jordan
(962-6) 832-237

PAKISTAN

Dr. A. Samad Shera
WHO Collaborating Centre for
   Treatment, Education and
   Research in Diabetes
Diabetic Association of Pakistan
5-E/3 Nazimabad
Karachi 74600
Pakistan
(92 21) 661-6890

EUROPE

BELGIUM

WHO Collaborating Center for
   the Development of the Biology
   of Endocrine Pancreas (centre
   collaborateur de l'OMS pour le
   developpment de la biologie du
   pancreas endocrine)
Faculty of Sciences
Catholic University of Louvain
5, place Croix du Sud
B-1348 Louvain-la-Neuve
Belgium
(32 10) 473 405/473 003

CROATIA

Dr. Z. Metelko
WHO Collaborating Centre for
   Development of Appropriate
   Technology in the Control of
   Diabetes Mellitus
University Clinic for Diabetes,
   Endocrinology and Metabolic
   Disease
Vuk Vrhovac Institute

Dugi dol 4a
41000 Zagreb
Croatia
(385-1) 232-222

CZECH REPUBLIC

Professor Jaroslaw Rybka
WHO Collaborating Centre for
   Development, Management
   and Evaluation of the
   National Diabetes Control
   Programme
Internal Clinic of the Postgraduate
   Medical Institute
Havlickovo Nabrezi 600
Czech Republic
762 75 Zlin
(42-67) 28 235

DENMARK

Dr. K. Borch-Johnsen
WHO Collaborating Centre for
   Research and Training on
   the Pathogenesis of Diabetes
   Mellitus
Steno Diabetes Center
Niels Steensens Vej 2
DK-2820 Gentofte
Denmark
(45 31) 68 0800

FRANCE

Dr. Eveline Eschewege
WHO Collaborating Centre for
   Coordination of and Training
   in Clinical Research and
   Epidemiology in Diabetes
INSERM-Unite 21
16 Avenue Paul Vaillant-Couturier
F-94807 Villejuif Cedex
France
22 1 4677 2469

Professor Michel Pinget
WHO Collaborating Centre for
   the Prevention and Control of
   Diabetes
Centre European d'Etude du
   Diabetes (CeeD)
Service d'Endocrinologie et des
   Maladies de la Nutrition
1 place de l'hôpital
F-67091 Strasbourg
France
(33-1) 88 16 11 49

GERMANY

Professor Michael Berger
WHO Collaborating Centre for
   Diabetes Prevention
Department of Metabolic Diseases
   and Nutrition
Heinrich Heine Univ. Dusseldorf
Mooren Strasse 6
D-40225 Düsseldorf
Germany
(49 211) 811 7812

ISRAEL

Professor Z. Laron
WHO Collaborating Centre for
   the Study of Diabetes in Youth
Endocrinology & Diabetes
   Research Unit
Schneider Children's Medical
   Center of Israel (CMCI)
14 Kaplan Street, Petach-Tiqva
Israel
(972-3) 939 3610

ITALY

Professor P. Brunetti
WHO Collaborating Centre for
   Improvement of Quality of
   Care in Diabetes According to
   the St. Vincent Declaration
Department of Internal Medicine,
   Endocrinology and Metabolic
   Disorders Faculty of Medicine
University of Perugia
Via E. dal Pozzo
1-06126 Perugia
Italy
(39 75) 5721 366-5723 623

Professor Massimo Porta
WHO Collaborating Centre for
   Blindness
Universita degli Studio di Torino
Centro Retinopatia Diabetica
University of Torino
Corso Achilee Mario Dogliotti, 14
I-10126 Torino
Italy
(39-11) 663 5318

RUSSIAN FEDERATION

Professor A. S. Ametorv
WHO Collaborating Centre for
   Diabetes Education and
   Informatics

Russian Academy for Advanced
   Medical Studies (RAAMS)
20 Chassoraya Street
125315 Moscow
Russia
(7-095) 152-1982

SWITZERLAND

Dr. J. Assal
WHO Collaborating Centre for
   Reference and Research in
   Diabetes Education
Division of Therapeutic Education
   for Chronic Diseases–3HL
Faculty of Medicine
Hôpital Cantonal Universitaire
1211 Geneva
Switzerland
(41 22) 3729702

UNITED KINGDOM

Professor Harry Keen
WHO Collaborating Centre for
   the Study and Control of
   Long-Term Complications of
   Diabetes Mellitus
Unit for Metabolic Medicine
Division of Medicine Guy's
   Hospital
London SE1 9RT
England
(44-171) 955-5000

Professor K. Alberti
WHO Collaborating Centre for
   Training, Evaluation and
   Research in Diabetes
Department of Medicine
The University of Newcastle-
   upon-Tyne
Floor 4-Clinical Block
The Medical School
Framlington Place
Newcastle upon Tyne NE2 4HH
England
(44 91) 222 7020

SOUTHEAST ASIA

BANGLADESH

Dr. Hajera Mahtab
WHO Collaborating Centre for
   Research and Training for
   Prevention and Control of
   Diabetes Mellitus
Bangladesh Institute of Research
   and Rehabilitation in Diabetes,
   Endocrine and Metabolic
   Disorders (BIRDEM)
122, Kazi Nazrul Islan Avenue
Dhaka 1000
Bangladesh
(880-2) 866-641-50

WESTERN PACIFIC

AUSTRALIA

Professor Paul Zimmet
WHO Collaborating Centre for
   the Epidemiology of Diabetes
   Mellitus and Health Promotion
   for Noncommunicable
   Diseases Control
International Diabetes Institute
P.O. Box 185
260 Kooyong Road
Caulfield VIC 3162
Australia
(61-3) 925-85049

JAPAN

Dr. Hideshi Kuzuya
WHO Collaborating Centre for
   Diabetes Treatment and
   Education
Diabetes Center
Institute of Endocrinology and
   Metabolic Disease
Kyoto National Hospital
Fukakusa, Makaihata-cho
   Fushimu-ku
Kyoto 612-8555
Japan
(81 75) 641 9161

APPENDIX VII
WEB SITES THAT INCLUDE DIABETES INFORMATION

Alzheimer's Association
www.alz.org

American Academy of Family
Physicians
www.aafp.org

American Academy of
Ophthalmology
www.eyenet.org

American Academy of Pediatrics
www.aap.org

American Association of Clinical
Endocrinologists
www.aace.com

American Association of Diabetes
Educators
www.aadenet.org

The American College of Foot
and Ankle Surgeons (ACFAS)
www.acfas.org

American Diabetes Association
www.diabetes.org

Association of Asian Pacific Community Health Organizations
www.aapcho.org

Children with Diabetes On-Line
Community
www.childrenwithdiabetes.com

Division of Diabetes Translation
National Center for Chronic
Disease Prevention and
Health Promotion
Centers for Disease Control and
Prevention
www.cdc.gov/diabetes

American Heart Association
www.americanheart.org

Diabetes UK (United Kingdom)
www.diabetes.org.uk

The Glaucoma Foundation
www.glaucoma-foundation.org
www.osteo.org

The National Institute on Aging
www.aoa.dhhs.gov

National Institute on Alcohol
Abuse and Alcoholism (NIAA)
www.niaaa.nih.gov

National Institute of Diabetes and
Digestive and Kidney Diseases
(NIDDK)
www.niddk.nih.gov/health/
diabetes/diabetes.htm

National Stroke Association
www.stroke.org

National Women's Health
Information Center
www.4woman.gov/faq/
hormone.htm.

Nutrition and Health for Older
Americans
www.eatright.org/olderamericans

United States Renal Data System
(USRDS) Coordinating Center
www.usrds.org

U.S. Veterans Administration
www.va.gov

Visiting Nurses Association of
America
www.vnaa.org

APPENDIX VIII
IMPORTANT BUT OFTEN OVERLOOKED KEY ISSUES IN DIABETES

This appendix lists frequently overlooked points and advice that should be considered by people with diabetes and their families.

1. Not only should people with diabetes receive immunizations against flu or pneumonia, but experts also recommend that family members of individuals with diabetes be immunized as well. This will help protect both the family member and the person with diabetes.

2. Medicare and many other health plans provide once a year coverage for therapeutic shoes for patients with diabetes. Patients need to obtain a prescription for the shoes from their physician.

3. People with diabetes should not get new glasses or contact lenses until their glucose levels have been stable for four to six weeks.

4. A medical identification bracelet is very important for everyone who has diabetes. Symptoms of diabetes are often confused with other illnesses.

5. Everyone with diabetes should have an emergency plan for what to do if blood glucose levels swing out of control.

6. Some people with diabetes should have an exercise stress test before undergoing any moderate or intensive exercise program in order to rule out cardiovascular disease. These include people who fit any one or more of the following groups: over age 35; had Type 2 diabetes for more than 10 years; had Type 1 diabetes for more than 15 years; have kidney disease; have proliferative retinopathy; have peripheral vascular disease; have autonomic neuropathy; or have any other risk factors for coronary artery disease.

7. People with diabetes should check their feet daily, making a foot inspection as much a part of the daily routine as teeth brushing. They should also wear comfortable shoes that were bought at the end of the day when the feet are usually the most swollen.

8. Excellent glycemic control levels are as follows:
   Pre-meal: 80–120
   Pre-bedtime: 100–140

9. Adolescents are most at risk to develop Type 2 diabetes if there is a family history of diabetes and if the adolescents are overweight and inactive.

10. Among people with Type 2 diabetes, the key factor that predicted hospitalization was elevated blood glucose levels in the 2–3 weeks prior to admission.

APPENDIX IX
MEDICATIONS USED TO TREAT TYPE 2 DIABETES

(See INSULIN entry in text for insulin information.)

I. INSULIN SECRETAGOGUES

	1st Generation	2nd Generation
A. Sulfonylureas	Tolbutamide	Glyburide/ Micronized Glyburide
	Tolazamide	Glipizide
	Chlorpropramide	Glimepride
B. Meglitinide	Repaglinide (Prandin)	
C. Phenylalanine Derivatives	Nateglinide (Starlix)	
II. Thiazolidinediones (TZDs)	Rosiglitazone (Avandia)	
	Pioglitazone (Actos)	
III. Alpha Glucosidase Inhibitors	Acarbose (Precose)	
	Miglitol (Glyset)	
IV. Biguanide	Metformin (Glucophage)	

SULFONYLUREA MEDICATIONS AND TYPICAL DOSING

Generic Name	Trade Name	Number of Daily Doses	Typical Daily Dose
Tolbutamide	Orinase	2–3	500–3000 mg/day
Acetohexamide	Dymelor	1–2	250–500 mg/1–2 a day
Tolazamide	Tolinase	1–2	100–1000 mg/day
Chlorpropamide	Diabinese	1	100–500 mg/day
Glyburide	Diabeta Micronase	1	1.25–20 mg/day
Micronized glyburide	Glynase PresTab	1	1.5–12 mg/day
Glipizide	Glucotrol	1	2.5–40 mg/day
Glipizide GITS	Glucotrol XL	1	2.5–20 mg/day
Glimepiride	Amaryl	1	0.5–8 mg/day

SECRETAGOGUE MEDICATIONS AND TYPICAL DOSING

Generic Name	Trade Name	Typical Dosing
Repaglinide	Prandin	1.5–16 mg, 3 or 4/day
Nateglinide	Starlix	180–360 mg/day

TZD MEDICATIONS AND TYPICAL DOSING

Generic Name	Trade Name	Typical Dosing
Rosiglitazone	Avandia	2–8 mg/day, 1–2/day
Pioglitazone	Actos	15–45 mg/day

ALPHA GLUCOSIDE INHIBITOR MEDICATIONS AND TYPICAL DOSING

Generic Name	Trade Name	Typical Doses
Miglitol	Glyset	75–300 mg/day
Acarbose	Precose	75–300 mg/day

APPENDIX X
BODY MASS INDEX CHARTS AND CURVES FOR CHILDREN AND YOUNG ADULTS UNDER AGE 20

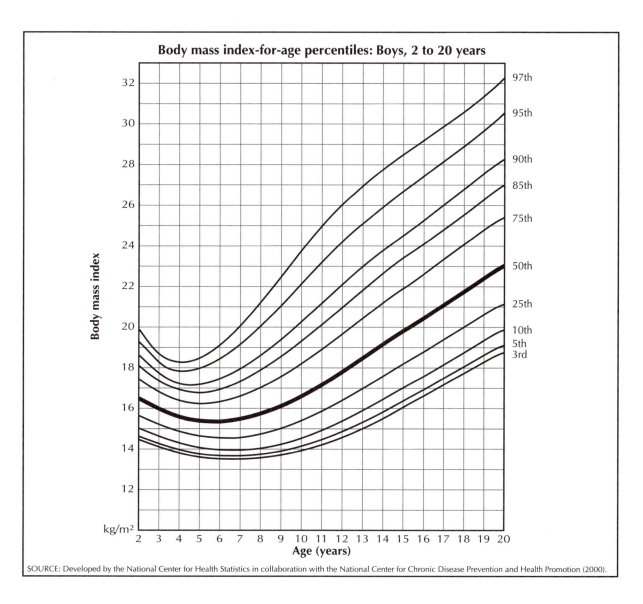

Body mass index-for-age percentiles: Boys, 2 to 20 years

SOURCE: Developed by the National Center for Health Statistics in collaboration with the National Center for Chronic Disease Prevention and Health Promotion (2000).

Body mass index-for-age percentiles: Girls, 2 to 20 years

SOURCE: Developed by the National Center for Health Statistics in collaboration with the National Center for Chronic Disease Prevention and Health Promotion (2000).

CALCULATED BODY MASS INDEX   29"–37" AND 18 LBS.–26 LBS.

Height		Weight																
Cm	In (Kg)	8.2	8.4	8.6	8.8	9.1	9.3	9.5	9.8	10.0	10.2	10.4	10.7	10.9	11.1	11.3	11.6	11.8
	(Lb)	18	18.5	19	19.5	20	20.5	21	21.5	22	22.5	23	23.5	24	24.5	25	25.5	26
73.7	29	15.0	15.5	15.9	16.3	16.7	17.1	17.6	18.0	18.4	18.8	19.2	19.6	20.1	20.5	20.9	21.3	21.7
74.9	29.5	14.5	14.9	15.3	15.8	16.2	16.6	17.0	17.4	17.8	18.2	18.6	19.0	19.4	19.8	20.2	20.6	21.0
76.2	30	14.1	14.5	14.8	15.2	15.6	16.0	16.4	16.8	17.2	17.6	18.0	18.4	18.7	19.1	19.5	19.9	20.3
77.5	30.5	13.6	14.0	14.4	14.7	15.1	15.5	15.9	16.2	16.6	17.0	17.4	17.8	18.1	18.5	18.9	19.3	19.7
78.7	31	13.2	13.5	13.9	14.3	14.6	15.0	15.4	15.7	16.1	16.5	16.8	17.2	17.6	17.9	18.3	18.7	19.0
80.0	31.5		13.1	13.5	13.8	14.2	14.5	14.9	15.2	15.6	15.9	16.3	16.7	17.0	17.4	17.7	18.1	18.4
81.3	32			13.0	13.4	13.7	14.1	14.4	14.8	15.1	15.4	15.8	16.1	16.5	16.8	17.2	17.5	17.9
82.6	32.5					13.3	13.6	14.0	14.3	14.6	15.0	15.3	15.6	16.0	16.3	16.6	17.0	17.3
83.8	33						13.2	13.6	13.9	14.2	14.5	14.8	15.2	15.5	15.8	16.1	16.5	16.8
85.1	33.5							13.2	13.5	13.8	14.1	14.4	14.7	15.0	15.3	15.7	16.0	16.3
86.4	34								13.1	13.4	13.7	14.0	14.3	14.6	14.9	15.2	15.5	15.8
87.6	34.5										13.3	13.6	13.9	14.2	14.5	14.8	15.1	15.4
88.9	35											13.2	13.5	13.8	14.1	14.3	14.6	14.9
90.2	35.5												13.1	13.4	13.7	13.9	14.2	14.5
91.4	36													13.0	13.3	13.6	13.8	14.1
92.7	36.5															13.2	13.5	13.7
94.0	37																13.1	13.4

Whenever a child's specific height or weight measurement is not listed, round to the closest number in the table.

CALCULATED BODY MASS INDEX   29"–43" AND 26.5 LBS.–34.5 LBS.

Weight

Height Cm	In	Kg 12.0 / Lb 26.5	12.2 / 27	12.5 / 27.5	12.7 / 28	12.9 / 28.5	13.2 / 29	13.4 / 29.5	13.6 / 30	13.8 / 30.5	14.1 / 31	14.3 / 31.5	14.5 / 32	14.7 / 32.5	15.0 / 33	15.2 / 33.5	15.4 / 34	15.6 / 34.5
73.7	29	22.2	22.6	23.0	23.4	23.8	24.2	24.7	25.1	25.5	25.9	26.3	26.8	27.2	27.6	28.0	28.4	28.8
74.9	29.5	21.4	21.8	22.2	22.6	23.0	23.4	23.8	24.2	24.6	25.0	25.4	25.9	26.3	26.7	27.1	27.5	27.9
76.2	30	20.7	21.1	21.5	21.9	22.3	22.7	23.0	23.4	23.8	24.2	24.6	25.0	25.4	25.8	26.2	26.6	27.0
77.5	30.5	20.0	20.4	20.8	21.2	21.5	21.9	22.3	22.7	23.1	23.4	23.8	24.2	24.6	24.9	25.3	25.7	26.1
78.7	31	19.4	19.8	20.1	20.5	20.9	21.2	21.6	21.9	22.3	22.7	23.0	23.4	23.8	24.1	24.5	24.9	25.2
80.0	31.5	18.8	19.1	19.5	19.8	20.2	20.5	20.9	21.3	21.6	22.0	22.3	22.7	23.0	23.4	23.7	24.1	24.4
81.3	32	18.2	18.5	18.9	19.2	19.6	19.9	20.3	20.6	20.9	21.3	21.6	22.0	22.3	22.7	23.0	23.3	23.7
82.6	32.5	17.6	18.0	18.3	18.6	19.0	19.3	19.6	20.0	20.3	20.6	21.0	21.3	21.6	22.0	22.3	22.6	23.0
83.8	33	17.1	17.4	17.8	18.1	18.4	18.7	19.0	19.4	19.7	20.0	20.3	20.7	21.0	21.3	21.6	22.0	22.3
85.1	33.5	16.6	16.9	17.2	17.5	17.9	18.2	18.5	18.8	19.1	19.4	19.7	20.0	20.4	20.7	21.0	21.3	21.6
86.4	34	16.1	16.4	16.7	17.0	17.3	17.6	17.9	18.2	18.5	18.9	19.2	19.5	19.8	20.1	20.4	20.7	21.0
87.6	34.5	15.7	15.9	16.2	16.5	16.8	17.1	17.4	17.7	18.0	18.3	18.6	18.9	19.2	19.5	19.8	20.1	20.4
88.9	35	15.2	15.5	15.8	16.1	16.4	16.6	16.9	17.2	17.5	17.8	18.1	18.4	18.7	18.9	19.2	19.5	19.8
90.2	35.5	14.8	15.1	15.3	15.6	15.9	16.2	16.5	16.7	17.0	17.3	17.6	17.9	18.1	18.4	18.7	19.0	19.2
91.4	36	14.4	14.6	14.9	15.2	15.5	15.7	16.0	16.3	16.5	16.8	17.1	17.4	17.6	17.9	18.2	18.4	18.7
92.7	36.5	14.0	14.2	14.5	14.8	15.0	15.3	15.6	15.8	16.1	16.4	16.6	16.9	17.2	17.4	17.7	17.9	18.2
94.0	37	13.6	13.9	14.1	14.4	14.6	14.9	15.2	15.4	15.7	15.9	16.2	16.4	16.7	16.9	17.2	17.5	17.7
95.3	37.5	13.2	13.5	13.7	14.0	14.2	14.5	14.7	15.0	15.2	15.5	15.7	16.0	16.2	16.5	16.7	17.0	17.2
96.5	38		13.1	13.4	13.6	13.9	14.1	14.4	14.6	14.9	15.1	15.3	15.6	15.8	16.1	16.3	16.6	16.8
97.8	38.5			13.0	13.3	13.5	13.8	14.0	14.2	14.5	14.7	14.9	15.2	15.4	15.7	15.9	16.1	16.4
99.1	39					13.2	13.4	13.6	13.9	14.1	14.3	14.6	14.8	15.0	15.3	15.5	15.7	15.9
100.3	39.5						13.1	13.3	13.5	13.7	14.0	14.2	14.4	14.6	14.9	15.1	15.3	15.5
101.6	40								13.2	13.4	13.6	13.8	14.1	14.3	14.5	14.7	14.9	15.2
102.9	40.5									13.1	13.3	13.5	13.7	13.9	14.1	14.4	14.6	14.8
104.1	41											13.2	13.4	13.6	13.8	14.0	14.2	14.4
105.4	41.5												13.1	13.3	13.5	13.7	13.9	14.1
106.7	42														13.2	13.4	13.6	13.8
108.0	42.5															13.0	13.2	13.4
109.2	43																	13.1

Whenever a child's specific height or weight measurement is not listed, round to the closest number in the table.

CALCULATED BODY MASS INDEX   29″–43″ AND 35 LBS.–43 LBS

Height Cm	In	Weight Kg 15.9 Lb 35	16.1 35.5	16.3 36	16.6 36.5	16.8 37	17.0 37.5	17.2 38	17.5 38.5	17.7 39	17.9 39.5	18.1 40	18.4 40.5	18.6 41	18.8 41.5	19.1 42	19.3 42.5	19.5 43
73.7	29	29.3	29.7	30.1	30.5	30.9	31.3	31.8	32.2	32.6	33.0	33.4	33.9	34.3	34.7			
74.9	29.5	28.3	28.7	29.1	29.5	29.9	30.3	30.7	31.1	31.5	31.9	32.3	32.7	33.1	33.5	33.9	34.3	34.7
76.2	30	27.3	27.7	28.1	28.5	28.9	29.3	29.7	30.1	30.5	30.9	31.2	31.6	32.0	32.4	32.8	33.2	33.6
77.5	30.5	26.5	26.8	27.2	27.6	28.0	28.3	28.7	29.1	29.5	29.9	30.2	30.6	31.0	31.4	31.7	32.1	32.5
78.7	31	25.6	26.0	26.3	26.7	27.1	27.4	27.8	28.2	28.5	28.9	29.3	29.6	30.0	30.4	30.7	31.1	31.5
80.0	31.5	24.8	25.2	25.5	25.9	26.2	26.6	26.9	27.3	27.6	28.0	28.3	28.7	29.1	29.4	29.8	30.1	30.5
81.3	32	24.0	24.4	24.7	25.1	25.4	25.7	26.1	26.4	26.8	27.1	27.5	27.8	28.2	28.5	28.8	29.2	29.5
82.6	32.5	23.3	23.6	24.0	24.3	24.6	25.0	25.3	25.6	26.0	26.3	26.6	27.0	27.3	27.6	28.0	28.3	28.6
83.8	33	22.6	22.9	23.2	23.6	23.9	24.2	24.5	24.9	25.2	25.5	25.8	26.1	26.5	26.8	27.1	27.4	27.8
85.1	33.5	21.9	22.2	22.6	22.9	23.2	23.5	23.8	24.1	24.4	24.7	25.1	25.4	25.7	26.0	26.3	26.6	26.9
86.4	34	21.3	21.6	21.9	22.2	22.5	22.8	23.1	23.4	23.7	24.0	24.3	24.6	24.9	25.2	25.5	25.8	26.2
87.6	34.5	20.7	21.0	21.3	21.6	21.9	22.2	22.4	22.7	23.0	23.3	23.6	23.9	24.2	24.5	24.8	25.1	25.4
88.9	35	20.1	20.4	20.7	20.9	21.2	21.5	21.8	22.1	22.4	22.7	23.0	23.2	23.5	23.8	24.1	24.4	24.7
90.2	35.5	19.5	19.8	20.1	20.4	20.6	20.9	21.2	21.5	21.8	22.0	22.3	22.6	22.9	23.2	23.4	23.7	24.0
91.4	36	19.0	19.3	19.5	19.8	20.1	20.3	20.6	20.9	21.2	21.4	21.7	22.0	22.2	22.5	22.8	23.1	23.3
92.7	36.5	18.5	18.7	19.0	19.3	19.5	19.8	20.1	20.3	20.6	20.8	21.1	21.4	21.6	21.9	22.2	22.4	22.7
94.0	37	18.0	18.2	18.5	18.7	19.0	19.3	19.5	19.8	20.0	20.3	20.5	20.8	21.1	21.3	21.6	21.8	22.1
95.3	37.5	17.5	17.7	18.0	18.2	18.5	18.7	19.0	19.2	19.5	19.7	20.0	20.2	20.5	20.7	21.0	21.2	21.5
96.5	38	17.0	17.3	17.5	17.8	18.0	18.3	18.5	18.7	19.0	19.2	19.5	19.7	20.0	20.2	20.4	20.7	20.9
97.8	38.5	16.6	16.8	17.1	17.3	17.6	17.8	18.0	18.3	18.5	18.7	19.0	19.2	19.4	19.7	19.9	20.2	20.4
99.1	39	16.2	16.4	16.6	16.9	17.1	17.3	17.6	17.8	18.0	18.3	18.5	18.7	19.0	19.2	19.4	19.6	19.9
100.3	39.5	15.8	16.0	16.2	16.4	16.7	16.9	17.1	17.3	17.6	17.8	18.0	18.2	18.5	18.7	18.9	19.2	19.4
101.6	40	15.4	15.6	15.8	16.0	16.3	16.5	16.7	16.9	17.1	17.4	17.6	17.8	18.0	18.2	18.5	18.7	18.9
102.9	40.5	15.0	15.2	15.4	15.6	15.9	16.1	16.3	16.5	16.7	16.9	17.1	17.4	17.6	17.8	18.0	18.2	18.4
104.1	41	14.6	14.8	15.1	15.3	15.5	15.7	15.9	16.1	16.3	16.5	16.7	16.9	17.1	17.4	17.6	17.8	18.0
105.4	41.5	14.3	14.5	14.7	14.9	15.1	15.3	15.5	15.7	15.9	16.1	16.3	16.5	16.7	16.9	17.1	17.3	17.6
106.7	42	13.9	14.1	14.3	14.5	14.7	14.9	15.1	15.3	15.5	15.7	15.9	16.1	16.3	16.5	16.7	16.9	17.1
108.0	42.5	13.6	13.8	14.0	14.2	14.4	14.6	14.8	15.0	15.2	15.4	15.6	15.8	16.0	16.2	16.3	16.5	16.7
109.2	43	13.3	13.5	13.7	13.9	14.1	14.3	14.4	14.6	14.8	15.0	15.2	15.4	15.6	15.8	16.0	16.2	16.4

Whenever a child's specific height or weight measurement is not listed, round to the closest number in the table.

CALCULATED BODY MASS INDEX   43.5"–48" AND 35 LBS.–43 LBS.

Height		Weight																	
Cm	In	Kg 15.9	16.1	16.3	16.6	16.8	17.0	17.2	17.5	17.7	17.9	18.1	18.4	18.6	18.8	19.1	19.3	19.5
		Lb 35	35.5	36	36.5	37	37.5	38	38.5	39	39.5	40	40.5	41	41.5	42	42.5	43
110.5	43.5	13.0	13.2	13.4	13.6	13.7	13.9	14.1	14.3	14.5	14.7	14.9	15.0	15.2	15.4	15.6	15.8	16.0
111.8	44		13.1	13.1	13.3	13.4	13.6	13.8	14.0	14.2	14.3	14.5	14.7	14.9	15.1	15.3	15.4	15.6
113.0	44.5				13.3	13.1	13.3	13.5	13.7	13.8	14.0	14.2	14.4	14.6	14.7	14.9	15.1	15.3
114.3	45					13.1	13.0	13.2	13.4	13.5	13.7	13.9	14.1	14.2	14.4	14.6	14.8	14.9
115.6	45.5								13.1	13.2	13.4	13.6	13.8	13.9	14.1	14.3	14.4	14.6
116.8	46										13.1	13.3	13.5	13.6	13.8	14.0	14.1	14.3
118.1	46.5											13.0	13.2	13.3	13.5	13.7	13.8	14.0
119.4	47													13.0	13.2	13.4	13.5	13.7
120.7	47.5															13.1	13.2	13.4
121.9	48																	13.1

Whenever a child's specific height or weight measurement is not listed, round to the closest number in the table.

CALCULATED BODY MASS INDEX   30"–44" AND 43.5 LBS.–51.5 LBS.

Height		Weight																
Cm	In	Kg 19.7	20.0	20.2	20.4	20.6	20.9	21.1	21.3	21.5	21.8	22.0	22.2	22.5	22.7	22.9	23.1	23.4
		Lb 43.5	44	44.5	45	45.5	46	46.5	47	47.5	48	48.5	49	49.5	50	50.5	51	51.5
76.2	30	34.0	34.4	34.8														
77.5	30.5	32.9	33.3	33.6	34.0	34.4	34.8											
78.7	31	31.8	32.2	32.6	32.9	33.3	33.7	34.0	34.4	34.8								
80.0	31.5	30.8	31.2	31.5	31.9	32.2	32.6	32.9	33.3	33.7	34.0	34.4	34.7					
81.3	32	29.9	30.2	30.6	30.9	31.2	31.6	31.9	32.3	32.6	33.0	33.3	33.6	34.0	34.3	34.7		
82.6	32.5	29.0	29.3	29.6	30.0	30.3	30.6	31.0	31.3	31.6	32.0	32.3	32.6	32.9	33.3	33.6	33.9	34.3
83.8	33	28.1	28.4	28.7	29.1	29.4	29.7	30.0	30.3	30.7	31.0	31.3	31.6	32.0	32.3	32.6	32.9	33.2
85.1	33.5	27.3	27.6	27.9	28.2	28.5	28.8	29.1	29.4	29.8	30.1	30.4	30.7	31.0	31.3	31.6	32.0	32.3
86.4	34	26.5	26.8	27.1	27.4	27.7	28.0	28.3	28.6	28.9	29.2	29.5	29.8	30.1	30.4	30.7	31.0	31.3
87.6	34.5	25.7	26.0	26.3	26.6	26.9	27.2	27.5	27.8	28.1	28.4	28.6	28.9	29.2	29.5	29.8	30.1	30.4
88.9	35	25.0	25.3	25.5	25.8	26.1	26.4	26.7	27.0	27.3	27.5	27.8	28.1	28.4	28.7	29.0	29.3	29.6
90.2	35.5	24.3	24.5	24.8	25.1	25.4	25.7	25.9	26.2	26.5	26.8	27.1	27.3	27.6	27.9	28.2	28.5	28.7
91.4	36	23.6	23.9	24.1	24.4	24.7	25.0	25.2	25.5	25.8	26.0	26.3	26.6	26.9	27.1	27.4	27.7	27.9
92.7	36.5	23.0	23.2	23.5	23.7	24.0	24.3	24.5	24.8	25.1	25.3	25.6	25.9	26.1	26.4	26.7	26.9	27.2
94.0	37	22.3	22.6	22.9	23.1	23.4	23.6	23.9	24.1	24.4	24.7	24.9	25.2	25.4	25.7	25.9	26.2	26.4
95.3	37.5	21.7	22.0	22.2	22.5	22.7	23.0	23.2	23.5	23.7	24.0	24.2	24.5	24.7	25.0	25.2	25.5	25.7
96.5	38	21.2	21.4	21.7	21.9	22.2	22.4	22.6	22.9	23.2	23.4	23.6	23.9	24.1	24.3	24.6	24.8	25.1
97.8	38.5	20.6	20.9	21.1	21.3	21.6	21.8	22.1	22.3	22.5	22.8	23.0	23.2	23.5	23.7	24.0	24.2	24.4
99.1	39	20.1	20.3	20.6	20.8	21.0	21.3	21.5	21.7	22.0	22.2	22.4	22.6	22.9	23.1	23.3	23.6	23.8
100.3	39.5	19.6	19.8	20.1	20.3	20.5	20.7	21.0	21.2	21.4	21.6	21.9	22.1	22.3	22.5	22.8	23.0	23.2
101.6	40	19.1	19.3	19.6	19.8	20.0	20.2	20.4	20.7	20.9	21.1	21.3	21.5	21.8	22.0	22.2	22.4	22.6
102.9	40.5	18.6	18.9	19.1	19.3	19.5	19.7	19.9	20.1	20.4	20.6	20.8	21.0	21.2	21.4	21.6	21.9	22.1
104.1	41	18.2	18.4	18.6	18.8	19.0	19.2	19.4	19.7	19.9	20.1	20.3	20.5	20.7	20.9	21.1	21.3	21.5
105.4	41.5	17.8	18.0	18.2	18.4	18.6	18.8	19.0	19.2	19.4	19.6	19.8	20.0	20.2	20.4	20.6	20.8	21.0
106.7	42	17.3	17.5	17.7	17.9	18.1	18.3	18.5	18.7	18.9	19.1	19.3	19.5	19.7	19.9	20.1	20.3	20.5
108.0	42.5	16.9	17.1	17.3	17.5	17.7	17.9	18.1	18.3	18.5	18.7	18.9	19.1	19.3	19.5	19.7	19.9	20.0
109.2	43	16.5	16.7	16.9	17.1	17.3	17.5	17.7	17.9	18.1	18.3	18.4	18.6	18.8	19.0	19.2	19.4	19.6
110.5	43.5	16.2	16.3	16.5	16.7	16.9	17.1	17.3	17.5	17.6	17.8	18.0	18.2	18.4	18.6	18.8	18.9	19.1
111.8	44	15.8	16.0	16.2	16.3	16.5	16.7	16.9	17.1	17.2	17.4	17.6	17.8	18.0	18.2	18.3	18.5	18.7

Whenever a child's specific height or weight measurement is not listed, round to the closest number in the table.

CALCULATED BODY MASS INDEX — 44.5"–51" AND 43.5 LBS.–51.5 LBS.

Height		Weight																
Cm	In	Kg 19.7	20.0	20.2	20.4	20.6	20.9	21.1	21.3	21.5	21.8	22.0	22.2	22.5	22.7	22.9	23.1	23.4
		Lb 43.5	44	44.5	45	45.5	46	46.5	47	47.5	48	48.5	49	49.5	50	50.5	51	51.5
110.5	43.5	13.0	13.2	13.4	13.6	13.7	13.9	14.1	14.3	14.5	14.7	14.9	15.0	15.2	15.4	15.6	15.8	16.0
113.0	44.5	15.4	15.6	15.8	16.0	16.2	16.3	16.5	16.7	16.9	17.0	17.2	17.4	17.6	17.8	17.9	18.1	18.3
114.3	45	15.1	15.3	15.5	15.6	15.8	16.0	16.1	16.3	16.5	16.7	16.8	17.0	17.2	17.4	17.5	17.7	17.9
115.6	45.5	14.8	14.9	15.1	15.3	15.5	15.6	15.8	16.0	16.1	16.3	16.5	16.6	16.8	17.0	17.2	17.3	17.5
116.8	46	14.5	14.6	14.8	15.0	15.1	15.3	15.5	15.6	15.8	15.9	16.1	16.3	16.4	16.6	16.8	16.9	17.1
118.1	46.5	14.1	14.3	14.5	14.6	14.8	15.0	15.1	15.3	15.4	15.6	15.8	15.9	16.1	16.3	16.4	16.6	16.7
119.4	47	13.8	14.0	14.2	14.3	14.5	14.6	14.8	15.0	15.1	15.3	15.4	15.6	15.8	15.9	16.1	16.2	16.4
120.7	47.5	13.6	13.7	13.9	14.0	14.2	14.3	14.5	14.6	14.8	15.0	15.1	15.3	15.4	15.6	15.7	15.9	16.0
121.9	48	13.3	13.4	13.6	13.7	13.9	14.0	14.2	14.3	14.5	14.6	14.8	15.0	15.1	15.3	15.4	15.6	15.7
124.5	49			13.0	13.2	13.3	13.5	13.6	13.8	13.9	14.1	14.2	14.3	14.5	14.6	14.8	14.9	15.1
127.0	50							13.1	13.2	13.4	13.5	13.6	13.8	13.9	14.1	14.2	14.3	14.5
129.5	51											13.1	13.2	13.4	13.5	13.7	13.8	13.9
132.1	52														13.0	13.1	13.3	13.4

Whenever a child's specific height or weight measurement is not listed, round to the closest number in the table.

CALCULATED BODY MASS INDEX   47″–56″ AND 52 LBS.–60 LBS.

Height		Weight																
Cm	In	Kg 23.6	23.8	24.0	24.3	24.5	24.7	24.9	25.2	25.4	25.6	25.9	26.1	26.3	26.5	26.8	27.0	27.2
		Lb 52	52.5	53	53.5	54	54.5	55	55.5	56	56.5	57	57.5	58	58.5	59	59.5	60
119.4	47	16.6	16.7	16.9	17.0	17.2	17.3	17.5	17.7	17.8	18.0	18.1	18.3	18.5	18.6	18.8	18.9	19.1
120.7	47.5	16.2	16.4	16.5	16.7	16.8	17.0	17.1	17.3	17.5	17.6	17.8	17.9	18.1	18.2	18.4	18.5	18.7
121.9	48	15.9	16.0	16.2	16.3	16.5	16.6	16.8	16.9	17.1	17.2	17.4	17.5	17.7	17.9	18.0	18.2	18.3
124.5	49	15.2	15.4	15.5	15.7	15.8	16.0	16.1	16.3	16.4	16.5	16.7	16.8	17.0	17.1	17.3	17.4	17.6
127.0	50	14.6	14.8	14.9	15.0	15.2	15.3	15.5	15.6	15.7	15.9	16.0	16.2	16.3	16.5	16.6	16.7	16.9
129.5	51	14.1	14.2	14.3	14.5	14.6	14.7	14.9	15.0	15.1	15.3	15.4	15.5	15.7	15.8	15.9	16.1	16.2
132.1	52	13.5	13.7	13.8	13.9	14.0	14.2	14.3	14.4	14.6	14.7	14.8	15.0	15.1	15.2	15.3	15.5	15.6
134.6	53	13.0	13.1	13.3	13.4	13.5	13.6	13.8	13.9	14.0	14.1	14.3	14.4	14.5	14.6	14.8	14.9	15.0
137.2	54					13.0	13.1	13.3	13.4	13.5	13.6	13.7	13.9	14.0	14.1	14.2	14.3	14.5
139.7	55									13.0	13.1	13.2	13.4	13.5	13.6	13.7	13.8	13.9
142.2	56													13.0	13.1	13.2	13.3	13.5

Whenever a child's specific height or weight measurement is not listed, round to the closest number in the table.

CALCULATED BODY MASS INDEX   35.5"–51" AND 61 LBS.–77 LBS.

Height Cm	In	| Weight																
		Kg 27.7	28.1	28.6	29.0	29.5	29.9	30.4	30.8	31.3	31.8	32.2	32.7	33.1	33.6	34.0	34.5	34.9
		Lb 61	62	63	64	65	66	67	68	69	70	71	72	73	74	75	76	77
90.2	35.5	34.0	34.6															
91.4	36	33.1	33.6	34.2	34.7													
92.7	36.5	32.2	32.7	33.2	33.8	34.3	34.8											
94.0	37	31.3	31.8	32.4	32.9	33.4	33.9	34.4	34.9									
95.3	37.5	30.5	31.0	31.5	32.0	32.5	33.0	33.5	34.0	34.5	35.0							
96.5	38	29.7	30.2	30.7	31.2	31.6	32.1	32.6	33.1	33.6	34.1	34.6						
97.8	38.5	28.9	29.4	29.9	30.4	30.8	31.3	31.8	32.3	32.7	33.2	33.7	34.2	34.6				
99.1	39	28.2	28.7	29.1	29.6	30.0	30.5	31.0	31.4	31.9	32.4	32.8	33.3	33.7	34.2	34.7		
100.3	39.5	27.5	27.9	28.4	28.8	29.3	29.7	30.2	30.6	31.1	31.5	32.0	32.4	32.9	33.3	33.8	34.2	34.7
101.6	40	26.8	27.2	27.7	28.1	28.6	29.0	29.4	29.9	30.3	30.8	31.2	31.6	32.1	32.5	33.0	33.4	33.8
102.9	40.5	26.1	26.6	27.0	27.4	27.9	28.3	28.7	29.1	29.6	30.0	30.4	30.9	31.3	31.7	32.1	32.6	33.0
104.1	41	25.5	25.9	26.3	26.8	27.2	27.6	28.0	28.4	28.9	29.3	29.7	30.1	30.5	31.0	31.4	31.8	32.2
105.4	41.5	24.9	25.3	25.7	26.1	26.5	26.9	27.4	27.8	28.2	28.6	29.0	29.4	29.8	30.2	30.6	31.0	31.4
106.7	42	24.3	24.7	25.1	25.5	25.9	26.3	26.7	27.1	27.5	27.9	28.3	28.7	29.1	29.5	29.9	30.3	30.7
108.0	42.5	23.7	24.1	24.5	24.9	25.3	25.7	26.1	26.5	26.9	27.2	27.6	28.0	28.4	28.8	29.2	29.6	30.0
109.2	43	23.2	23.6	24.0	24.3	24.7	25.1	25.5	25.9	26.2	26.6	27.0	27.4	27.8	28.1	28.5	28.9	29.3
110.5	43.5	22.7	23.0	23.4	23.8	24.2	24.5	24.9	25.3	25.6	26.0	26.4	26.8	27.1	27.5	27.9	28.2	28.6
111.8	44	22.2	22.5	22.9	23.2	23.6	24.0	24.3	24.7	25.1	25.4	25.8	26.1	26.5	26.9	27.2	27.6	28.0
113.0	44.5	21.7	22.0	22.4	22.7	23.1	23.4	23.8	24.1	24.5	24.9	25.2	25.6	25.9	26.3	26.6	27.0	27.3
114.3	45	21.2	21.5	21.9	22.2	22.6	22.9	23.3	23.6	24.0	24.3	24.7	25.0	25.3	25.7	26.0	26.4	26.7
115.6	45.5	20.7	21.1	21.4	21.7	22.1	22.4	22.8	23.1	23.4	23.8	24.1	24.5	24.8	25.1	25.5	25.8	26.1
116.8	46	20.3	20.6	20.9	21.3	21.6	21.9	22.3	22.6	22.9	23.3	23.6	23.9	24.3	24.6	24.9	25.3	25.6
118.1	46.5	19.8	20.2	20.5	20.8	21.1	21.5	21.8	22.1	22.4	22.8	23.1	23.4	23.7	24.1	24.4	24.7	25.0
119.4	47	19.4	19.7	20.1	20.4	20.7	21.0	21.3	21.6	22.0	22.3	22.6	22.9	23.2	23.6	23.9	24.2	24.5
120.7	47.5	19.0	19.3	19.6	19.9	20.3	20.6	20.9	21.2	21.5	21.8	22.1	22.4	22.7	23.1	23.4	23.7	24.0
121.9	48	18.6	18.9	19.2	19.5	19.8	20.1	20.4	20.8	21.1	21.4	21.7	22.0	22.3	22.6	22.9	23.2	23.5
124.5	49	17.9	18.2	18.4	18.7	19.0	19.3	19.6	19.9	20.2	20.5	20.8	21.1	21.4	21.7	22.0	22.3	22.5
127.0	50	17.2	17.4	17.7	18.0	18.3	18.6	18.8	19.1	19.4	19.7	20.0	20.2	20.5	20.8	21.1	21.4	21.7
129.5	51	16.5	16.8	17.0	17.3	17.6	17.8	18.1	18.4	18.7	18.9	19.2	19.5	19.7	20.0	20.3	20.5	20.8

Whenever a child's specific height or weight measurement is not listed, round to the closest number in the table.

CALCULATED BODY MASS INDEX   52"–64" AND 61 LBS.–77 LBS.

Height		Weight																
Kg		27.7	28.1	28.6	29.0	29.5	29.9	30.4	30.8	31.3	31.8	32.2	32.7	33.1	33.6	34.0	34.5	34.9
Cm	**Lb / In**	61	62	63	64	65	66	67	68	69	70	71	72	73	74	75	76	77
132.1	52	15.9	16.1	16.4	16.6	16.9	17.2	17.4	17.7	17.9	18.2	18.5	18.7	19.0	19.2	19.5	19.8	20.0
134.6	53	15.3	15.5	15.8	16.0	16.3	16.5	16.8	17.0	17.3	17.5	17.8	18.0	18.3	18.5	18.8	19.0	19.3
137.2	54	14.7	14.9	15.2	15.4	15.7	15.9	16.2	16.4	16.6	16.9	17.1	17.4	17.6	17.8	18.1	18.3	18.6
139.7	55	14.2	14.4	14.6	14.9	15.1	15.3	15.6	15.8	16.0	16.3	16.5	16.7	17.0	17.2	17.4	17.7	17.9
142.2	56	13.7	13.9	14.1	14.3	14.6	14.8	15.0	15.2	15.5	15.7	15.9	16.1	16.4	16.6	16.8	17.0	17.3
144.8	57	13.2	13.4	13.6	13.8	14.1	14.3	14.5	14.7	14.9	15.1	15.4	15.6	15.8	16.0	16.2	16.4	16.7
147.3	58			13.2	13.4	13.6	13.8	14.0	14.2	14.4	14.6	14.8	15.0	15.3	15.5	15.7	15.9	16.1
149.9	59					13.1	13.3	13.5	13.7	13.9	14.1	14.3	14.5	14.7	14.9	15.1	15.3	15.6
152.4	60							13.1	13.3	13.5	13.7	13.9	14.1	14.3	14.5	14.6	14.8	15.0
154.9	61									13.0	13.2	13.4	13.6	13.8	14.0	14.2	14.4	14.5
157.5	62												13.2	13.4	13.5	13.7	13.9	14.1
160.0	63														13.1	13.3	13.5	13.6
162.6	64																13.0	13.2

Whenever a child's specific height or weight measurement is not listed, round to the closest number in the table.

CALCULATED BODY MASS INDEX   40.5"–60" AND 78 LBS.–94 LBS.

Height Cm	In	Weight Kg 35.4 / Lb 78	35.8 / 79	36.3 / 80	36.7 / 81	37.2 / 82	37.6 / 83	38.1 / 84	38.6 / 85	39.0 / 86	39.5 / 87	39.9 / 88	40.4 / 89	40.8 / 90	41.3 / 91	41.7 / 92	42.2 / 93	42.6 / 94
101.6	40	34.3	34.7															
102.9	40.5	33.4	33.9	34.3	34.7													
104.1	41	32.6	33.0	33.5	33.9	34.3	34.7											
105.4	41.5	31.8	32.2	32.7	33.1	33.5	33.9	34.3	34.7									
106.7	42	31.1	31.5	31.9	32.3	32.7	33.1	33.5	33.9	34.3	34.7							
108.0	42.5	30.4	30.8	31.1	31.5	31.9	32.3	32.7	33.1	33.5	33.9	34.3	34.6					
109.2	43	29.7	30.0	30.4	30.8	31.2	31.6	31.9	32.3	32.7	33.1	33.5	33.8	34.2	34.6	35.0		
110.5	43.5	29.0	29.4	29.7	30.1	30.5	30.8	31.2	31.6	32.0	32.3	32.7	33.1	33.4	33.8	34.2	34.6	34.9
111.8	44	28.3	28.7	29.1	29.4	29.8	30.1	30.5	30.9	31.2	31.6	32.0	32.3	32.7	33.0	33.4	33.8	34.1
113.0	44.5	27.7	28.0	28.4	28.8	29.1	29.5	29.8	30.2	30.5	30.9	31.2	31.6	32.0	32.3	32.7	33.0	33.4
114.3	45	27.1	27.4	27.8	28.1	28.5	28.8	29.2	29.5	29.9	30.2	30.6	30.9	31.2	31.6	31.9	32.3	32.6
115.6	45.5	26.5	26.8	27.2	27.5	27.8	28.2	28.5	28.9	29.2	29.5	29.9	30.2	30.6	30.9	31.2	31.6	31.9
116.8	46	25.9	26.2	26.6	26.9	27.2	27.6	27.9	28.2	28.6	28.9	29.2	29.6	29.9	30.2	30.6	30.9	31.2
118.1	46.5	25.4	25.7	26.0	26.3	26.7	27.0	27.3	27.6	28.0	28.3	28.6	28.9	29.3	29.6	29.9	30.2	30.6
119.4	47	24.8	25.1	25.5	25.8	26.1	26.4	26.7	27.1	27.4	27.7	28.0	28.3	28.6	29.0	29.3	29.6	29.9
120.7	47.5	24.3	24.6	24.9	25.2	25.6	25.9	26.2	26.5	26.8	27.1	27.4	27.7	28.0	28.4	28.7	29.0	29.3
121.9	48	23.8	24.1	24.4	24.7	25.0	25.3	25.6	25.9	26.2	26.5	26.9	27.2	27.5	27.8	28.1	28.4	28.7
124.5	49	22.8	23.1	23.4	23.7	24.0	24.3	24.6	24.9	25.2	25.5	25.8	26.1	26.4	26.6	26.9	27.2	27.5
127.0	50	21.9	22.2	22.5	22.8	23.1	23.3	23.6	23.9	24.2	24.5	24.7	25.0	25.3	25.6	25.9	26.2	26.4
129.5	51	21.1	21.4	21.6	21.9	22.2	22.4	22.7	23.0	23.2	23.5	23.8	24.1	24.3	24.6	24.9	25.1	25.4
132.1	52	20.3	20.5	20.8	21.1	21.3	21.6	21.8	22.1	22.4	22.6	22.9	23.1	23.4	23.7	23.9	24.2	24.4
134.6	53	19.5	19.8	20.0	20.3	20.5	20.8	21.0	21.3	21.5	21.8	22.0	22.3	22.5	22.8	23.0	23.3	23.5
137.2	54	18.8	19.0	19.3	19.5	19.8	20.0	20.3	20.5	20.7	21.0	21.2	21.5	21.7	21.9	22.2	22.4	22.7
139.7	55	18.1	18.4	18.6	18.8	19.1	19.3	19.5	19.8	20.0	20.2	20.5	20.7	20.9	21.2	21.4	21.6	21.8
142.2	56	17.5	17.7	17.9	18.2	18.4	18.6	18.8	19.1	19.3	19.5	19.7	20.0	20.2	20.4	20.6	20.8	21.1
144.8	57	16.9	17.1	17.3	17.5	17.7	18.0	18.2	18.4	18.6	18.8	19.0	19.3	19.5	19.7	19.9	20.1	20.3
147.3	58	16.3	16.5	16.7	16.9	17.1	17.3	17.6	17.8	18.0	18.2	18.4	18.6	18.8	19.0	19.2	19.4	19.6
149.9	59	15.8	16.0	16.2	16.4	16.6	16.8	17.0	17.2	17.4	17.6	17.8	18.0	18.2	18.4	18.6	18.8	19.0
152.4	60	15.2	15.4	15.6	15.8	16.0	16.2	16.4	16.6	16.8	17.0	17.2	17.4	17.6	17.8	18.0	18.2	18.4

Whenever a child's specific height or weight measurement is not listed, round to the closest number in the table.

CALCULATED BODY MASS INDEX   61"–71" AND 78 LBS.–94 LBS.

Height		Weight																
Cm	In	Kg 35.4	35.8	36.3	36.7	37.2	37.6	38.1	38.6	39.0	39.5	39.9	40.4	40.8	41.3	41.7	42.2	42.6
		Lb 78	79	80	81	82	83	84	85	86	87	88	89	90	91	92	93	94
154.9	61	14.7	14.9	15.1	15.3	15.5	15.7	15.9	16.1	16.2	16.4	16.6	16.8	17.0	17.2	17.4	17.6	17.8
157.5	62	14.3	14.4	14.6	14.8	15.0	15.2	15.4	15.5	15.7	15.9	16.1	16.3	16.5	16.6	16.8	17.0	17.2
160.0	63	13.8	14.0	14.2	14.3	14.5	14.7	14.9	15.1	15.2	15.4	15.6	15.8	15.9	16.1	16.3	16.5	16.7
162.6	64	13.4	13.6	13.7	13.9	14.1	14.2	14.4	14.6	14.8	14.9	15.1	15.3	15.4	15.6	15.8	16.0	16.1
165.1	65		13.1	13.3	13.5	13.6	13.8	14.0	14.1	14.3	14.5	14.6	14.8	15.0	15.1	15.3	15.5	15.6
167.6	66				13.1	13.2	13.4	13.6	13.7	13.9	14.0	14.2	14.4	14.5	14.7	14.8	15.0	15.2
170.2	67							13.2	13.3	13.5	13.6	13.8	13.9	14.1	14.3	14.4	14.6	14.7
172.7	68									13.1	13.2	13.4	13.5	13.7	13.8	14.0	14.1	14.3
175.3	69												13.1	13.3	13.4	13.6	13.7	13.9
177.8	70														13.1	13.2	13.3	13.5
180.3	71																	13.1

Whenever a child's specific height or weight measurement is not listed, round to the closest number in the table.

CALCULATED BODY MASS INDEX — 44"–68" AND 95 LBS.–112 LBS.

Weight (Kg / Lb)

Height (Cm)	(In)	43.1 / 95	43.5 / 96	44.0 / 97	44.5 / 98	44.9 / 99	45.4 / 100	45.8 / 101	46.3 / 102	46.7 / 103	47.2 / 104	47.6 / 105	48.1 / 106	48.5 / 107	49.0 / 108	49.4 / 109	49.9 / 110	50.8 / 112
111.8	44	34.5	34.9															
113.0	44.5	33.7	34.1	34.4	34.8													
114.3	45	33.0	33.3	33.7	34.0	34.4	34.7											
115.6	45.5	32.3	32.6	32.9	33.3	33.6	34.0	34.3	34.6	35.0								
116.8	46	31.6	31.9	32.2	32.6	32.9	33.2	33.6	33.9	34.2	34.6	34.9						
118.1	46.5	30.9	31.2	31.5	31.9	32.2	32.5	32.8	33.2	33.5	33.8	34.1	34.5	34.8				
119.4	47	30.2	30.6	30.9	31.2	31.5	31.8	32.1	32.5	32.8	33.1	33.4	33.7	34.1	34.4	34.7		
120.7	47.5	29.6	29.9	30.2	30.5	30.8	31.2	31.5	31.8	32.1	32.4	32.7	33.0	33.3	33.7	34.0	34.3	34.9
121.9	48	29.0	29.3	29.6	29.9	30.2	30.5	30.8	31.1	31.4	31.7	32.0	32.3	32.7	33.0	33.3	33.6	34.2
124.5	49	27.8	28.1	28.4	28.7	29.0	29.3	29.6	29.9	30.2	30.5	30.7	31.0	31.3	31.6	31.9	32.2	32.8
127.0	50	26.7	27.0	27.3	27.6	27.8	28.1	28.4	28.7	29.0	29.2	29.5	29.8	30.1	30.4	30.7	30.9	31.5
129.5	51	25.7	25.9	26.2	26.5	26.8	27.0	27.3	27.6	27.8	28.1	28.4	28.7	28.9	29.2	29.5	29.7	30.3
132.1	52	24.7	25.0	25.2	25.5	25.7	26.0	26.3	26.5	26.8	27.0	27.3	27.6	27.8	28.1	28.3	28.6	29.1
134.6	53	23.8	24.0	24.3	24.5	24.8	25.0	25.3	25.5	25.8	26.0	26.3	26.5	26.8	27.0	27.3	27.5	28.0
137.2	54	22.9	23.1	23.4	23.6	23.9	24.1	24.4	24.6	24.8	25.1	25.3	25.6	25.8	26.0	26.3	26.5	27.0
139.7	55	22.1	22.3	22.5	22.8	23.0	23.2	23.5	23.7	23.9	24.2	24.4	24.6	24.9	25.1	25.3	25.6	26.0
142.2	56	21.3	21.5	21.7	22.0	22.2	22.4	22.6	22.9	23.1	23.3	23.5	23.8	24.0	24.2	24.4	24.7	25.1
144.8	57	20.6	20.8	21.0	21.2	21.4	21.6	21.9	22.1	22.3	22.5	22.7	22.9	23.2	23.4	23.6	23.8	24.2
147.3	58	19.9	20.1	20.3	20.5	20.7	20.9	21.1	21.3	21.5	21.7	21.9	22.2	22.4	22.6	22.8	23.0	23.4
149.9	59	19.2	19.4	19.6	19.8	20.0	20.2	20.4	20.6	20.8	21.0	21.2	21.4	21.6	21.8	22.0	22.2	22.6
152.4	60	18.6	18.7	18.9	19.1	19.3	19.5	19.7	19.9	20.1	20.3	20.5	20.7	20.9	21.1	21.3	21.5	21.9
154.9	61	17.9	18.1	18.3	18.5	18.7	18.9	19.1	19.3	19.5	19.7	19.8	20.0	20.2	20.4	20.6	20.8	21.2
157.5	62	17.4	17.6	17.7	17.9	18.1	18.3	18.5	18.7	18.8	19.0	19.2	19.4	19.6	19.8	19.9	20.1	20.5
160.0	63	16.8	17.0	17.2	17.4	17.5	17.7	17.9	18.1	18.2	18.4	18.6	18.8	19.0	19.1	19.3	19.5	19.8
162.6	64	16.3	16.5	16.6	16.8	17.0	17.2	17.3	17.5	17.7	17.9	18.0	18.2	18.4	18.5	18.7	18.9	19.2
165.1	65	15.8	16.0	16.1	16.3	16.5	16.6	16.8	17.0	17.1	17.3	17.5	17.6	17.8	18.0	18.1	18.3	18.6
167.6	66	15.3	15.5	15.7	15.8	16.0	16.1	16.3	16.5	16.6	16.8	16.9	17.1	17.3	17.4	17.6	17.8	18.1
170.2	67	14.9	15.0	15.2	15.3	15.5	15.7	15.8	16.0	16.1	16.3	16.4	16.6	16.8	16.9	17.1	17.2	17.5
172.7	68	14.4	14.6	14.7	14.9	15.1	15.2	15.4	15.5	15.7	15.8	16.0	16.1	16.3	16.4	16.6	16.7	17.0

Whenever a child's specific height or weight measurement is not listed, round to the closest number in the table.

CALCULATED BODY MASS INDEX   69"–77" AND 95 LBS.–112 LBS.

Height		Weight																
Cm	**In**	Kg 43.1	43.5	44.0	44.5	44.9	45.4	45.8	46.3	46.7	47.2	47.6	48.1	48.5	49.0	49.4	49.9	50.8
		Lb 95	96	97	98	99	100	101	102	103	104	105	106	107	108	109	110	112
175.3	69	14.0	14.2	14.3	14.5	14.6	14.8	14.9	15.1	15.2	15.4	15.5	15.7	15.8	15.9	16.1	16.2	16.5
177.8	70	13.6	13.8	13.9	14.1	14.2	14.3	14.5	14.6	14.8	14.9	15.1	15.2	15.4	15.5	15.6	15.8	16.1
180.3	71	13.2	13.4	13.5	13.7	13.8	13.9	14.1	14.2	14.4	14.5	14.6	14.8	14.9	15.1	15.2	15.3	15.6
182.9	72		13.0	13.2	13.3	13.4	13.6	13.7	13.8	14.0	14.1	14.2	14.4	14.5	14.6	14.8	14.9	15.2
185.4	73					13.1	13.2	13.3	13.5	13.6	13.7	13.9	14.0	14.1	14.2	14.4	14.5	14.8
188.0	74								13.1	13.2	13.4	13.5	13.6	13.7	13.9	14.0	14.1	14.4
190.5	75											13.1	13.2	13.4	13.5	13.6	13.7	14.0
193.0	76													13.0	13.1	13.3	13.4	13.6
195.6	77																13.0	13.3

Whenever a child's specific height or weight measurement is not listed, round to the closest number in the table.

CALCULATED BODY MASS INDEX   48"–76" AND 114 LBS.–146 LBS.

Weight (top numbers in each weight column are **Kg**, lower numbers are **Lb**)

Height Cm	In	51.7 / 114	52.6 / 116	53.5 / 118	54.4 / 120	55.3 / 122	56.2 / 124	57.2 / 126	58.1 / 128	59.0 / 130	59.9 / 132	60.8 / 134	61.7 / 136	62.6 / 138	63.5 / 140	64.4 / 142	65.3 / 144	66.2 / 146
121.9	48	34.8																
124.5	49	33.4	34.0	34.6														
127.0	50	32.1	32.6	33.2	33.7	34.3	34.9											
129.5	51	30.8	31.4	31.9	32.4	33.0	33.5	34.1	34.6									
132.1	52	29.6	30.2	30.7	31.2	31.7	32.2	32.8	33.3	33.8	34.3	34.8						
134.6	53	28.5	29.0	29.5	30.0	30.5	31.0	31.5	32.0	32.5	33.0	33.5	34.0	34.5				
137.2	54	27.5	28.0	28.5	28.9	29.4	29.9	30.4	30.9	31.3	31.8	32.3	32.8	33.3	33.8	34.2	34.7	
139.7	55	26.5	27.0	27.4	27.9	28.4	28.8	29.3	29.7	30.2	30.7	31.1	31.6	32.1	32.5	33.0	33.5	33.9
142.2	56	25.6	26.0	26.5	26.9	27.4	27.8	28.2	28.7	29.1	29.6	30.0	30.5	30.9	31.4	31.8	32.3	32.7
144.8	57	24.7	25.1	25.5	26.0	26.4	26.8	27.3	27.7	28.1	28.6	29.0	29.4	29.9	30.3	30.7	31.2	31.6
147.3	58	23.8	24.2	24.7	25.1	25.5	25.9	26.3	26.8	27.2	27.6	28.0	28.4	28.8	29.3	29.7	30.1	30.5
149.9	59	23.0	23.4	23.8	24.2	24.6	25.0	25.4	25.9	26.3	26.7	27.1	27.5	27.9	28.3	28.7	29.1	29.5
152.4	60	22.3	22.7	23.0	23.4	23.8	24.2	24.6	25.0	25.4	25.8	26.2	26.6	27.0	27.3	27.7	28.1	28.5
154.9	61	21.5	21.9	22.3	22.7	23.1	23.4	23.8	24.2	24.6	24.9	25.3	25.7	26.1	26.5	26.8	27.2	27.6
157.5	62	20.9	21.2	21.6	21.9	22.3	22.7	23.0	23.4	23.8	24.1	24.5	24.9	25.2	25.6	26.0	26.3	26.7
160.0	63	20.2	20.5	20.9	21.3	21.6	22.0	22.3	22.7	23.0	23.4	23.7	24.1	24.4	24.8	25.2	25.5	25.9
162.6	64	19.6	19.9	20.3	20.6	20.9	21.3	21.6	22.0	22.3	22.7	23.0	23.3	23.7	24.0	24.4	24.7	25.1
165.1	65	19.0	19.3	19.6	20.0	20.3	20.6	21.0	21.3	21.6	22.0	22.3	22.6	23.0	23.3	23.6	24.0	24.3
167.6	66	18.4	18.7	19.0	19.4	19.7	20.0	20.3	20.7	21.0	21.3	21.6	22.0	22.3	22.6	22.9	23.2	23.6
170.2	67	17.9	18.2	18.5	18.8	19.1	19.4	19.7	20.0	20.4	20.7	21.0	21.3	21.6	21.9	22.2	22.6	22.9
172.7	68	17.3	17.6	17.9	18.2	18.5	18.9	19.2	19.5	19.8	20.1	20.4	20.7	21.0	21.3	21.6	21.9	22.2
175.3	69	16.8	17.1	17.4	17.7	18.0	18.3	18.6	18.9	19.2	19.5	19.8	20.1	20.4	20.7	21.0	21.3	21.6
177.8	70	16.4	16.6	16.9	17.2	17.5	17.8	18.1	18.4	18.7	18.9	19.2	19.5	19.8	20.1	20.4	20.7	20.9
180.3	71	15.9	16.2	16.5	16.7	17.0	17.3	17.6	17.9	18.1	18.4	18.7	19.0	19.2	19.5	19.8	20.1	20.4
182.9	72	15.5	15.7	16.0	16.3	16.5	16.8	17.1	17.4	17.6	17.9	18.2	18.5	18.7	19.0	19.3	19.5	19.8
185.4	73	15.0	15.3	15.6	15.8	16.1	16.4	16.6	16.9	17.2	17.4	17.7	17.9	18.2	18.5	18.7	19.0	19.3
188.0	74	14.6	14.9	15.2	15.4	15.7	15.9	16.2	16.4	16.7	17.0	17.2	17.5	17.7	18.0	18.2	18.5	18.7
190.5	75	14.2	14.5	14.7	15.0	15.2	15.5	15.7	16.0	16.2	16.5	16.7	17.0	17.2	17.5	17.7	18.0	18.2
193.0	76	13.9	14.1	14.4	14.6	14.9	15.1	15.3	15.6	15.9	16.1	16.3	16.6	16.8	17.0	17.3	17.5	17.8
195.6	77	13.5	13.8	14.0	14.2	14.5	14.7	14.9	15.2	15.4	15.7	15.9	16.1	16.4	16.6	16.8	17.1	17.3
198.1	78	13.2	13.4	13.6	13.9	14.1	14.3	14.6	14.8	15.0	15.3	15.5	15.7	15.9	16.2	16.4	16.6	16.9

Whenever a child's specific height or weight measurement is not listed, round to the closest number in the table.

CALCULATED BODY MASS INDEX 55"–78" AND 148 LBS.–180 LBS.

Height Cm	Height In	Kg 67.1 / Lb 148	68.0 / 150	68.9 / 152	69.9 / 154	70.8 / 156	71.7 / 158	72.6 / 160	73.5 / 162	74.4 / 164	75.3 / 166	76.2 / 168	77.1 / 170	78.0 / 172	78.9 / 174	79.8 / 176	80.7 / 178	81.6 / 180
139.7	55	34.4	34.9															
142.2	56	33.2	33.6	34.1	34.5	35.0												
144.8	57	32.0	32.5	32.9	33.3	33.8	34.2	34.6										
147.3	58	30.9	31.3	31.8	32.2	32.6	33.0	33.4	33.9	34.3								
149.9	59	29.9	30.3	30.7	31.1	31.5	31.9	32.3	32.7	33.1	33.5	33.9	34.3	34.7				
152.4	60	28.9	29.3	29.7	30.1	30.5	30.9	31.2	31.6	32.0	32.4	32.8	33.2	33.6	34.0	34.4	34.8	
154.9	61	28.0	28.3	28.7	29.1	29.5	29.9	30.2	30.6	31.0	31.4	31.7	32.1	32.5	32.9	33.3	33.6	34.0
157.5	62	27.1	27.4	27.8	28.2	28.5	28.9	29.3	29.6	30.0	30.4	30.7	31.1	31.5	31.8	32.2	32.6	32.9
160.0	63	26.2	26.6	26.9	27.3	27.6	28.0	28.3	28.7	29.1	29.4	29.8	30.1	30.5	30.8	31.2	31.5	31.9
162.6	64	25.4	25.7	26.1	26.4	26.8	27.1	27.5	27.8	28.2	28.5	28.8	29.2	29.5	29.9	30.2	30.6	30.9
165.1	65	24.6	25.0	25.3	25.6	26.0	26.3	26.6	27.0	27.3	27.6	28.0	28.3	28.6	29.0	29.3	29.6	30.0
167.6	66	23.9	24.2	24.5	24.9	25.2	25.5	25.8	26.1	26.5	26.8	27.1	27.4	27.8	28.1	28.4	28.7	29.1
170.2	67	23.2	23.5	23.8	24.1	24.4	24.7	25.1	25.4	25.7	26.0	26.3	26.6	26.9	27.3	27.6	27.9	28.2
172.7	68	22.5	22.8	23.1	23.4	23.7	24.0	24.3	24.6	24.9	25.2	25.5	25.8	26.2	26.5	26.8	27.1	27.4
175.3	69	21.9	22.2	22.4	22.7	23.0	23.3	23.6	23.9	24.2	24.5	24.8	25.1	25.4	25.7	26.0	26.3	26.6
177.8	70	21.2	21.5	21.8	22.1	22.4	22.7	23.0	23.2	23.5	23.8	24.1	24.4	24.7	25.0	25.3	25.5	25.8
180.3	71	20.6	20.9	21.2	21.5	21.8	22.0	22.3	22.6	22.9	23.2	23.4	23.7	24.0	24.3	24.5	24.8	25.1
182.9	72	20.1	20.3	20.6	20.9	21.2	21.4	21.7	22.0	22.2	22.5	22.8	23.1	23.3	23.6	23.9	24.1	24.4
185.4	73	19.5	19.8	20.1	20.3	20.6	20.8	21.1	21.4	21.6	21.9	22.2	22.4	22.7	23.0	23.2	23.5	23.7
188.0	74	19.0	19.3	19.5	19.8	20.0	20.3	20.5	20.8	21.1	21.3	21.6	21.8	22.1	22.3	22.6	22.9	23.1
190.5	75	18.5	18.7	19.0	19.2	19.5	19.7	20.0	20.2	20.5	20.7	21.0	21.2	21.5	21.7	22.0	22.2	22.5
193.0	76	18.0	18.3	18.5	18.7	19.0	19.2	19.5	19.7	20.0	20.2	20.4	20.7	20.9	21.2	21.4	21.7	21.9
195.6	77	17.6	17.8	18.0	18.3	18.5	18.7	19.0	19.2	19.4	19.7	19.9	20.2	20.4	20.6	20.9	21.1	21.3
198.1	78	17.1	17.3	17.6	17.8	18.0	18.3	18.5	18.7	19.0	19.2	19.4	19.6	19.9	20.1	20.3	20.6	20.8

Whenever a child's specific height or weight measurement is not listed, round to the closest number in the table.

CALCULATED BODY MASS INDEX   61"–78" AND 182 LBS.–214 LBS.

Height			Weight																
		Kg	82.6	83.5	84.4	85.3	86.2	87.1	88.0	88.9	89.8	90.7	91.6	92.5	93.4	94.3	95.3	96.2	97.1
Cm	In	Lb	182	184	186	188	190	192	194	196	198	200	202	204	206	208	210	212	214
154.9	61		34.4	34.8															
157.5	62		33.3	33.7	34.0	34.4	34.8												
160.0	63		32.2	32.6	32.9	33.3	33.7	34.0	34.4	34.7									
162.6	64		31.2	31.6	31.9	32.3	32.6	33.0	33.3	33.6	34.0	34.3	34.7						
165.1	65		30.3	30.6	31.0	31.3	31.6	32.0	32.3	32.6	32.9	33.3	33.6	33.9	34.3	34.6	34.9		
167.6	66		29.4	29.7	30.0	30.3	30.7	31.0	31.3	31.6	32.0	32.3	32.6	32.9	33.2	33.6	33.9	34.2	34.5
170.2	67		28.5	28.8	29.1	29.4	29.8	30.1	30.4	30.7	31.0	31.3	31.6	32.0	32.3	32.6	32.9	33.2	33.5
172.7	68		27.7	28.0	28.3	28.6	28.9	29.2	29.5	29.8	30.1	30.4	30.7	31.0	31.3	31.6	31.9	32.2	32.5
175.3	69		26.9	27.2	27.5	27.8	28.1	28.4	28.6	28.9	29.2	29.5	29.8	30.1	30.4	30.7	31.0	31.3	31.6
177.8	70		26.1	26.4	26.7	27.0	27.3	27.5	27.8	28.1	28.4	28.7	29.0	29.3	29.6	29.8	30.1	30.4	30.7
180.3	71		25.4	25.7	25.9	26.2	26.5	26.8	27.1	27.3	27.6	27.9	28.2	28.5	28.7	29.0	29.3	29.6	29.8
182.9	72		24.7	25.0	25.2	25.5	25.8	26.0	26.3	26.6	26.9	27.1	27.4	27.7	27.9	28.2	28.5	28.8	29.0
185.4	73		24.0	24.3	24.5	24.8	25.1	25.3	25.6	25.9	26.1	26.4	26.7	26.9	27.2	27.4	27.7	28.0	28.2
188.0	74		23.4	23.6	23.9	24.1	24.4	24.7	24.9	25.2	25.4	25.7	25.9	26.2	26.4	26.7	27.0	27.2	27.5
190.5	75		22.7	23.0	23.2	23.5	23.7	24.0	24.2	24.5	24.7	25.0	25.2	25.5	25.7	26.0	26.2	26.5	26.7
193.0	76		22.2	22.4	22.6	22.9	23.1	23.4	23.6	23.9	24.1	24.3	24.6	24.8	25.1	25.3	25.6	25.8	26.0
195.6	77		21.6	21.8	22.1	22.3	22.5	22.8	23.0	23.2	23.5	23.7	24.0	24.2	24.4	24.7	24.9	25.1	25.4
198.1	78		21.0	21.3	21.5	21.7	22.0	22.2	22.4	22.6	22.9	23.1	23.3	23.6	23.8	24.0	24.3	24.5	24.7

Whenever a child's specific height or weight measurement is not listed, round to the closest number in the table.

CALCULATED BODY MASS INDEX   66″–78″ AND 216 LBS.–250 LBS.

Height Cm	Height In	Weight Kg 98.0 / Lb 216	98.9 / 218	99.8 / 220	100.7 / 222	101.6 / 224	102.5 / 226	103.4 / 228	104.3 / 230	105.2 / 232	106.1 / 234	107.0 / 236	108.0 / 238	108.9 / 240	109.8 / 242	110.7 / 244	111.6 / 246	112.5 / 248	113.4 / 250
167.6	66	34.9																	
170.2	67	33.8	34.1	34.5	34.8														
172.7	68	32.8	33.1	33.5	33.8	34.1	34.4	34.7	35.0										
175.3	69	31.9	32.2	32.5	32.8	33.1	33.4	33.7	34.0	34.3	34.6	34.9							
177.8	70	31.0	31.3	31.6	31.9	32.1	32.4	32.7	33.0	33.3	33.6	33.9	34.1	34.4	34.7				
180.3	71	30.1	30.4	30.7	31.0	31.2	31.5	31.8	32.1	32.4	32.6	32.9	33.2	33.5	33.8	34.0	34.3	34.6	34.9
182.9	72	29.3	29.6	29.8	30.1	30.4	30.7	30.9	31.2	31.5	31.7	32.0	32.3	32.5	32.8	33.1	33.4	33.6	33.9
185.4	73	28.5	28.8	29.0	29.3	29.6	29.8	30.1	30.3	30.6	30.9	31.1	31.4	31.7	31.9	32.2	32.5	32.7	33.0
188.0	74	27.7	28.0	28.2	28.5	28.8	29.0	29.3	29.5	29.8	30.0	30.3	30.6	30.8	31.1	31.3	31.6	31.8	32.1
190.5	75	27.0	27.2	27.5	27.7	28.0	28.2	28.5	28.7	29.0	29.2	29.5	29.7	30.0	30.2	30.5	30.7	31.0	31.2
193.0	76	26.3	26.5	26.8	27.0	27.3	27.5	27.8	28.0	28.2	28.5	28.7	29.0	29.2	29.5	29.7	29.9	30.2	30.4
195.6	77	25.6	25.9	26.1	26.3	26.6	26.8	27.0	27.3	27.5	27.7	28.0	28.2	28.5	28.7	28.9	29.2	29.4	29.6
198.1	78	25.0	25.2	25.4	25.7	25.9	26.1	26.3	26.6	26.8	27.0	27.3	27.5	27.7	28.0	28.2	28.4	28.7	28.9

Whenever a child's specific height or weight measurement is not listed, round to the closest number in the table.

APPENDIX XI
AFFILIATES TO JOSLIN DIABETES CENTER

CONNECTICUT

New Britain General Hospital
100 Grand Street
New Britain, CT 06050
(888) 4JOSLIN (toll free) or
    (860) 224-5672

Charlotte Hungerford Hospital
Hungerford Building
540 Litchfield Street
Torrington, CT 06790
(860) 489-0661

Lawrence & Memorial Hospital
50 Faire Harbor Place
Suite 2E
New London, CT 06320
(877) JOSLIN-1

FLORIDA

Mease Countryside Hospital
3231 McMullen Booth Road
MS 586
Safety Harbor, FL 34695
(727) 725-6283

Morton Plant Mease Health Care
455 Pinellas Street
Clearwater, FL 34616
(727) 461-8300

INDIANA

Floyd Memorial Hospital &
    Health Services
1850 State Street
New Albany, IN 47150
(812) 949-5700 or
    (888) 77-FMHHS

MARYLAND

North Arundel Hospital
301 Hospital Drive
Glen Burnie, MD 21042
(410) 787-4940

University of Maryland
    Medical System
22 South Greene Street—
    N6W100
Baltimore, MD 21202-1595
(410) 328-6584 or
    (888) JOSLIN-8

MASSACHUSETTS

Falmouth Affiliate
210 Jones Road
Falmouth, MA 02540
(508) 548-1944

Mercy Hospital
299 Carew Street
Springfield, MA 01104
(413) 748-7000 or
    (877) JOSLIN-8

NEW JERSEY

Saint Barnabas Ambulatory
    Care Center
200 South Orange Avenue
Livingston, NJ 07039
(973) 322-7200

St. Barnabas Medical Center
    (Satellite of Saint Barnabas)
Community Medical Center
    Division
368 Lakehurst Road
Suite 305
Toms River, NJ 08753
(732) 349-5757

Kimball Medical Center
    (Satellite of Saint Barnabas)
600 River Avenue
Room 1050, South One
Lakewood, NJ 08701
(973) 886-4748

NEW YORK

Arnot Ogden Medical Center
600 Fitch Street
Suite 203
Elmira, NY 14905

Hudson Valley Hospital Center
224 Veterans Road
Suite 201
Yorktown Heights, NY 10598
(888) HVHC-JOSLIN or (914)
    962-1320

SUNY Upstate Medical
    University
90 Presidential Plaza
Syracuse, NY 13202
(315) 464-5726

Sound Shore Medical Center
16 Guion Place
New Rochelle, NY 10801
(914) 633-9680

Westchester Medical Center
Outpatient Department
Macy Pavilion
100 Grassland Road
Room 1197-B
Valhalla, NY 10595
(800) 456-7546

PENNSYLVANIA

Western Pennsylvania Hospital
5140 Liberty Avenue
Pittsburgh, PA 15224
(412) 578-1724

Forbes Regional Hospital
Forbes Lifestyle Center
Professional Office Building 2
2580 Haymaker Road

Suite 403
Monroeville, PA 15146
(412) 578-1724

SOUTH CAROLINA

McLeod Regional Medical
    Center
555 East Cheves Street
Florence, SC 25901
(888) 777-6965

TENNESSEE

Memorial Hospital
2525 de Sales Avenue
Chattanooga, TN 37404-3322
(423) 495-7970

WASHINGTON

Swedish Medical Center
910 Boylston Avenue
Seattle, WA 98104-0999
(206) 215-2440 or (888) JOSLIN1

WEST VIRGINIA

St. Mary's Hospital
2900 First Avenue
Huntington, WV 25702
(304) 526-8363

BIBLIOGRAPHY

"Acromegaly: Genetically Modified Growth Hormone May Offer Hope for Treatment." *Drug Week* (May 1, 2000): No page numbers provided.

Adler, Amanda I., M.D., Ph.D. "Lower-Extremity Amputation in Diabetes." *Diabetes Care* 22, no. 7 (July 1999): 1029–1035.

Adlerberth, Annika M., M.D. "Diabetes and Long-Term Risk of Mortality from Coronary and Other Causes in Middle-Aged Swedish Men." *Diabetes Care* 21, no. 4 (April 1998): 539–545.

Ahroni, Jessie H., Ph.D. A.R.N.P., C.D.E. *101 Foot Care Tips for People with Diabetes* (New York: McGraw Hill, 2000).

Aiello, Joan H. "Preventing Diabetic Nephropathy: The Role of Primary Care." *The Nurse Practitioner* x, no. x (February 1998): 12–13, 17–18, 23–24.

"ALF Overview Preview." *Contemporary Longterm Care* 23, no. 6 (June 2000): 9.

"Alzheimer's Disease: Seeking New Ways to Preserve Brain Function: An Interview with Kenneth L. Davis." *Geriatrics* 54, no. 2 (February 1, 1999): 42–47.

American Academy of Family Physicians. "The Benefits and Risks of Controlling Blood Glucose Levels in Patients with Type 2 Diabetes Mellitus: A Review of the Evidence and Recommendations." American Diabetes Association, released August 1999.

American Academy of Pediatrics. "Screening for Retinopathy in the Pediatric Patient with Type 1 Diabetes Mellitus." *Pediatrics* 101, no. 2 (February 1998): 313–314.

American Diabetes Association. "Position Statement: Aspirin Therapy in Diabetes." *Diabetes Care* 24, Supp. 1 (2001): S62–S63.

American Diabetes Association. "Position Statement: Diabetes Mellitus and Exercise." *Diabetes Care* 24, Supp. 1 (2001): S51–S55.

American Diabetes Association. "Position Statement: Management of Dyslipidemia in Adults with Diabetes." *Diabetes Care* 24, Supp. 1 (2001): S58–S61.

American Diabetes Association. "Preventive Foot Care in People with Diabetes." *Diabetes Care* 24, Supp. 1, Clinical Practice Recommendations, 2001. S56–S57.

American Diabetes Association. "Hypoglycemia and Employment/Licensure." *Diabetes Care* 24, Supp. 1: S118.

American Diabetes Association. "Continuous Subcutaneous Insulin Infusion." *Diabetes Care* 22, Supp. 1 (1999): S76–S77.

American Diabetes Association. "Gestational Diabetes Mellitus." *Diabetes Care* 24, Supp. 1 (January 2001): S77–S79.

American Diabetes Association. "Tests of Glycemia in Diabetes." *Diabetes Care* 22, Supp. 1 (1999): S107–S112.

American Diabetes Association. "Type 2 Diabetes in Children and Adolescents." *Pediatrics* 105, no. 3 (March 2000): 671–680.

"The Americans with Disabilities Act: What It Means to You." *Diabetes Forecast* 47, no. 9 (1994): 59.

Annese, V., et al. "Gastrointestinal Motor Dysfunction, Symptoms, and Neuropathy in Noninsulin-Dependent (Type 2) Diabetes Mellitus." *Journal of Clinical Gastroenterology* 29, no. 2 (September 1999): 171–177.

Apgar, Barbara. "Spontaneous Vaginal Delivery and Risk of Erb's Palsy." *American Family Physician* 58, no. 4 (1998): 973–976.

Arfken, Cynthia L., Ph.D., et al. "Development of Proliferative Diabetic Retinopathy in African-Americans and Whites with Type 1 Diabetes." *Diabetes Care* 21, no. 5 (May 1998): 792–795.

Arent, Shereen. "Supreme Court Decisions Make It More Difficult for People with Diabetes to Fight Discrimination." *Diabetes Forecast* 52, no. 9 (September 1999): 33–35.

Bakker, S. J. L., et al. "Thiamine Supplementation to Prevent Induction of Low Birth Weight by Conventional Therapy for Gestational Diabetes Mellitus." *Medical Hypotheses* (July 2000): 88–90.

Bakris, George L., M.D., et al. "Preserving Renal Function in Adults with Hypertension and Diabetes: A Consensus Approach." *American Journal of Kidney Diseases* 36, no. 3 (September 2000): 646–661.

Barbour, Marilyn M., Pharm.D. "Hormone Replacement Therapy Should Not Be Used as Secondary Prevention of Coronary Heart Disease." *Pharmacotherapy* 20, no. 9 (2000): 1021–1027.

Bardsley, Joan K., M.B.A., C.D.E., and Passaro, Maureen, M.D. "The Alphabet Soup of Diabetes Research Studies." *Diabetes Spectrum* 14, no. 1 (2001): 44–48.

Barnett, Jeffrey L. "Gut Reactions. (How Diabetes Can Affect the Gastrointestinal Tract.)" *Diabetes Forecast* 50, no. 8 (August 1997): 26–30.

Bassili, Amal, Dr.P.H., et al. "Quality of Care of Children with Chronic Diseases in Alexandria, Egypt: The Models of Asthma, Type 1 Diabetes, Epilepsy, and Rheumatic Heart Disease". *Pediatrics* 106, no. 1 (July 2000): 106.

Baumer, J. H. "Social Disadvantage, Family Composition and Diabetes." *Archives of Disease in Childhood* 79 (1998): 427–430.

Beckles, G. L. A., and Thompson-Reid, P. E., eds. *Diabetes and Women's Health Across the Life Stages: A Public Health Perspective.* Conference Edition. Atlanta: U.S. Department of Health and Human Services, Centers for Disease Control and Prevention, National Center for Chronic Disease Prevention and Health Promotion, Division of Diabetes Translation, 2001.

Begue, Rodolfo E., et al. "Helicobacter Pylori Infection and Insulin Requirement among Children with Type 1 Diabetes Mellitus." *Pediatrics* 103, no. 6 (June 1999): 103–109.

Bell, David S. H., M.B., and Ovalle, Fernando, M.D. "Diabetes as a Risk Factor for Ischemic Heart Disease." *Clinical Reviews* (Spring 2000): 88–92.

Bell, David S. H., M.B., and Ovalle, Fernando, M.D. "Management of Type 2 Diabetes." *Clinical Reviews* (Spring 2000): 93–96.

Benbow, S. J., et al. "Diabetic Peripheral Neuropathy and Quality of Life." *QJM: Monthly Journal of the Association of Physicians* 91, no. 11 (1998): 733–737.

Bernstein, Gerald, M.D., "The Diabetic Stomach: Management Strategies for Clinicians and Patients." *Diabetes Spectrum* 12 (2000): 11–20.

Bird, Elizabeth, editor and compiler. "The Diabetic Mother and Breastfeeding." La Leche League International, 1999.

Black, Sandra A., Ph.D. "Increased Health Burden Associated with Comorbid Depression in Older Diabetic Mexican Americans: Results from the Hispanic Established Population for the Epidemiologic Study of the Elderly Survey." *Diabetes Care* 22, no. 1 (January 1999): 56–64.

Bloomgarden, Zachary T., M.D. "Cardiovascular Disease in Type 2 Diabetes." *Diabetes Care* 22, no. 10 (October 1999): 1739–1744.

Boland, E., et al. "A Primer on the Use of Insulin Pumps in Adolescents." *The Diabetes Educator* 24, no. 1 (1998): 78–86.

Borch-Johnsen, Knut. "Improving Prognosis of Type 1 Diabetes: Mortality, Accidents, and Impact on Insurance." *Diabetes Care* 22, Supp. 2 (March 1999): B1–B3.

Brancati, Frederick L., M.D., M.H.S., et al. "Incident Type 2 Diabetes Mellitus in African American and White Adults." *Journal of the American Medical Association* 283, no. 17 (May 3, 2000): 2253–2259.

Bryden, Kathryn S., R.N. "Eating Habits, Body Weight, and Insulin Misuse." *Diabetes Care* 22, no. 12 (December 1999): 1956–1960.

Burke, James P., Ph.D., et al. "A Quantitative Scale of Acanthosis Nigricans." *Diabetes Care* 22, no. 10 (October 1999): 2655–2659.

Cassell, Dana K., and David H. Gleaves, Ph.D. *The Encyclopedia of Obesity and Eating Disorders* (New York: Facts On File, Inc., 2000).

Castelli, William P., M.D., and Griffin, Glen C., M.D. *Good Fat, Bad Fat: Reduce Your Heart-Attack Odds* (Tucson, Ariz.: Fisher Books, 1997).

Centers for Disease Control and Prevention, U.S. Department of Health and Human Services. *CDC Fact Book 2000/2001.* September 2000.

Centers for Disease Control and Prevention, U.S. Department of Health and Human Services. "Chronic Diseases and Their Risk Factors: The Nation's Leading Causes of Death." December 1999.

Chalew, S. A., et al. "Predictors of Glycemic Control in Children with Type 1 Diabetes: The Importance of Race." *Journal of Diabetes Complications* 4, no. 2 (March–April 2000): 71–77.

Chin, Marshall H., M.D., M.P.H. "Diabetes in the African-American Medicare Population: Morbidity, Quality of Care, and Resource Utilization." *Diabetes Care* 21, no. 7 (July 1998): 1090–1095.

Chiu, Ken C., M.D., F.A.C.E. "Insulin Sensitivity Differs Among Ethic Groups with Compensatory Response in ß Cell Function." *Diabetes Care* 23, no. 9 (September 2000): 1353–1358.

Clark, Wayne. "Pumped Up: But Is It for Everyone?" *JDF International Countdown* 18, no. 2 (1997): 20–21, 24, 26–28.

Clarke, William L., M.D. "Advocating for the Child with Diabetes." *Diabetes Spectrum* 12, no. 4 (1999): 230–235.

Cobin, Rhoda H., M.D., F.A.C.E., Chairman. "AACE Medical Guidelines for Clinical Practice for Management of Menopause." *Endocrine Practice* 5, no. 6 (November/December 1999): 354–366.

Colberg, Sheri R., Ph.D. "Exercise and Diabetes Control." *Physician & Sportsmedicine,* 28, no. 4 (April 2000). www.physsportmed.com/issues/2000/04_00/colberg.htm

Colton, Patricia A., et al. "Eating Disturbances in Young Women with Type 1 Diabetes Mellitus: Mechanisms and Consequences." *Psychiatric Annals* 29, no. 4 (April 1, 1999): 213–218.

Cooper, James W., ed. *Diabetes Mellitus in the Elderly* (New York: The Haworth Press, 1999).

Cooper, Nancy, R.D., C.D.E. "Using Herbal Therapies Safely." *Diabetes Self-Management* 16, no. 3: 6–8, 10–13.

Cooper, Stephanie, M.D., and Caldwell, James H., M.D. "Coronary Artery Disease in People with Diabetes: Diagnostic and Risk Factor Evaluation." *Clinical Diabetes* 17, no. 2 (1999): 58–72.

Corrigan, J., and Larsen, P. "Tips for Toddler Care." *Diabetes Self-Management* 13, no. 4 (1996): 26–28, 31.

Cox, Daniel J., Ph.D., et al. "Biopsychobehavioral Model of Severe Hypoglycemia II: Understanding the Risk of Severe Hypoglycemia." *Diabetes Care* 22, no. 12 (December 1999): 2018–2025.

Culleton, John L., M.D. "Preventing Diabetic Foot Complications." *Postgraduate Medicine* 106, no. 1 (July 1999): 74–78, 83.

Cummings, Jennifer, M.D., et al. "A Review of the DIGAMI Study: Intensive Insulin Therapy During and After Myocardial Infarctions in Diabetic Patients," from *Diabetes Spectrum* 12, no. 2 (1999), in *Annual Review of Diabetes 2000* (Alexandria, Va: American Diabetes Association, 2000).

Cundy, T., et al. "Perinatal Mortality in Type 2 Diabetes Mellitus," *Diabetic Medicine: A Journal of the British Diabetic Association* 17, no. 1 (January 2000): 33–39.

Cutfield, Wayne S., et al. "Incidence of Diabetes Mellitus and Impaired Glucose Tolerance in Children and Adolescents Receiving Growth-Hormone Treatment." *The Lancet* 355, no. 9204 (February 2000): 610–613.

Dabelea, Dana, et al. "Effect of Diabetes in Pregnancy on Offspring: Follow-up Research in the Pima Indians." *Journal of Maternal-Fetal Medicine* 9, no. 1 (January–February 2000): 83–88.

Daneman, Denis, M.B., B.Ch., F.R.C.P.C., Frank, Marcia, R.N., M.H.Sc., C.D.E., and Perlman, Kusiel, M.D., F.R.C.P.C. *When a Child Has Diabetes* (New York: Firefly Books, 1999).

Davidson, Maryanne, et al. "Teaching Teens to Cope: Coping Skills Training for Adolescents with Adolescent-Dependent Diabetes Mellitus." *Journal of the Society of Pediatric Nurses* 2, no. 2 (April–June 1997): 65–73.

Davidson, Mayer B., M.D. "It's Time to Change the Paradigm for Delivery Diabetes Care." *Clinical Diabetes* 18, no. 2 (Spring 2000).

Davies, M. J., Raymond, N. T., Day, J.L., et al. "Impaired Glucose Tolerance and Fasting Hyperglycemia Have Different Characteristics." *Diabetes Medicine* 17 (2000): 433–440.

Davis, Catherine L. "History of Gestational Diabetes, Insulin Resistance and Coronary Risk." *Journal of Diabetes Complications* 13, no. 4 (August 1999): 216–223.

Daviss, W. Burleson, et al. "Predicting Diabetic Control from Competence, Adherence, Adjustment, and Psychopathology." *Journal of the American Academy of Child and Adolescent Psychiatry* 34, no. 12 (December 1995): 1629–1637.

De Alva, Maria L. "Education: A Liberating Tool." *Diabetes Spectrum* 12, no. 3 (1999): 132–135.

Davis, D. L., et al. "History of Gestational Diabetes, Insulin Resistance and Coronary Risk." *Journal of Diabetes Complications* 13, no. 4 (July–August 1999): 216–223.

Deedwania, Prakash C., M.D. "Hypertension and Diabetes." *Archives of Internal Medicine* 160, no. 11 (June 12, 2000): 1585–1594.

Dendinger, M. J. "Traveling with Diabetes: Business as Usual." *Diabetes Self-Management* 15, no. 3 (1998): 7–8, 11–13.

De Vegt, Femmie, M.S.C., et al. "Similar 9-Year Mortality Risks and Reproducibility for the World Health Organization and American Diabetes Association Glucose Tolerance Categories." *Diabetes Care* 23, no. 1 (January 2000): 40–44.

Dey, Jayant, M.D., et al. "Factors Influencing Patient Acceptability of Diabetes Treatment Regimens. *Clinical Diabetes* 18, no. 2 (Spring 2000): 61–67.

"Diabetes, Head Trauma, Marriage and Dementia." *Psychiatric Medicine in Primary Care Archives* (March 1, 2000).

The Diabetes Control and Complications Trial Research Group. "A Comparison of the Study Populations in the Diabetes Control and Complications Trial and the Wisconsin Epidemiologic Study of Diabetic Retinopathy." *Archives of Internal Medicine* 155 (April 10, 1995): 745–754.

The Diabetes Control and Complications Trial Research Group. "Adverse Events and Their Association with Treatment Regimens in the Diabetes Control and Complications Trial." *Diabetes Care* 18, no. 11 (November 1995): 1415–1427.

Diabetes Control and Complications Research Group. "Baseline Analysis of Renal Function in the Diabetes Control and Complications Research Trial." *Kidney International* 43 (1993): 668–674.

Diabetes Control and Complications Research Group. "Clustering of Long-Term Complications in Families with Diabetes in the Diabetes Control and Complications Trial." *Diabetes* 46 (November 1997): 1829–1839.

The Diabetes Control and Complications Trial Research Group. "Early Worsening of Diabetic Retinopathy in the Diabetes Control and Complications Trial." *The Archives of Ophthalmology* 116 (1998): 874–886.

Diabetes Control and Complications Research Group. "Effect of Intensive Diabetes Management on Macrovascular Events and Risk Factors in the Diabetes Control and Complications Trial." *The American Journal of Cardiology* 75 (May 1, 1995): 894–903.

Diabetes Control and Complications Research Group. "Effect of Intensive Diabetes Treatment on the Development and Progression of Long-Term Complications in Adolescents with Insulin-Dependent Diabetes Mellitus: Diabetes Control and Complications Trial." *The Journal of Pediatrics* 125, no. 2 (August 1994): 177–188.

Diabetes Control and Complications Research Group. "The Effect of Intensive Treatment of Diabetes on the Development and Progression of Long-Term Complications in Insulin-Dependent Diabetes Mellitus." *The New England Journal of Medicine* 329 (September 30, 1993): 977–986.

Diabetes Control and Complications Research Group. "Effect of Intensive Therapy on the Development and Progression of Diabetic Nephropathy in the Diabetes Control and Complications Trial." *Kidney International* 47 (1995): 1703–1720.

Diabetes Control and Complications Research Group. "The Effect of Intensive Diabetes Therapy on the Development and Progression of Neuropathy." *Annals of Internal Medicine* 122, no. 8 (April 15, 1995): 561–568.

The Diabetes Control and Complications Trial Research Group. "Effect of Intensive Diabetes Management on Macrovascular Events and Risk Factors in the Diabetes Control and Complications Trial." *The American Journal of Cardiology* 75 (May 1, 1995): 36–51.

The Diabetes Control and Complications Trial Research Group. "The Effect of Intensive Diabetes Therapy on Measures of Autonomic Nervous System Function in the Diabetes Control and Complications Trial (DCCT)." *Diabetologia* 41 (1998): 416–423.

The Diabetes Control and Complications Trial Research Group. "Effect of Intensive Diabetes Treatment on Nerve Conduction in the Diabetes Control and Complications Trial." *Annals of Neurology* 38, no. 6 (December 1995): 869–880.

The Diabetes Control and Complications Trial Research Group. "Effects of Intensive Diabetes Therapy on Neuropsychological Function in Adults in the Diabetes Control and Complications Trial." *Annals of Internal Medicine* 124 (1996): 379–388.

Diabetes Control and Complications Research Group. "Epidemiology of Severe Hypoglycemia in the Diabetes Control and Complications Research Trial." *The American Journal of Medicine* 90 (April 1991): 450–459.

Diabetes Control and Complications Research Group. "Expanded Role of the Dietitian in the Diabetes Control and Complications Trial: Implications for Clinical Practice." *Journal of the American Dietetic Association* 93 (July 1993): 758–764.

Diabetes Control and Complications Research Group. "Factors in Development of Diabetic Neuropathy: Baseline Analysis of Neuropathy in Feasibility Phase of Diabetes Control and Complications Trial (DCCT)." *Diabetes* 37 (April 1998): 476–481.

Diabetes Control and Complications Research Group. "Hypoglycemia in the Diabetes Control and Complications Trial." *Diabetes* 46 (February 1997): 271–286.

Diabetes Control and Complications Research Group, "Progression of Retinopathy with Intensive versus Conventional Treatment in the Diabetes Control and Complications Trial," *Ophthalmology* 102, no. 4 (April 1995): 647–661.

The Diabetes Control and Complications Trial Research Group. "Effects of Intensive Diabetes Therapy on Neuropsychological Function in Adults in the Diabetes Control and Complications Trial." *Annals of Internal Medicine* 124, no. 4 (February 15, 1996): 379–388.

The Diabetes Control and Complications Trial Research Group. "Expanded Role of the Dietitian in the Diabetes Control and Complications Trial: Implications for Clinical Practice." *Journal of the American Dietetic Association* 93, no. 7 (July 1993): 758–764, 767.

The Diabetes Control and Complications Trial Research Group. "Epidemiology of Diabetes Interventions and Complications (EDIC)." *Diabetes Care* 22, no. 1 (January 1999): 99–111.

The Diabetes Control and Complications Trial Research Group. "Hypoglycemia in the Diabetes Control and Complications Trial." *Diabetes* 46 (February 1997): 271–286.

The Diabetes Control and Complications Trial Research Group. "Influence of Intensive Diabetes Treatment on Quality-of-Life Outcomes in the Diabetes Control and Complications Trial." *Diabetes Care* 19, no. 3 (March 1996): 195–203.

The Diabetes Control and Complications Trial Research Group. "Lifetime Benefits and Costs of Intensive Therapy as Practiced in the Diabetes Control and Complications Trial." *Journal of the American Medical*

Association 276, no. 17 (November 6, 1996): 1409–1415.

The Diabetes Control and Complications Trial Research Group. "Nutrition Interventions for Intensive Therapy in the Diabetes Control and Complications Trial." *Journal of the American Dietetic Association* 93, no. 7 (July 1993): 768–772.

The Diabetes Control and Complications Trial Research Group. "Pregnancy Outcomes in the Diabetes Control and Complications Trial." *American Journal of Obstetrics & Gynecology* 174 (1996): 1343–1353.

The Diabetes Control and Complications Trial Research Group. "Progression of Retinopathy with Intensive versus Conventional Treatment in the Diabetes Control and Complications Trial." *Ophthalmology* 102, no. 4 (April 1995): 647–661.

The Diabetes Control and Complications Trial Research Group. "Diabetes Control and Complications Trial Research Group (DCCT): Update." *Diabetes Care* 13, no. 4 (April 1990): 427–433.

The Diabetes Control and Complications Trial Research Group. "The Relationship of Glycemic Exposure (HbA1C) to the Risk of Development and Progression of Retinopathy in the Diabetes Control and Complications Trial." *Diabetes* 44 (August 1995): 968–983.

Doughty, Geoffrey, et al. "Home-Based Management Can Achieve Intensification Cost-Effectively in Type 1 Diabetes." *Pediatrics* 103, no. 1 (January 1999): 122–128.

Dune, F. P., et al. "Pre-conception Diabetes Care in Insulin-Dependent Diabetes Mellitus." *QJM: Monthly Journal of the Association of Physicians* 92, no n. (1999): 175–176.

Dyck, Peter James, M.D., et al. "Risk Factors for Severity of Diabetic Polyneuropathy." *Diabetes Care* 22, no. 9 (September 1999): 1479–1486.

Ecker, J. L., et al. "Gestational Diabetes." *New England Journal of Medicine* 342, no. 12 (March 23, 2000): 896–897.

Economies, Panaylotis A., M.D., et al. "Assessment of Physician Responses to Abnormal Results of Bone Densitometry Studies." *Endocrine Practice* 6, no. 5 (September/October 2000): 351–356.

Edelwich, Jerry, L.C.S.W., and Brodsky, Archie. *Diabetes: Caring for Your Emotions as Well as Your Health* (Reading, Mass.: Perseus Books, 1998).

Egeland, Grace M., et al. "Birth Characteristics of Women Who Develop Gestational Diabetes: Population Based Study." *British Medical Journal* 321, no. 7250 (September 2000): 546–547.

Ehm, Margaret Gelder, et al. "Genomewide Search for Type 2 Diabetes Susceptibility Genes in Four American Populations." *American Journal of Human Genetics* 66 (2000): 1871–1881.

Elam, Marshall B., Ph.D., M.D., et al. "Effect of Niacin on Lipid and Lipoprotein Levels and Glycemic Control in Patients with Diabetes and Peripheral Arterial Disease: The ADMIT Study: A Randomized Trial." *Journal of the American Medical Association* 284, no. 13 (2000): 1263–1270.

Emanuele, Nicholas V., M.D., et al. "Consequences of Alcohol Use in Diabetics." *Alcohol Health & Research World* 22, no. 3 (1998): 211–219.

"End-Stage Renal Disease Attributed to Diabetes among American Indians/Alaska Natives with Diabetes—United States, 1990–1999." *Morbidity and Mortality Weekly Report* 49, no. 42 (October 27, 2000): 959–962.

Engelgau, Michael M., M.D., M.S., et al. "Screening for Type 2 Diabetes." *Diabetes Care* 23, no. 10 (October 2000): 1563–1580.

Epidemiology of Diabetes Interventions and Complications (EDIC) Research Group. "Epidemiology of Diabetes Interventions and Complications (EDIC)." *Diabetes Care* 22, no. 1 (January 1999): 99–111.

Espeland, Mark A., Ph.D., et al. "Effect of Postmenopausal Hormone Therapy on Glucose and Insulin Concentrations." *Diabetes Care* 21, no. 10 (October 1998): 1589–1595.

Estacio, Reymond O., M.D., et al. "Effect of Blood Pressure Control on Diabetic Microvascular Complications in Patients with Hypertension and Type 2 Diabetes." *Diabetes Care* 23, Supp. 2 (April 2000): B54–B64.

Evans, Josie M., M., Ph.D., et al. "Impact of Type 1 and Type 2 Diabetes on Patterns and Costs of Drug Prescribing." *Diabetes Care* 23, no. 6 (June 2000): 770–774.

Evans, Timothy C., M.D., et al. "Diabetic Nephropathy." *Clinical Diabetes,* 18, no. 1 (Winter 2000): 278–285.

Fagot-Campagna, Anne, K. M., Venkat Narayan, and Giuseppina Imperatore, "Type 2 Diabetes in Children." *British Medical Journal* 322 (2001): 377–378.

Fagot-Campagna, Anne, M.D., Ph.D., et al. "Type 2 Diabetes among North American Children and Adolescents: An Epidemiological Review and a Public Health Perspective." *Journal of Pediatrics* 136, no. 5 (May 2000): 664–672.

Feld, Stanley, M.D., F.A.C.P., M.A.C.E., et al. "The American Association of Clinical Endocrinologists Medical Guidelines for the Management of Diabetes Mellitus: The AACE System of Intensive Diabetes Self-Management—2000 Update." *Endocrine Practice* 6, no. 1 (January–February 2000): 43–84.

Ford, Earl S., M.D., "Diabetes and Serum Ferritin Concentration Among U.S. Adults." *Diabetes Care* 22, no. 12 (December 1999): 1978–1983.

Fisher, Lawrence, and Weihs, Karen L. "Can Addressing Family Relationships Improve Outcomes in Chronic Disease?" *Journal of Family Practice* 49, no. 6 (June 2000): 561–566.

Fisher, Lawrence, Ph.D. "The Family and Disease Management in Hispanic and European-American Patients with Type 2 Diabetes." *Diabetes Care* 23, no. 3 (March 2000): 267–272.

Fong, Donald S., M.D., M.P.H., and Ross, Robin Deem, M.D. *The Diabetes Eye Care Sourcebook* (Chicago, Ill.: Lowell House, 1999).

Fong, Donald, S., et al. "Impaired Color Vision Associated with Diabetic Retinopathy: Early Treatment Diabetic Retinopathy Study report No. 15." *American Journal of Ophthalmology* (November 1, 1999): 612–617.

Ford, Earl S., M.D., and Cogswell, Mary E., Dr.P.H., "Diabetes and Serum Ferritin Concentration among U.S. Adults." *Diabetes Care* 22, no. 12 (December 1999): 1978–1983.

Franklin, Frank A., Jr., M.D., Ph.D., and Franklin, Cynthia C., M.P.H., R.N., C.P.N.P. "Dyslipidemia in Children" *Clinical Reviews* (no volume or number listed) (Spring 2000): 58–61.

Fukui, Michiaki, et al. "Growth-Hormone Treatment and Risk of Diabetes." *The Lancet* 355, no. 9218 (May 2000): 1913–1914.

Gary, Tiffany, M.H.S., et al. "Depressive Symptoms and Metabolic Control in African-Americans with Type 2 Diabetes." *Diabetes Care* 23, no. 1 (January 2000): 23–29.

Giacco, Rosalba, M.D., et al. "Long-Term Dietary Treatment with Increased Amounts of Fiber-Rich Low-Glycemic Index Natural Foods Improves Blood Glucose Control and Reduces the Number of Hypoglycemic Events in Type 1 Diabetic Patients." *Diabetes Care* 23, no. 10 (October 2000): 1461–1466.

"Giant Leap." *Chemist & Druggist,* October 16, 1999.

Gill, Geoffrey, et al. "Painless Stress Fractures in Diabetic Neuropathic Feet." *Postgraduate Medical Journal* 73 (1997): 241–242.

Gillum, Richard F., M.D., et al. "Diabetes Mellitus, Coronary Heart Disease Incidence, and Death from All Causes in African American and European American Women: The NHANES I Epidemiologic Follow-up Study." *Journal of Clinical Epidemiology* 53, no. 5 (May 2000): 511–518.

Gregg, Edward, Ph.D. "Diabetes and Physical Disability Among Older U.S. Adults." *Diabetes Care* 23, no. 9 (September 2000): 1272–1277.

Gregg, E. W., et al. "Is Diabetes Associated with Cognitive Impairment and Cognitive Decline among Older Women?" *Archives of Internal Medicine* 160 (2000): 174–180.

Grey, Margaret, Dr.P.H., F.A.A.N., et al. "Short-Term Effects of Coping Skills Training as Adjunct to Intensive Therapy in Adolescents." *Diabetes Care* 21, no. 6 (June 1998): 902–908.

Grinslade, Susan, and Buck, Elizabeth A. "Clinical Care: Diabetic Ketoacidosis: Implications for the Medical-Surgical Nurse." *Medsurg Nursing* 8, no. 1 (February 1, 1999): 37–45.

Gu, Ken, Ph.D. "Mortality in Adults with and without Diabetes in a National Cohort of the U.S. Population, 1971–1993." *Diabetes Care* 21, no. 7 (July 1998): 1138–1145.

Hadden, Dr. R., and McCance, D. R. "Advances in Management of Type 1 Diabetes and Pregnancy." *Current Opinions in Obstetrics & Gynecology* 11, no. 6 (December 1999): 557–562.

Haire-Joshu, Debra, Ph.D., "Smoking and Diabetes: Technical Review." *Diabetes Care* 22, no. 11 (November 1999): 1887–1898.

Hansen, James R., M.D., et al. "Type 2 Diabetes Mellitus in Youth: A Growing Challenge." *Clinical Diabetes* 18, no. 2 (Spring 2000): 52–60.

Hampson, Sarah E., Ph.D., et al. "Behavioral Interventions for Adolescents with Type 1 Diabetes." *Diabetes Care* 23, no. 9 (September 2000): 1416–1422.

Harris, Maureen I., Ph.D., M.P.H. "Is the Risk of Diabetic Retinopathy Greater in Non-Hispanic Blacks and Mexican Americans Than in Non-Hispanic Whites with Type 2 Diabetes?" *Diabetes Care* 21, no. 8 (August 1998): 1230–1235.

Harris, Maureen I., Ph.D., M.P.H. "Racial and Ethnic Differences in Health Insurance Coverage for Adults with Diabetes." *Diabetes Care* 22, no. 10 (October 1999): 1679–1682.

Harris, Michael A., and Lustman, Patrick J. "The Psychologist in Diabetes Care." *Clinical Diabetes* 16, no. 2 (April 1998): 91–94.

Harris, Stewart B., M.D., M.P.H., and Zinman, Bernard, M.D.C.M. "Editorial: Primary Prevention of Type 2 Diabetes in High-Risk Populations." *Diabetes Care* 23, no. 7 (July 2000): 879–881.

Herman, William H., M.D., M.P.H., and Charron-Prochownik, R.N., Ph.D. "Preconception Counseling: An Opportunity Not to Be Missed." *Clinical Diabetes* 18, no. 3 (Summer 2000): 122–123.

Herman, William H., M.D., M.P.H., and Engelgau, Michael, M., M.D., M.S. "Screening for Type 2 Diabetes Mellitus in Asymptomatic Adults." *Clinical Diabetes* 18, no. 2 (Spring 2000): 68.

Hermann, Robert, M.D., Ph.D., "Transient but Not Permanent Neonatal Diabetes Mellitus Is Associated with Paternal Uniparental Isodisomy of Chromosome 6." *Pediatrics* 105, no. 1 (January 2000): 49–52.

Hiltunen, Liisa. "Self-Perceived Health and Symptoms of Elderly Persons with Diabetes and Impaired Glucose Tolerance." *Age and Ageing* 25, no. 1 (January 1996): 59–67.

Hirsch, Irl B., M.D., ed. "Diabetic Nephropathy: Why Are We Seeing More." *Clinical Diabetes* 18, no. 1 (Winter 2000): 97–98.

Hirsch, Irl B., M.D. *12 Things You Must Know About Diabetes Care Right Now!* (Alexandria, Va: American Diabetes Association, 2000).

Hogg, Ronald J., M.D., et al. "Evaluation and Management of Proteinuria and Nephrotic Syndrome in Children: Recommendations from a Pediatric Nephrology Panel Established at the National Kidney Foundation Conference on Proteinuria, Albuminuria, Risk, Assessment, Detection, and Elimination (PARADE)." *Pediatrics* 105, no. 6 (June 2000): 1242–1249.

Holing, Emily V., Ph.D., et al. "Why Don't Women with Diabetes Plan Their Pregnancies?" *Diabetes Care* 21, no. 6 (June 1998): pp. 889–895.

Howard, Barbara V., Ph.D., et al. "Adverse Effects of Diabetes on Multiple Risk Factors in Women: The Strong Heart Study." *Diabetes Care* 21, no. 8 (August 1998): 1258–1265.

Hummel, Jeffrey. "Building a Computerized Disease Registry for Chronic Illness Management of Diabetes." *Clinical Diabetes* 18, no. 3 (Summer 2000): 107.

Hunt, Linda M., et al. "How Patients Adapt Diabetes Self-Care Recommendations to Everyday Life." *Journal of Family Practice* 46, no. 3 (March 1998): 207–216.

Hutchinson, Cindy. "Hypoglycemia: Making a Case for Glucose Gels and Tablets." *Nursing* (August 1, 1998): 68.

Hyponnen, Elina, M.S.C., M.P.H. "Infant Feeding, Early Weight Gain, and Risk of Type 1 Diabetes." *Diabetes Care* 22, no. 12 (December 1999): 1961–1965.

International Diabetes Institute, a World Health Organization Collaborating Centre for the Epidemiology of Diabetes and Health Promotion for Noncommunicable Disease, "The Asia-Pacific Perspective: Redefining Obesity and Its Treatment." February 2000, Australia.

Jacobs, Tikva S., M.D., and Kerstein, Morris D., M.D., "Is There a Difference in Outcome of Heel Ulcers in Diabetic and Non-Diabetic Patients?" *Wounds* 12, no. 4 (2000): 96–101.

Jellinger, Paul S., M.D., F.A.C.E. Chairman. "The American Association of Clinical Endocrinologists Medical Guidelines for Clinical Practice for the Diagnosis and Treatment of Dyslipidemia and Prevention of Atherogenesis." *Endocrine Practice* 6, no. 2 (March–April 2000): 162–213.

Jensen, D. M., et al. "Maternal and Perinatal Outcomes in 143 Danish Women with Gestational Diabetes Mellitus and 143 Controls with a Similar Risk Profile." *Diabetes Medicine* 17, no. 4 (April 2000): 281–286.

Jensen, Tonny, et al. "The HOPE Study and Diabetes." *The Lancet* 355, no. 9210 (April 2000): 1183–1184.

Johnson, Judith A. "Disease Funding and NIH Priority Setting." *CRS Report for Congress.* Updated September 10, 1998.

Johnson, Mary A., M.S., R.D., C.D.E., "Carbohydrate Counting for People with Type 2 Diabetes," *Diabetes Spectrum* 13, no. 3 (2000): 156–158.

Jonaitis, Mary Ann. "Complications During Pregnancy." *RN* 58, no. 10 (October 1995): 40–44.

Jones, Jennifer M., et al. "Eating Disorders in Adolescent Females with and without Type 1 Diabetes: Cross Sectional Study." *British Medical Journal* 320, no. 7249 (June 2000): 1563–1566.

Jones, Marion W., and Stone, Lisa C. "Management of the Woman with Gestational Diabetes Mellitus," *Journal of Perinatal & Neonatal Nursing.* (March 1, 1998): 13–24.

Joslin, Elliott P., M.D., M.A. *The Treatment of Diabetes Mellitus with Observations Upon the Disease Based Upon Thirteen Hundred Cases.* (Philadelphia, Pa.: Lea & Febiger, 1917).

Jovanovic, Lois, M.D. "Role of Diet and Insulin Treatment of Diabetes in Pregnancy." *Clinical Obstetrics and Gynecology* 43, no. 1 (March 2000): 46–55.

Kadohiro, Jane K., Dr.P.H., A.P.R.N., C.D.E. "Diabetes and Adolescents: From Research to Reality." *Diabetes Spectrum* 13, no. 2 (February 2000): 81.

Kahn, C. Ronald, M.D., Chairman of Diabetes Research Working Group. "Conquering Diabetes: A Strategic Plan for the 21st Century. A Report of the Congressionally-Established Diabetes Research Working Group, 1999." NIH Publication No. 99–4398, 1999.

Karlsen, Marie, et al. "Efficacy of Medical Nutrition Therapy: Are Your Patients Getting What They Need? *Clinical Diabetes* 14, no. 4 (May–June 1996): 54–61.

Karvonen, Marjatta, Ph.D., et al. "Incidence of Childhood Type 1 Diabetes Worldwide." *Diabetes Care* 23, no. 10 (October 2000): 1516.

Kaufman, F. "Preventing Hypoglycemia (Low Blood Glucose) in Children." *Diabetes Forecast* 52, no. 6 (1999): 77–79.

Kaye, Todd, M.D., "Muscoloskeletal Manifestations of Diabetes Mellitus." *Practical Diabetology* 14, no. 1 (1995): 2–4, 6.

King, Hilary, M.D., D.Sc., et al. "Global Burden of Diabetes, 1995–2025." *Diabetes Care* 21, no. 9 (September 1998): 1414–1431.

Kitzmiller, John L., M.D., et al. "Assessment of Costs and Benefits of Management of Gestational Diabetes Mellitus." *Diabetes Care* 21, Supp. 2 (1998): B123–B130.

Klein, Barbara E. K. "Incidence of Cataract Surgery in the Wisconsin Epidemiologic Study of Diabetic Retinopathy." *American Journal of Ophthalmology* 119, no. 3 (March 1995): 295–301.

Klein, Barbara E. K., M.D., et al. "Mortality and Hormone-Related Exposures in Women with Diabetes." *Diabetes Care* 22, no. 2 (February 1999): 248–252.

Klein, Ronald, M.D., M.P.H. "The 10-Year Incidence of Renal Insufficiency in People with Type 1 Diabetes." *Diabetes Care* 22, no. 5 (May 1999): 743–751.

Klonoff, D. C. "Noninvasive Blood Glucose Monitoring." *Clinical Diabetes* 16, no. 1 (1998): 43–45.

Knott, Laurence, G. P. "Diabetic Foot Problems: Targeting Those at Highest Risk." *Pulse* (no. v. or n.) (February 5, 2000): 59.

Komulainen, Jorma, M.D. "Clinical, Autoimmune, and Genetic Characteristics of Very Young Children with Type 1 Diabetes." *Diabetes Care* 22, no. 12 (December 1999): 1950–1955.

Konen, Joseph C., M.D., P.S.P.H., et al. "Racial Differences in Symptoms and Complications in Adults with Type 2 Diabetes." *Ethnicity and Health* 4, nos. 1–2 (February–May 1999): 39–49.

Kong, Marie-France, M.B. Ch.B., M.R.C.P. (U.K.), et al. "Natural History of Diabetic Gastroparesis." *Diabetes Care* 22, no. 2 (February 1999): 503–507.

Kovarik, J., and Mandel, T. E. "Islet Transplantation." *Transplantation Proceedings* 31, Supp. 1/2A (1999): 45S–48S.

Kripke, Clarissa C. "Gestational Diabetes: Screening in Low-Risk Women?" *American Family Physician* (February 15, 1999): 1004.

Kroop, Susan F., and Simon, Lee S. "Joint and Bone Manifestations of Diabetes Mellitus," in *Joslin's Diabetes Mellitus* (Philadelphia, Pa.: Lea & Febiger, 1994).

Krop, Julie S., M.D., et al. "Patterns of Expenditures and Use of Services among Older Adults with Diabetes." *Diabetes Care* 21, no. 5 (May 1998): 747–752.

Krop, Julie S., M.D., "Predicting Expenditures for Medicare Beneficiaries with Diabetes: A Prospective Cohort Study from 1994 to 1996." *Diabetes Care* 22, no. 10 (October 1999): 1660–1666.

Kruger, Davida F., M.S.N., R.N., C.S., C.D.E. *The Diabetes Travel Guide: How to Travel with Diabetes—Anywhere in the World* (Alexandria, Va.: American Diabetes Association, 2000).

Kruse, Ingrid, D.P.M. "How to Avoid Foot Problems If You Have Neuropathy." *Clinical Diabetes* 18, no. 3 (Summer 2000): 119–121.

Kulmala, Petri, et al. "Genetic Markers, Humoral Autoimmunity, and Prediction of Type 1 Diabetes in Siblings of Affected Children." *Diabetes* 49 (2000): 48–58.

Kurtenbach, Anne, et al. "Preretinopic Changes in the Colour Vision of Juvenile Diabetics." *British Journal of Ophthalmology* 83 (1999): 43–46.

Kumari, Meena, et al. "Minireview: Mechanisms by Which the Metabolic Syndrome and Diabetes Impair Memory." *Journals of Gerontology* 55 (May 1, 2000): B228–B232.

Laberge-Nadeau, Claiare, M.D., M.Sc., et al. "Impact of Diabetes on Crash Risks of Truck-Permit Holders and Commercial Drivers." *Diabetes Care* 23, no. 5 (May 2000): 612–617.

Lambing, Cheryl L., M.D., "Osteoporosis Prevention, Detection, and Treatment." *Postgraduate Medicine* 107, no. 7 (June 2000): 37–41.

Landon, M. B. "Obstetric Management of Pregnancies Complicated by Diabetes Mellitus." *Clinical Obstetrics & Gynecology* 43, no. 1 (March 2000): 65–74.

Lane, James D., Ph.D., et al. "Personality Correlates of Glycemic Control in Type 2 Diabetes." *Diabetes Care* 23 no. 9 (September 2000): 1321–1325.

Langer, O. "Management of Gestational Diabetes." *Clinical Obstetrics & Gynecology* 43, no. 1 (March 2000): 106–115.

Lauzzus, Finn, et al. "Diabetic Retinopathy in Pregnancy During Tight Metabolic Control." *Acta Obstretricia et Gynecologica Scandinavica* 79 (2000): 367–370.

Lee, Warren L., M.D., et al. "Impact of Diabetes on Coronary Artery Disease in Women and Men." *Diabetes Care* 23, no. 7 (July 2000): 962–968.

Leff, David N. "Many Are Fat But Few Are Diabetic: Analyzed by DNA Chips, Genes in Adipose Cells Aim to Predict Diabetes Onset Well in Advance." *BIOWORLD Today* (October 18, 2000): No page numbers.

Leichter, Steven B., M.D., F.A.C.P., F.A.C.E. "The Business of Diabetes Education Before and After New Medicare Regulations." *Clinical Diabetes* 17, no. 3 (1999): Available online at http://www.findarticles.com/cf_0/m0682/3-17/55396968/print.jhtml.

Leichter, Steven B., M.D., F.A.C.P., F.A.C.E. "Economic Considerations in the Application of Clinical Standards and Requirements in Diabetes Care. *Clinical Diabetes* 18, no. 2 (Spring 2000): 91–92.

"Levels of Diabetes-Related Preventive Care Practices—United States, 1997–1999." *Morbidity and Mortality Weekly Report* 49, no. 42 (October 27, 2000): 954–958.

Levetan, Claresa S., M.D., et al. "Effect of Physician Specialty on Outcomes in Diabetic Ketoacidosis." *Diabetes Care* 22, no. 11 (November 1999): 1790–1795.

Levetan, Claresa, M.D., "Mastering Diabetes at Medicare." *Clinical Diabetes* 18, no. 2 (Spring 2000) 74–79.

Levin, Marvin E., M.D., and Pfeiffer, Michael A., M.D., eds. *The Uncomplicated Guide to Diabetes Complications.* (Alexandria, Va: American Diabetes Association, 1998).

Levin, Seymour R., M.D. et al. "Effect of Intensive Glycemic Control on Microalbuminuria in Type 2 Diabetes." *Diabetes Care* 23, no. 10 (October 2000): 1478–1485.

Lindsay, Robert S., M.B., Ph.D., et al. "Secular Trends in Birth Weight, BMI, and Diabetes in the Offspring of Diabetic Mothers." *Diabetes Care* 23, no. 9 (September 2000) 1249–1254.

Lipton, Rebecca, B.S.N., M.P.H., Ph.D. "Ethnic Differences in Mortality from Insulin-Dependent Diabetes Mellitus among People Less Than 25 Years of Age." *Pediatrics* 103, no. 5 (May 1999): 952–956.

Liu, et al. "A Prospective Study of Whole-Grain Intake and Risk of Type 2 Diabetes Mellitus in U.S. Women." *American Journal of Public Health* 90, no. 9 (2000): 1409–1415.

Lodewick, Peter A., M.D. *A Diabetic Doctor Looks at Diabetes: His and Yours* (Los Angeles, Calif.: Lowell House, 1998).

Ludwig, David S., M.D., Ph.D. "High Glycemic Index Foods, Overeating, and Obesity." *Pediatrics* 103, no. 3 (March 1999): 103–106.

Ludwig, Endre, M.D., Ph.D. "Bacteriuria in Women with Diabetes Mellitus," *Infections in Urology* 13, Supp. 5A (2000): S3–S6.

Luna, Beatriz, Pharm.D., B.C.P.S., and Feinglos, Mark N., M.D., C.M. "Oral Agents in the Management of Type 2 Diabetes." *American Family Physician* 63, no. 9 (May 1, 2001): 1747–1756.

Lustman, Patrick J., Ph.D. "Fluoxetine for Depression in Diabetes." *Diabetes Care* 23 no. 5 (May 2000): 618–623.

McCleane, G. "Topical Application of Doxepin Hydrochloride, Capsaicin and a Combination of Both Produces Analgesia in Chronic Human Neuropathic Pain: A Randomized, Double-Blind, Placebo-Controlled Study." *British Journal of Clinical Pharmacology* 49, no. 6, (June 2000): 574–579.

McCulloch, David K., and Mazzaferri, Ernest L. "Comprehensive Management of Type 2 Diabetes/Commentary." *Hospital Practice* 35, no. 9 (Sept 15, 2000). www.hosppract.com/issues/2000/09/dmmmccu.htm

McGarry, Kelly A., M.D., et al. "Postmenopausal Osteoporosis." *Postgraduate Medicine* 108, no. 3 (Sept 2000): 79–82, 85–88, 91.

McKinlay, John, and Marceau, Lisa. "US Public Health and the 21st Century: Diabetes Mellitus." *The Lancet* 356, no. 9231 (August 26, 2000): 757–761.

McLaughlin, Tracey, M.D., and Reaven, Gerald, M.D. "Insulin Resistance and Hypertension: Patients in Double Jeopardy for Cardiovascular Disease," *Geriatrics* 55, no. 6 (June 2000): 28ff.

McNamara, Damian. "Overcoming Juvenile Diabetes with a Little Planning and High Tech." *FDA Consumer* 34, no. 4 (July 2000): 28.

McWin, Jr. Gerald, Ph.D., et al. "Diabetes and Automobile Crashes in the Elderly." *Diabetes Care* 22, no. 2 (February 1999): 220–227.

"Diabetes During Pregnancy—United States, 1993–1005." *Morbidity and Mortality Weekly Report* 47, no. 20 (May 29, 1998): 408–414.

Marks, Jennifer B., M.D. "Diabetes Management in the Future: A Whiff and a Long Shot?" *Clinical Diabetes* 16, no. 3 (1998): 140–141.

Marre, Michel, M.D. Ph.D. "Genetics and the Prediction of Complications in Type 1 Diabetes." *Diabetes Care* 22, Supp. 2 (1998): B53–B58.

Marre, M., et al. "Hereditary Factors in the Development of Diabetic Renal Disease." *Diabetes Metabolism* 26, Supp. 4 (July 2000): 30–36.

Mathiesen, Bent, MD, and Borch-Johnsen, Knut, M.D., "Diabetes and Accident Insurance." *Diabetes Care* 20, no. 11 (November 1997): 1781–1784.

Matyka, K. A., et al. "Genetic Testing for Maturity Onset Diabetes of the Young in Childhood Hyperglycaemia." *Archives of Disease in Childhood* 78 (1998): 552–554.

Mayfield, Jennifer A., M.D., M.P.H. "Technical Review: Preventive Foot Care in People with Diabetes." *Diabetes Care* 21, no. 12 (December 1998): 2161–2177.

Mayfield, Jennifer A., M.D., M.P.H., et al. "Work Disability and Diabetes." *Diabetes Care* 22 (July 1999): 1105–1109.

Mehta, Shruti, H., M.P.H., et al. "Prevalence of Type 2 Diabetes Mellitus among Persons with Hepatitis C Virus Infection in the United States." *Annals of Internal Medicine* 133 (2000): 592–599.

Meltzer, David, M.D., Ph.D., et al. "Effect of Future Costs on Cost-Effectiveness of Medical Interventions Among Young Adults: The Example of Intensive Therapy for Type 1 Diabetes Mellitus." *Medical Care* 38, no. 6 (June 2000): 679–685.

Meltzer, Lisa J., M.S., et al. "Disordered Eating, Body Mass, and Glycemic Control in Adolescents with Type 1 Diabetes." *Diabetes Care* 24 (2001): 678–682.

Mesiya, Sikander A., M.D., and Anil Minocha, M.D., F.A.C.P., F.A.C.G. "Gastrointestinal Disease in Diabetes Mellitus." *Clinical Reviews* (Winter 1998/1999): 33–38.

Metterburg, J. "Breaking the Skin Barrier." *JDF International Countdown* 19, no. 4 (1998): 12–14, 16, 18.

Michalek, Arthur M., et al. "Hypothyroidism and Diabetes Mellitus in an American Indian Population." *Journal of Family Practice* 49, no. 7 (July 2000): 638.

Mokdad, Ali H., Ph.D., et al. "Diabetes Trends in the U.S.: 1990–1998." *Diabetes Care* 23, no. 9 (September 2000): 1278–1283.

Mollema, Eline D., M.Sc., et al. "Diabetes Fear of Injecting and Self-Testing Questionnaire." *Diabetes Care* 23, no. 6 (June 2000): 765–769.

Montague, Carl T. "The Perils of Portliness." *Diabetes* 49, no. 6 (2000): 883–888.

Montori, Victor M., M.D., et al. "Fish Oil Supplementation in Type 2 Diabetes." *Diabetes Care* 23, no. 9 (September 2000): 1407–1415.

Mooradian, Arshag D., M.D., et al. "Diabetes Care for Older Adults." *Diabetes Spectrum* 12, no. 2 (1999): 70–77.

Moore, Lynn L., M.D., et al. "A Prospective Study of the Risk of Congenital Defects Associated with Maternal Obesity and Diabetes Mellitus." *Epidemiology* 11, no. 6 (November 2000): 689–694.

Morgan, Christopher, et al. "Relationship Between Diabetes and Mortality." *Diabetes Care* 23, no. 8 (August 2000): 1103–1107.

Morley, John E. "Editorial: Diabetes Mellitus: A Major Disease of Older Persons." *The Journals of Gerontology. Series A, Biological Sciences and Medical Sciences* 55, no. 5 (May 2000): M255–M256.

Morelli, Vincent, and Zoorob, Roger J., "Depression, Diabetes, Obesity." *American Family Physician* 62, no. 5 (September 2000): 1051–1064.

Morris, Andrew, et al. "Adherence to Insulin Treatment, Glycaemic Control, and Ketoacidosis in Insulin-Dependent Diabetes Mellitus." *The Lancet* 350, no. 9090 (November 22, 1997): 1505–1510.

Moses, Robert G., F.R.A.C.P. "Gestational Diabetes: Is A Higher Cesarean Section Rate Inevitable?" *Diabetes Care* 23, no. 1 (January 2000): 15–17.

Moss, Scot, E., M.A. "The 14-Year Incidence of Lower-Extremity Amputations in a Diabetic Population." *Diabetes Care* 22, no. 6 (June 1999): 951–959.

Moss, S. E., et al. "Risk Factors for Hospitalization in People with Diabetes." *Archives of Internal Medicine* 159 (1999): 2053–2057.

Mrena, Samy, M.B., et al. "Staging of Preclinical Type 1 Diabetes in Siblings of Affected Children." *Pediatrics* 104, no. 4, (October 1999): 925–930.

Nardino, Robert J., M.D. "Alpha-Lipoic Acid for the Prevention and Treatment of Diabetic Neuropathy." *Alternative Medicine Alert Archives* 3 (July 2000): 73–77.

Nash, J. Madeleine, reported by Alice Park/New York, "Health/The New Science of Alzheimer's: The New Science of Alzheimer's Racing against Time—And One Another—Researchers Close In on the Aging Brain's Most Heartbreaking Disorder." *Time International* 56, no. 4 (July 24, 2000). www.time.com/time/europe/magazine/2000/0724/alzheimers2.html

National Center for Chronic Disease Prevention and Health Promotion. "Diabetes among Older Adults: A Heavy Burden and a Great Public Health Opportunity." *Chronic Disease Notes & Reports* 12, no. 3 (Fall 1999): 7–9.

National Heart, Lung, and Blood Institute, National Institutes of Health. "Clinical Guidelines on the Identification, Evaluation, and Treatment of Overweight and Obesity in Adults: The Evidence Report." NIH Publication No. 98-4083, September 1998.

National Institutes of Health, National Institute of Diabetes and Digestive and Kidney Diseases. "Diabetes in America," 2nd edition, National Diabetes Data Group, NIH Publication No. 95-1468, 1995.

National Institutes of Health. "21: Oral Health," in *Healthy People 2010.* National Institutes of Health, 2000.

Nicolucci, Antonio, M.D., et al. "Stratifying Patients at Risk of Diabetic Complications." *Diabetes Care* 21, no. 9 (September 1998): 1439–1444.

Nichols, Gregory A., M.B.A., Ph.D., et al. "Predictors of Glycemic Control in Insulin-Using Adults with Type 2 Diabetes." *Diabetes Care* 23, no. 3 (March 2000): 273–277.

Nichols, Gregory, Ph.D. "Type 2 Diabetes: Incremental Medical Care Costs During the 8 Years Preceding Diagnosis." *Diabetes Care* 23, no. 11 (November 2000): 1654–1659.

Nettle, S. L., et al. "Age-Independent Oxidative Stress in Elderly Patients with Non-Insulin-Dependent Diabetes Mellitus." *QJM: Monthly Journal of the Association of Physicians* 92 (1999): 33–38.

O'Brien, Judith A., B.S.P.A., et al. "Direct Medical Costs of Complications Resulting from Type 2 Diabetes in the U.S." *Diabetes Care* 21, no. 7 (July 1998): 1122–1128.

Ollendorf, Daniel A., M.P.H. "Potential Economic Benefits of Lower-Extremity Amputation Prevention Strategies in Diabetes." *Diabetes Care* 21, no. 8 (August 1998): 1240–1245.

Oman, Douglas, and Reed, Dwayne. "Religion and Mortality among the Community-Dwelling Elderly." *American Journal of Public Health* 88, no. 10 (1998): 1469–1475.

Ott, A. et al. "Diabetes Mellitus and the Risk of Dementia: The Rotterdam Study." *Neurology* 53 (1999): 1937–1942.

Paauw, Douglas S., M.D., F.A.C.P. "Infectious Emergencies in Patients with Diabetes." *Clinical Diabetes* 18, no. 3 (Summer 2000): 102–106.

Padgett, Deborah L., Ph.D., et al. "Managing Diabetes in the Workplace: Critical Factors." *Diabetes Spectrum* 9, no. 1 (1996): 13–20.

Parving, Hans-Henrik, M.D., D.M.Sc. "Diabetic Hypertensive Patients: Is This a Group in Need of Particular Care and Attention?" *Diabetes Care* 22, Supp. 2 (1999).

Pascot, Agnes, M.Sc., et al. "Age-Related Increase in Visceral Adipose Tissue and Body Fat and the Metabolic Risk Profile of Premenopausal Women." *Diabetes Care* 22, no. 9 (September 1999): 1471–1478.

Peragallo-Dittko, V. "Planes, Trains, and Diabetes: A Guide to Safe Travel." *Diabetes Self-Management* 14, no. 3 (1997): 32–33, 35, 38–40.

Perrin, Ellen C., M.D., et al. "Shared Vision: Concordance among Fathers, Mothers, and Pediatricians About Unmet Needs of Children with Chronic Health Conditions." *Pediatrics* 105, no. 1 (January 2000): 277–285.

Peters, Anne, M.D. (reviewer). "Landmark Studies: Hope for the Diabetic Heart." *Clinical Diabetes* 18, no. 3 (Summer 2000): 130–131.

Petit, Jr., William, M.D. "Management of Diabetes Mellitus During Pregnancy." In *Self-Assessment Profile in Endocrinology and Metabolism.* Palumbo, Pasquale J., M.D., M.A.C.E., Chair. (Washington, D.C.: The American Association of Clinical Endocrinologists and the American College of Endocrinology) 2001: 102–107.

Petrella, Robert J., M.D., Ph.D., "Exercise for Older Patients with Chronic Disease." *Physician & Sportsmedicine* 27, no. 11. www.physsportmed.com/issues/1999/10_15_99/petrella.htm.

Petterson, Tim, M.R.C.P., et al. "Well-Being and Treatment Satisfaction in Older People with Diabetes." *Diabetes Care* 21, no. 6 (June 1998): 930–935.

Pfeiffer, Michael A., M.D. "Brittle Diabetes." *Diabetes Forecast* 53, no. 11 (November 2000): 13.

Pham, Hau, D.P.M., et al. "Screening Techniques to Identify People at High Risk for Diabetic Foot Ulceration." *Diabetes Care* 23, no. 5 (May 2000): 606–611.

Piette, John D., Ph.D. "Lifestyle and Behavior: Interactive Resources for Patient Education and Support." *Diabetes Spectrum* 13, no. 2 (2000): 110.

Pinkowish, Mary Desmond. "Diabetes and CVD Risks in African American Children: The Role of Insulin Metabolism." *Patient Care* 34, no. 9 (May 15, 2000). www.findarticles.com/cf_0/m3233/9_34/62450760/print.jhtml.

Poirier, Steven J. "Preserving the Diabetic Kidney." *Journal of Family Practice* 46, no. 1 (January 1998): 21–28.

Pollock, Myrna, et al. "Eating Disorders and Maladaptive Dietary/Insulin Management among Youths with Childhood-Onset Insulin-Dependent Diabetes Mellitus." *Journal of the American Academy of Child and Adolescent Psychiatry* 34, no. 3 (March 1995): 291–297.

Ponder, Stephen W., M.D., C.D.E., et al. "Type 2 Diabetes Mellitus in Teens." *Diabetes Spectrum* 13, no. 2 (2000): 95–105.

Porte, Daniel, Jr., M.D., and Sherwin, Robert S., M.D. *Ellenberg & Rifkin's Diabetes Mellitus* (Stamford, Conn.: Appleton & Lange, 1997).

Position Statement: Smoking and Diabetes. *Diabetes Care* 24, Supplement no. 1 (January 2001): 564–565.

"Pre-Pregnancy Microalbuminuria Predicts Pre-Eclampsi in Insulin-Dependent Diabetes Mellitus." *The Lancet* 354 (January 30, 1000): 377.

Rajala, Ulla, Ph.D., et al. "High Cardiovascular Disease Mortality in Subjects with Visual Impairment Caused by Diabetic Retinopathy." *Diabetes Care* 23, no. 7 (July 2000): 957–961.

Ramsey, Scott, D. M.D., Ph.D., et al. "Incidence, Outcomes, and Cost of Foot Ulcers in Patients with Diabetes." *Diabetes Care* 22, no. 3 (March 1999): 382–387.

Ratner Kaufman, Francie, M.D., et al. "Association between Diabetes Control and Visits to a Multidisciplinary Pediatric Diabetes Clinic." *Pediatrics* 103, no. 5 (May 1999): 948–951.

Reader, Diane, R.D., L.D., C.D.E. "Carbohydrate Counting for Pregnant Women." *Diabetes Spectrum* 13, no. 3 (2000): 152–153.

Reaven, Peter, M.D., et al. "Cardiovascular Disease Insulin Risk in Mexican-American and Anglo-American Children and Mothers." *Pediatrics* 101, no. 4 (April 1998): 101–105.

Reaven, Gerald M. "Pathophysiciology of Insulin Resistance in Human Disease." *Physiological Reviews* 75, no. 3 (July 1995): 473–487.

Regan, Timothy J. "Moderate Alcohol Consumption and Risk of Coronary Heart Disease among Women with Type 2 Diabetes Mellitus." *Circulation* 102, no. 5 (August 2000): 487–488.

Resnick, Helaine, E., Ph.D., M.P.H., et al. "American Diabetes Association Diabetes Diagnostic Criteria, Advancing Age, and Cardiovascular Risk Profiles: Results from the Third National Health and Nutrition Examination Survey." *Diabetes Care* 23, no. 2 (February 2000): 176–180.

Rickabaugh, Tim E. "Knowledge and Attitudes Related to Diabetes and Exercise Guidelines for Diabetic Children, Their Parents, and Physical Education Teachers." *Research Quarterly for Exercise and Sport* 70, no. 4 (December 1999): 389–394.

Ritz, Eberhard, M.D., et al. "How Can We Improve Prognosis I Diabetic Patients with End-Stage Renal Disease." *Diabetes Care* 22, Supp. 2 (March 1999): B80–B83.

Roberts, Ralph, M.B.B.Ch., M.R.C.P., M.R.C.O.G., M.D., "Hypertension in Women with Gestational Diabetes." *Diabetes Care* 21, Supp. 2 (1998): B27–B32.

Robertson, R. Paul, M.D., et al. "Pancreas and Islet Transplantation for Patients with Diabetes." *Diabetes Care* 23, no. 1 (January 2000): 112–116.

Robertson, R. Paul, M.D. "Successful Islet Transplantation for Patients with Diabetes—Fact or Fantasy?" *The New England Journal of Medicine* 343, no. 4 (July 27, 2000): 289–290.

Roffe, Christine. "Ageing of the Heart." *British Journal of Biomedical Science* 55, no. 2 (June 1, 1998): 136–148.

Rosenn, Barak, M., and Miodovnik, Menachem. "Glycemic Control in the Diabetic Pregnancy: Is Tighter Always Better?" *Journal of Maternal-Fetal Medicine* 9 (2000): 29–34.

Rosenn, B. M., and Miodovnik, M. "Medical Complications of Diabetes Mellitus in Pregnancy." *Clinical Obstetrics & Gynecology* 43, no. 1 (March 2000): 17–31.

Rosilio, Myriam, M.D., et al. "Factors Associated with Glycemic Control: A Cross-Sectional Nationwide Study in 2,579 French Children with Type 1 Diabetes." *Diabetes Care* 21, no. 7 (July 1998): 1146–1153.

Roumain, Janine, M.D., M.P.H., et al. "The Relationship of Menstrual Irregularity to Type 2 Diabetes in Pima Indian Women." *Diabetes Care* 21, no. 3 (March 1998): 346–349.

Roy, Monique, S., M.D. "Diabetic Retinopathy in African Americans with Type 1 Diabetes: The New Jersey 725." *Archives of Ophthalmology* 118, no. 1 (January 2000): 105–115.

Rubin, Richard R., Ph.D., C.D.E., and Peyrot, Mark, Ph.D. "Men and Diabetes: Psychosocial and Behavioral Issues." *Diabetes Spectrum* 11, no. 2 (1998): 81–87.

Rutledge, K. Suchari, M.D., et al. "Effectiveness of Postprandial Humalog in Toddlers with Diabetes." *Pediatrics* 100, no. 6 (December 1997): 968–972.

Sadur, Craig N., M.D., et al. "Diabetes Management in a Health Maintenance Organization: Efficacy of Care Management Using Cluster Visits." *Diabetes Care* 22, no. 12 (December 1999): 2011–2017.

Saffel-Shrier, Susan, M.S., R.D., C.D., Certified Gerontologist. "Carbohydrate Counting for Older Patients." *Diabetes Spectrum* 13, no. 3 (2000): 158–162.

Samaras, Katherine, M.B.B.S., F.R.A.C.P., et al. "Effects of Postmenopausal Hormone Replacement Therapy on Central Abdominal Fat, Glycemic Control, Lipid Metabolism, and Vascular Factors in Type 2 Diabetes." *Diabetes Care* 22, no. 9 (September 1999): 1401–1407.

Samaras, Katherine, M.B.B.S., F.R.A.C.P. "Genes Versus Environment: The Relationship between Dietary Fat and Total and Central Abdominal Fat." *Diabetes Care* 21, no. 12 (December 1998): 2069–2076.

Santoro, N., Col. N.F., Eckman, M.H., et al. "Therapeutic controversy: hormone replacement—where are we going." *J. Clin Endocrinol Metab* 84, no. 6 (1999): 1798–1812.

Scavini, Marina, M.D., and Schade, David S., M.D. "Implantable Insulin Pumps." *Clinical Diabetes* 14, no. 2 (1996): 30–35.

Schafer, Lorraine, C., Ph.D. "Fostering Quality of Life in Individuals with Diabetes." *Diabetes Spectrum* 13, (2000): 50–55.

Scheen, Andre J., M.D., Ph.D., and Lefebvre, Pierre, J., M.D., Ph.D., F.R.C.P., M.A.E. "Management of the Obese Diabetic Patient," from *Diabetes Reviews* 7, no. 2, 1999. In *Annual Review of Diabetes 2000* (Alexandria, Va: American Diabetes Association, 2000).

Schreiner, Barb, R.N., M.N., C.D.E., et al. "Management Strategies for the Adolescent Lifestyle." *Diabetes Spectrum* 13, no. 2 (2000): 83–87.

Schroeder, Betsy, et al. "Correlation between Glycemic Control and Menstruation in Diabetic Adolescents." *Journal of Reproductive Medicine* 45, no. 1 (January 2000): 1–5.

Scott, Carla R., et al. "Characteristics of Youth-Onset Noninsulin-Dependent Diabetes Mellitus and Insulin-Dependent Diabetes Mellitus at Diagnosis." *Pediatrics* 100, no. 1 (July 1997): 84–91.

Sekhri, Neelam K. "Managed Care: The U.S. Experience." *Bulletin of the World Health Organization* 78, no. 6 (June 2000): 830.

"Self-Reported Prevalence of Diabetes among Hispanics—United States, 1994–1997." *Morbidity and Mortality Weekly Report* 48, no. 1 (January 15, 1999): 8–12.

Shapiro, A.M. James, et al. "Islet Transplantation in Seven Patients with Type 1 Diabetes Mellitus Using a Glucocorticoid-Free Immunosuppressive Regimen." *The New England Journal of Medicine* 343, no. 4 (July 27, 2000): 230–238.

Shatin, Deborah, Ph.D., et al. "Health Care Utilization by Children with Chronic Illnesses: A Comparison of Medicaid and Employer Insured Managed Care." *Pediatrics* 102, no. 4 (October 1998): 102–105.

Shaw, Jonathan E., M.R.C.P., et al. "Type 2 Diabetes Worldwide According to the New Classification and Criteria." *Diabetes Care* 23, Supp. 2 (April 2000): B5–B10.

Shirey, Lee et al. "Diabetes: A Drain on U.S. Resources." *Challenges for the 21st Century: Chronic and Disabling Conditions* 1, no. 6 (April 2000): 1–6.

Sinai, B. M. "Risk Factors, Pregnancy Complications, and Prevention of Hypertensive Disorders in Women with Pregravid Diabetes Mellitus." *Journal of Maternal Fetal Medicine* 9, no. 1 (January–February 2000): 62–65.

Simmons, D., F.R.A.C.P., M.D., et al. "Can Medication Packaging Improve Glycemic Control and Blood Pressure in Type 2 Diabetes?" *Diabetes Care* 23, no. 2 (February 2000): 153–156.

Simmons, Zachary, M.D., and Feldman, Eva L., M.D., Ph.D. "The Pharmacological Treatment of Painful Diabetic Neuropathy." *Clinical Diabetes* 18, no. 3 (Summer 2000): 116–118.

Skinner, T. Chas Ph.D., and Sarah E. Hampson, Ph.D. "Personal Models of Diabetes in Relation to Self-Care, Well-Being, and Glycemic Control: A Prospective Study in Adolescence." *Diabetes Care* 24, no. 5 (May 2001): 828–833.

Smith, Stephen H. "Conquering Diabetes: A Report from the Diabetes Research Working Group." *Diabetes Spectrum* 12, no. 4 (1999): 243–249.

Smith, Steven A., M.D., and Poland, Gregory A., M.D. "Technical Review: Use of Influenza and Pneumococcal Vaccines in People with Diabetes." *Diabetes Care* 23, no. 1 (January 2000): 95–108.

Slyper, Arnold H. "Childhood Obesity, Adipose Tissue Distribution, and the Pediatric Practitioner." *Pediatrics* 102, no. 1 (July 1998): 102.

Snoek, Frank J., M.A., Ph.D. "Quality of Life: A Closer Look at Measuring Patients' Well-Being." *Diabetes Spectrum* 13 (2000) in *Annual Review of Diabetes 2000* (Alexandria, Va: American Diabetes Association, 2000): 223–229.

South Dakota Diabetes Control Program and South Dakota Diabetes Advisory Council. "Basic Practice Guidelines for Diabetes Mellitus." February 1999.

Strachan, Mark, et al. "Recovery of Cognitive Function and Mood After Severe Hypoglycemia in Adults with Insulin-Treated Diabetes." *Diabetes Care* 23, no. 3 (March 2000): 305–312.

Stellato, Rebecca K. S.M. "Testosterone, Sex Hormone-Binding Globulin, and the Development of Type 2 Diabetes in Middle-Aged Men." *Diabetes Care* 23, no. 4 (April 2000): 490–494.

Strano-Paul, Lisa, and Phanumas Strano-Paul. "Diabetes Management: Analysis of the American Diabetes Association's Clinical Practice Recommendations." *Geriatrics* 55, no. 4 (April 2000): 57–62.

Striker, Cecil, M.D., Compiler. *Famous Faces in Diabetes* (Boston, Mass.: G.K. Hall & Co., 1961).

Talbot, France, Ph.D., and Nouwen, Arie, Ph.D., "A Review of the Relationship between Depression and Diabetes in Adults." *Diabetes Care* 23, no. 10 (October 2000): 1556–1562.

Tarnow, Lise, M.D., et al. "Cardiovascular Morbidity and Early Mortality Cluster in Parents of Type 1 Diabetic Patients with Diabetic Nephropathy." *Diabetes Care* 23, no. 1 (January 2000): 30–33.

Ter Braak, Edith W. M. T., M.D., et al. "Clinical Characteristics of Type 1 Diabetic Patients with and without Severe Hypoglycemia." *Diabetes Care* 23, no. 10 (October 2000): 1467–1471.

Thaler, Leonard M., M.D., et al. "Diabetes in Urban African-Americans: XIX. Prediction of the Need for Pharmacological Therapy." *Diabetes Care* 23, no. 6 (June 2000): 820–825.

Thomas-Dobersen, Deborah, R.D., M.S., C.D.E., "Nutritional Management of Gestational Diabetes and Nutritional Management of Women with a History of Gestational Diabetes: Two Different Therapies or the Same?" *Clinical Diabetes* 17, no. 4 (1999). www.findarticles.com/cf_o/m0682/4_17/57562557/print.jhtml.

Tomar, Scott L., D.M.D., Dr.P.H., and Lester, Arlene, D.D.S., M.P.H. "Dental and Other Health Care Visits among U.S. Adults with Diabetes." *Diabetes Care* 23, no. 10 (October 2000): 1505–1510.

"Traveling with Diabetes." *Postgraduate Medicine* 105, no. 2 (1999): 233–234.

Travis, John. "Possible Alzheimer's Vaccine Seems Safe," *Science News* 158, no. 3 (July 15, 2000): 38.

Treiman, Gerald S., et al. "Management of Ischemic Heel Ulceration and Gangrene: An Evaluation of Factors Associated with Successful Healing." *Journal of Vascular Surgery* 31, no. 6 (June 2000): 1110–1118.

"Two Transition Metals Show Promise in Treating Diabetic Cats." *Veterinary Medicine* 95, no. 3 (March 1, 2000): 190–193.

Tuomilehto, Jaako M.D., Ph.D., et al. "Prevention of Type 2 Diabetes Mellitus by Changes in Lifestyle among Subjects with Impaired Glucose Tolerance." *New England Journal of Medicine* 344, no. 18 (May 3, 2001): 1343–1350.

Tumoninen, Jussi T., et al. "Bone Mineral Density in Patients with Type 1 and Type 2 Diabetes." *Diabetes Care* 22, no. 7 (July 1999): 1196–1200.

U.S. Department of Health and Human Services. *Physical Activity and Health: A Report of the Surgeon General.* Atlanta, Ga.: U.S. Department of Health and Human Services, Centers for Disease Control and Prevention, National Center for Chronic Disease Prevention and Health Promotion, 1996.

Vaarasmaki, M. S., et al. "Factors Predicting Peri- and Neonatal Outcome in Diabetic Pregnancy." *Early Human Development* 59 (July 2000): 61–70.

de Vegt, Femmie M.Sc., et al. "Similar 9-Year Mortality Risks and Reproducibility for the World Health Organization and American Diabetes Association Glucose Tolerance Categories: The Hoorn Study." *Diabetes Care* 23, no. 1 (January 2000): 40–44.

Vinik, Aaron, M.D., Ph.D., F.C.P., F.A.C.P., et al. "Gastrointestinal, Genitourinary, and Neurovascular Disturbances in Diabetes." *Diabetes Reviews* 7, no. 4 (1999): 346–366.

Vogt, Donna U. "Diabetes: Basic Information and Federal Funding." *CRS Report for Congress.* Updated July 15, 1998.

Wagner, Arnd. M.D., et al. "Therapy of Severe Diabetic Ketoacidosis: Zero-Mortality Under Very-Low-Dose Insulin Application." *Diabetes Care* 22, no. 5 (May 1999): 674–677.

Walker, Karen Z., Ph.D., et al. "Effects of Regular Walking on Cardiovascular Risk Factors and Body Composition in Normogylcemic Women and Women with Type 2 Diabetes." *Diabetes Care* 22, no. 4 (April 1999): 555–561.

Wallace, Jeffrey I. M.D., M.P.H. "Management of Diabetes in the Elderly," *Clinical Diabetes* 17, no. 1 (1999): 92–97.

Wallhagen, Margaret I., Ph.D., R.N., C.S., G.N.P. "Social Support in Diabetes." *Diabetes Spectrum* 12, no. 4 (1999): 254.

Wamala, Sarah P., Ph.D., et al. "Education and the Metabolic Syndrome in Women." *Diabetes Care* 22, no. 12 (December 1999): 1999–2003.

Wang, Yan, M.B.B.S., et al. "Dietary Variables and Glucose Tolerance in Pregnancy." *Diabetes Care* 23, no. 4 (April 2000): 460–464.

Ward, John Dale, M.D., F.R.C.P. "Improving Prognosis in Type 2 Diabetes." *Diabetes Care.* 22, Supp. 2 (1999): B84–B88.

Wei, Ming, M.D. "Alcohol Intake and Incidence of Type 2 Diabetes in Men." *Diabetes Care* 23, no. 1 (January 2000): 18–22.

Weiss, Peter A. M., M.D., et al. "Long-Term Follow-Up of Infants of Mothers with Type 1 Diabetes." *Diabetes Care* 23, no. 7 (July 2000): 905–911.

Weathermon, Ron, Pharm.D., and Crabb, David W., M.D. "Alcohol and Medication Interactions." *Alcohol Research & Health* 23, no. 1 (1999): 40–54.

Whitaker, Robert C., et al. "Gestational Diabetes and the Risk of Offspring Obesity." *Pediatrics* 101, no. 2 (February 1998): 101–103.

Wildin, Robert S., M.D., and Cogdell, David E., M.S. "Clinical Utility of Direct Mutation Testing for Congenital Nephrogenic Diabetes Insipidus in Families." *Pediatrics* 103, no. 3 (March 1999): 632–639.

Williams, Ann S., M.S.N., R.N., C.D.E. "Visual Aids: Independent Blood Glucose Testing." *Diabetes Self-Management* 16, no. 3 (1999): 45–46, 51–52.

Wing, Rena R., Ph.D., et al. "Lifestyle Intervention in Overweight Individuals with a Family History of Diabetes." *Diabetes Care* 21, no. 3 (March 1998): 350–359.

Wolosin, James D., M.D., F.A.C.P., and Edelman, Steven V., M.D., "Diabetes and the Gastrointestinal Tract." *Clinical Diabetes* 18, no. 4 (Fall 2000): 151.

World Health Organization, "Definition, Diagnosis and Classification of Diabetes Mellitus and Its Complications: Report of a WHO Consultation. Part 1: Diagnosis and Classification of Diabetes Mellitus." World Health Organization, Department of Noncommunicable Disease Surveillance, Geneva, Switzerland, WHO/NCD/NCS/99.2, 1999.

Wu, Patricia, M.D., F.A.C.E., F.R.C.P. "Thyroid Disease and Diabetes." *Diabetes Self-Management* 18, no. 3 (Winter 2000): 6–12.

Wunderlich, Robert P., D.P.M., et al. "Systemic Hyperbaric Oxygen Therapy: Lower-Extremity Wound Healing and the Diabetic Foot." *Diabetes Care* 23, no. 10 (October 2000): 1551–1555.

Yager, Joel, "Weighty Perspectives: Contemporary Challenges in Obesity and Eating Disorders." *American Journal of Psychiatry* 157, no. 6 (June 1, 2000): 851–853.

Zielke, J. "Alcohol: A Primer: How Does Alcohol Affect Diabetes?" *Diabetes Forecast* 52, no. 3 (1999): 64–66.

INDEX

DATE DUE